THE MAKING
OF THE
IDEAL
PHYSICIAN

THE MAKING OF THE *IDEAL* PHYSICIAN

Edward C. Rosenow III, MD
J. Keith Mansel, MD
Walter R. Wilson, MD

Foreword by Robert R. Waller, MD

With a Chapter by Adamarie Multari, MD

On the cover: *The Doctor* (1887) by Sir Luke Fildes

Words can't completely describe what Fildes accomplishes in his painting, but the artwork does send a message in all languages to all health-care providers and their patients. The doctor has spent the night caring for the sick child and providing a gentle touch. In the presence of the child's family, the doctor compounds elixirs, which are of little medicinal value but bring them a bit of peace and hope while waiting for the fever to break.

The very presence of the physician in a room can be a powerful force in healing and relieving suffering.

The doctor is attending the patient, watching and waiting—just being there is the epitome of the *ideal* physician. The essence of Fildes' painting is the depiction of the quality of patient centeredness, which is the essential feature of the contemporary doctor-patient relationship. *The needs of the patient come first* (Mayo Clinic's primary value).

The Doctor reminds contemporary physicians of the crucial importance of the doctor-patient relationship and the value of a patient-centered approach to care.

Copy Editor: Tamara Dawson Bonnicksen
Graphic Designer: Jane Swanson
Cover design by Jim Postier, Postier Studios

Print information available on the last page.

ISBN: 978-1-4907-8370-3 (sc)
ISBN: 978-1-4907-8371-0 (e)
Library of Congress Control Number: 2017911573

Order this book online at www.trafford.com or email orders@trafford.com. Most Trafford titles also are available at major online book retailers.

Trafford rev. 12/06/2017

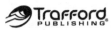
www.trafford.com
North America and International
Toll-free: 888-232-4444 (USA and Canada)
Fax: 812-355-4082

This book is dedicated to all professional health-care providers whose skills and passion for the Art of Medicine will help restore the trust the medical profession has lost. We hope the information in this book will help in that endeavor.

The Platinum Rule of Medicine:

Treat every patient like you would want a member of your family treated.

It's fun to be kind!

Contents

Chapter

Foreword

In 2003, Dr. Edward C. Rosenow III, former Arthur M. and Gladys D. Gray Professor of Medicine at Mayo Clinic, wrote *The Art of Living ... The Art of Medicine: The Wit and Wisdom of Life and Medicine: A Physician's Perspective*. Dr. Rosenow, who has been a great friend and mentor to me and many others who have served on the Mayo staff, characterized that writing as a "how-to book" for young physicians and our health-care colleagues who were in the process of learning the essential elements of professionalism and, while doing so, also learning how to best maintain balance in their lives. Since 2003, I have read his book from cover to cover at least ten times and requested dozens of additional copies to give to students, trainees, family members, and friends.

And now, Dr. Rosenow, along with coauthors Dr. J. Keith Mansel and Dr. Walter R. Wilson, two distinguished Mayo* physicians of the highest order, have written this book, *The Making of the Ideal Physician*, which builds on the approach to Dr. Rosenow's earlier book. The authors take to the next level the essence of what professionalism really means in the practice of medicine in today's world. They have succeeded in putting the Art of Medicine in proper perspective with the science and, throughout each chapter, provide lessons for living.

We read and hear too much these days about how to "fix" the world of health care. The authors describe beautifully the core values that must be woven into the fabric of our lives as we go forward to repair health-care systems: respect for others, civility, total honesty, compassion, equanimity, constancy of purpose, a sense of propriety, order, humor, and—especially—kindness. The authors all know—and teach—that joy abounds when kindness is linked to a life of service.

Anyone who has the privilege of service in health care would do well to own this book. Like Dr. Rosenow's first book, I will read every chapter many times over.

Robert R. Waller, MD, President and CEO of the Mayo Foundation, 1988–1999
Memphis, Tennessee
March 2017

*Dr. Mansel joined the staff of the University of Mississippi Medical Center after the book writing was completed.

Preface and Acknowledgments

This book is a compilation of subjects gathered from our combined 100-plus years of experience in medicine and medical education. We can't begin to name all the people we wish to thank for teaching us so much about the Art of Medicine—as well as the Science of Medicine. We learned not just by reading and attending lectures but also from our role models. And we are still learning—we'll never stop. Our goal is to educate young people and save them some time by discussing these subjects that took us many decades to learn. We also are passing along ideas to our practicing colleagues.

Working with young physicians and medical students is one of the most rewarding efforts any physician can undertake. We see it as an obligation—and one that offers tremendous rewards.

Some of the topics in this book relate to the responsibilities a health-care provider will encounter as he/she moves up the ladder of experience and responsibility. Throughout most of the chapters, we have stressed the importance of **caring** and **professionalism**, which is the reason for our frequent repetition of the importance of your own body language. We also talk about role models as being perhaps the most powerful method of learning. In different parts of the book, we also have stressed the importance of the Art of Medicine, which encompasses relating to your patients and coworkers, your passion for medicine and the patient's care, work-life balance, burnout/stress, mentoring, and powerful healing actions. We hope that future doctors will think of this book as a reference manual that they can return to later in their careers.

The physician's power to heal is just that: powerful. But we think the most important aspect of a physician's healing abilities is the Platinum Rule of Medicine:

Treat every patient like you would want a member of your family treated.

We are extremely grateful to the Clinton Family Fund and an anonymous donor for their support of this effort. A special thanks to Tamara Dawson Bonnicksen, our copy editor, who was immensely helpful in checking the details that we authors might tend to overlook or accept as accurate. We couldn't have completed the book without her: "She isn't just any copy editor." Thanks also to Jane Swanson for her wonderful talent in designing this book.

As you read the book, please note that we use Mayo Clinic as an example in different scenarios based on our careers and experiences there.

Chapter One

So You Want to Be a Physician

Many of you decided you wanted to be a physician or nurse when you were younger than five years old. This came about after witnessing a physician give comfort care to a family member, and you remembered how much he or she appreciated it and the family's frequent conversations about it. Over the years, you found that you had no one to talk to about what it takes to be a member of the medical profession. You haven't needed anything but routine care from your family physician(s) and never really got to talk to them. You formed some impressions from what you saw on TV or in the movies! Or you have talked to counselors in high school and college. We have found that many college counselors don't have very good insight or knowledge about medical and osteopathic schools and what it takes to get into them—let alone what being a physician entails. It is always helpful to talk to a physician who might agree to be your mentor.

Applicants to medical schools are finding that even if they have outstanding grades, they may not be accepted into some programs because they've done little or no volunteer work aiding the underserved. Volunteering is very important to many admissions committees. Have a separate résumé for your volunteer work going back to grade school. Describe and document what you have done with a short paragraph for each project—go by the motto: *If it isn't documented, it didn't happen!* This résumé is more for your records than for submission, but you may want letters from some of your volunteer-work supervisors. It also can be a good source of material for your Personal Statement, which is mostly about "Why I want to be a doctor." Mention your number of blood donations. Have you signed up to be an organ donor? Your interviewer may be a transplant physician. It is better to volunteer for a few organizations over a long period rather than for multiple ones for a few weeks at a time. This amounts to a "continuity of caring."

You don't need to go out of the country to volunteer—although a number of medical schools emphasize global medicine to their students—but it is a maturing experience. Admissions committee members don't view building hospitals or schools outside the country as rewarding as volunteering by directly helping people, e.g., visiting the homebound elderly, working in a hospice or homeless shelter, and on and on. There is no limit to the opportunities.

Process

I (author ECR) have been on the Mayo Medical School (MMS) admissions committee, and I can say that comparing our authors' admissions experiences of three to five or more decades ago to today's process is like comparing night and day. I'm sure I filled out a short application, but I don't remember being interviewed. I didn't take an MCAT. I don't recall an orientation of any kind, and there were no mentors before we started or once we were in medical school. The biggest difference is that any applicant will need to do at least some—how much likely depends on the medical school—volunteer work, even if he/she has a GPA of 4.0 and a high MCAT score. When I was on the admissions committee, the group interviewed several pre-med students who worked nearly full time to put themselves through college and minimize student loans and so didn't have time to do much volunteer work. We didn't penalize any of them for this. If this is your situation, a letter from your employer would be beneficial.

While I served on the admissions committee, we had about 4,500 applications for 50 positions in the freshman class! We could first reject about 1,000 applicants because of very low MCAT scores, incomplete applications, GPAs below our minimum expectation, visa problems, and so on. That left around 3,500 applications for review. Various members of the admissions executive committee screened these applicants to choose 300 to invite for an interview. The approximate twenty-two-member admissions committee included staff, emeriti, several medical students, and residents. Some schools accept up to 250 applicants for a position and have different admission criteria.

Important Resources

(Note that these resources may change over time.)

www.aamc.org
*Association of American Medical Colleges
(AAMC)*

www.aamc.org/students/applying/amcas
American Medical College Application Service

www.aacom.org/become-a-doctor/ applying
*American Association of Colleges of
Osteopathic Medicine (AACOM)
Application Service*

MCAT
Medical College Admission Test

MSAR
Medical School Admissions Requirements

Services.aamc.org/summerprograms
*Good source of ideas for summer programs,
such as the Summer Undergraduate
Research Fellowship (SURF)*

Canadian and Caribbean medical schools also may be resources for students.

Every week for about four to five months, each one of our seven executive-committee members reviewed twenty-five applications (given to us at random). It would take about fifteen to twenty minutes to review a few pages of background material, four to six letters of recommendation (two to five pages each), and the applicant's Personal Statement. Then I would vote to "invite" or "reject."

Most of the information you need regarding your application to medical and/or osteopathic school is on the websites listed on the opposite page. At the time of this writing, all medical-school applications go through the AAMC, and osteopathic-school applications go through AACOM. Always begin with these sources, and you can do this sometime in your mid-junior undergraduate year. The application process usually opens during the first week in June for the medical-school academic year beginning fifteen months later. You should be working on your application right away so that you can get it in as early as possible— perhaps the first two weeks in June. The application services collect and deliver your application information and exam scores to each school you choose.

You can apply to both medical and osteopathic schools. Before 1990 or so, a Doctor of Osteopathic Medicine (DO) practiced manipulative medicine, mostly of the spine. Today the DO is indistinguishable from a physician who has a medical degree (MD), and the training is the same. There are about thirty osteopathic schools in the United States that have education standards equivalent to United States medical schools. At this time, approximately one-third of medical-school graduates and two-thirds of osteopathic-school graduates go into primary care medicine. All schools require the MCAT, and you can take it up to three times. The MSAR can be purchased through aamc.org for a reasonable price, and it is worth it. It offers many details about each school's admission requirements. The MSAR also may be available in your college counseling office or library. (Keep in mind that some of these numbers and organizations may change.)

When you begin preparing your medical-school application, read the instructions thoroughly. **Proofread carefully**. A mentor who recently has been through the application process can be very helpful to you. Most, but not all, high school and college academic counselors also may be helpful. Students applying to a medical or osteopathic school likely will receive a "secondary" application if they are accepted for an interview. Some of these applications include a request for an essay.

The MCAT takes more than seven hours to complete. The essay portion has been dropped. There is a lot on psychology, sociology, inequality, etc. There are now eleven suggested prerequisite courses compared to eight previously. This will be in the MSAR.

There are two certifying boards: the American Osteopathic Association (AOA) and the Accreditation Council for Graduate Medical Education (ACGME). MD students take the ACGME, while DO students can take either.

As a side note, a homeopathic practitioner is totally unrelated to the DO and MD and practices alternative medicine, mostly with oral medicaments.

We were all urged to have no more than three or so "invites" out of our twenty-five because the total of 300 invitees added up quickly. Yet there were times I wanted to invite twenty of the twenty-five. These "kids," who were not much older than my grandkids, had worked so hard and exuded a passion for people, and I thought their enthusiasm was very genuine.

The whole committee met weekly to go over the "invites" and vote anonymously. The grading scale was "5" as the highest, and we could go down to "1" or "2," but almost never did. We had a lot of 3.5s to 4.9s. There could be several who had institutional actions, and a few would have misdemeanors. The applicants always had good explanations, knew they did wrong, and were very apologetic; ultimately, we didn't downgrade them for this. Applicants explained these infractions in a special area on the application. They may have gained maturity as a result of their wrongdoings or misdemeanors. It would be much more of a problem if an applicant did not list a misdemeanor and we found out—he/she would be dropped. Fortunately, this didn't happen.

We have drawn upon our experiences as past admissions committee members to create the following list of things to keep in mind when applying to medical school:

• Being a son or daughter of a physician didn't count, nor did being a legacy. We know of situations where wealthy potential donors offered to "donate" large amounts of money to the medical school—but this didn't help get their children accepted.

• Significant athletic or music skills didn't help (we had a number who were concert virtuosos). *(This has changed, and today the Mayo Clinic School of Medicine values athletics, artistic endeavors, and military service in the review process.)*

• We always looked for **passion** in the applicant. The fact we didn't sense it in an application didn't mean that it wasn't there, so we would probe an applicant a little bit along these lines during the interview. You can sense a quiet passion even if it is not obvious. Admissions committees can get a feel for this in your Letters of Reference (LOR).

• Does it help an applicant to have a Type A personality? Only—and we say only—if you also use it to maintain a balance in your life. A must.

• Do you have a **purpose** in life? Passion is today; purpose is your future—what you want to be and how you want to leave the world a little bit better. Physicians have a great opportunity to accomplish their goals and purpose. Incorporating your goals is something to consider in your personal letter that accompanies your application. But keep it within reason—curing cancer is noble, but it could be many decades before this happens.

• **Attitude**—a form of passion—is another quality that stands out. Many employers—without even knowing it—look for this in an applicant. Attitude and passion can be learned from role models. Who are your role models?

• On the flip side of having a good attitude, if your tendency is rudeness, medical schools don't want your application. You still have more growing up to do. We place a very high value on empathy, and arrogance is an absolute no-no! No medical school wants to find this out after you begin your first year.

• Some medical schools now offer half- to one-day sessions, commonly called "Med School 101," which focus on applications. These are usually held in the spring on a Saturday. Some pre-med students attend more than one of these sessions, so contact a medical school near you for a schedule. Schools often encourage students to bring their parents. Go to this early on—maybe your sophomore year—and then go back the next year to get questions answered that came up since your last visit. There also may be a finance officer there to explain scholarships, talk about incidental costs, and answer questions about student loans.

• Shadowing a physician on rounds can be enlightening and should be done maybe a half dozen times, but there isn't extra credit for doing more. It is recommended to help pre-med students get a better feel of the real world of a physician, but it has variable weight with admissions committees.

• Some applicants have worked with a researcher during off-quarters or even during a "gap" year after graduating from college. Publishing a paper with your research advisor(s) is looked on very favorably, providing you can document a significant contribution to it. Your advisor during the research can help you with this.

• Many applicants spoke two or more languages, which is nice, but of limited value regarding qualifying for admission. We suspect many schools in the United States might put some emphasis on speaking Spanish. In some major cities, a percentage of the population doesn't speak English.

• Surveys of college students disclose that one of their most important concerns is *time management* (this could begin in high school). To quote experts: time is everything. Managing your time could be one of the most important things you do—it is a form of *continuous improvement*. **There will always be someone who wants your time.** Begin keeping a time diary by recording everything you do in fifteen-minute periods, e.g., texting, watching TV, studying, class time, sleeping, etc., and do this for up to a week. Break the day into three blocks, such as morning, afternoon, and evening. Get academic work done during one of the blocks, and make sure you find time for extracurricular activities, such as volunteering and playing sports, and just having fun— even at work. These studies found that those who are involved in extracurricular activities are the happiest. Don't let your day become a blur of all your activities.

• Getting plenty of sleep is much more important than cramming into the night to study for a test or write a paper. *Pace yourself.* If you didn't learn this already, there are two things that college students want help with: *time management* and *access to good mentors.* I would add *networking.*

• When you are in the classroom, do not text or even look at your smartphone or tablet computer (unless you need it for the lecture). Maintain reasonable eye contact with the professor. Don't look bored. No talking or eating in class. College is serious business. And expensive!

• Ask good questions. This isn't buttering up the professor but a sign of intellectual curiosity (the professor can tell the difference). Or go up to the lecturer after the presentation or at a scheduled time. It was obvious in the Letters of Reference that professors like this, and it isn't an imposition. It's another sign that you want to learn. But don't ask inane questions just to get attention. If you are in the back half of the classroom, don't allow yourself to nod off—the professor can easily see this.

• You should have several mentors in college—a good mentor(s) can be a game changer. Talk to other students to find good mentors. But don't hesitate to change mentors if needed. Every so often, handwrite a nice thank-you note to your mentor (an email is not good enough). Ask several mentors to write reference letters for you.

• Being a teaching assistant (TA) can be rewarding to you and to your application.

• Experts will tell you to not let your parents advise on which courses to take and when. They also would advise you to not take all the heavy pre-med courses with labs in the first year. We recommend that you take a course in bioethics—this will be a good start to help you face problems you will encounter the rest of your life.

• Send in your application early—preferably in the first two weeks of June. The admissions committee secretary tells us that this is very important. Applications are reviewed in the order they are received, and they stay in this order. This doesn't mean that you will be ranked higher, but your invitation to an interview likely will occur sooner than those whose applications were received later.

• It is important to minimize or even avoid any credit card debt when applying to medical schools—even for travel and hotels. This lessens the load on your student debt.

• Some medical and osteopathic schools are requiring the completion of short-answer secondaries, which are questions about yourself, such as:

1. *What particular qualities do you feel you can bring to xxxxx school?*
2. *Why are you applying to an osteopathic school?*
3. *How have you familiarized yourself with the field of medicine, especially problems with health-care delivery?*
4. *How would you deal with a recalcitrant patient?*
5. *Who in your life has influenced you the most?*

These are just examples; most of them allow a limited number of words or characters.

Letters of Reference (LOR)

• Letters of Reference are extremely important, and all are read. Who should write the LOR? Anyone who knows you well, but follow the application guidelines for the school. Personal friends and family don't carry much, if any, weight.

• If you ask a professor or graduate student, including a TA who you worked closely with in a lab, to write a reference letter, it would be best that it be written toward the end of your association while you are still fresh in mind. He/she might just put it in your file until you are ready to begin your application process.

• While committee members read the multitude of LOR, a number commented on how some students quietly took on mentoring other classmates who weren't performing well. Some stuck with their "mentees" through two or three years. In some cases, the professor recognized that certain students were natural educators and asked them to help students having trouble. They commented on this in their letters.

• Educators have described a "new breed" of students—"the failing student." Their definition includes (1) sitting in the back of the room, (2) coming late, (3) missing class, and (4) being the first in the family to go to college. These students need special help, and this is where you could come in. Document what you do.

• Pre-med students sometimes wonder how to judge a medical school—they want to know if it will train them well enough to get into their preferred residency. We always say that it isn't what the school teaches but what the student puts in to getting an education and demonstrating excellent qualities and passion, which his/her dean and other letter writers point out in their LOR. Then it is up to the student to perform well in his/her interview.

Personal Letter

• This comes from the heart but shouldn't be a tearjerker! What do interviewers want to know about you that isn't in the rest of your application? Did you have an epiphany when you thought, "I am making the right decision on what I want to do with the rest of my life." Try to stick to a central theme but don't ramble. Use actual patient experiences, if applicable, and don't make anything up.

• Even if you are not applying for another year, you can begin to write your personal letter. You can revise as you go, but make this **your** letter, not your mother's or friend's. And **no** plagiarism! Some letters are computer-checked for plagiarism and, if found, will not be looked upon favorably.

• Always use spell-check and grammar check.

• How do you handle your stress? What do you like to read? Do you keep up, most likely via newspapers and weekly magazines including *Time* and *The Economist*, with the rapid changes in health-care delivery?

• Find a way to point out your **balance** in life. What do you do for fun? Do you have a sense of humor? It is important to mention what you do for fun in your personal letter. Maybe you are a leader in these activities. Don't wait until you are well along in whatever you do in your career before you realize the importance of balance. We authors have heard the following story (below) from patients in different variations (this is a composite). *But remember that doctors are patients, too, so this is relevant to everyone.*

> *I made the mistake of thinking (assuming) that my plans for my family would come true. But we have no control over the future. My plan was to work two jobs in order to have enough savings to support our daughter through college; she was the first family member who would be able to go. But since I was working two jobs, I didn't have time to attend her and her siblings' school events, and we didn't go on vacations since we were saving money. Looking back, I barely knew my kids. My worst fear happened: she has been given a diagnosis of terminal cancer. Our family is devastated. I am doing my best to care for her and the rest of my family during the time she has left, but how I wish I could go back in time. The future is never certain; I only wish I had better appreciated the time we had.*

• Although you are not asked to document your **leadership** qualities in your application, this is highly regarded, especially within your volunteer activities. When listing these activities, be sure to mention any leadership role.

The Interview

See the next chapter: *Tips on Being Interviewed for Medical or Osteopathic School.* We think this is one of the most important factors in your application to medical school or for any position that will require interactions with people. There are many tips to help you have a rewarding experience, which is especially important if your next interview could affect what you will be doing the rest of your life! An interview is analogous to *stage fright*! The more confidence you have in yourself, the better it will be. Nobody says this isn't stressful!

A general view of the process for applicants is (1) your academics will get your "foot in the door," (2) your experiences will get you an interview, and (3) your interview will get you the acceptance.

We appreciate the input of Gina Vitali-Rasanen for this chapter.

Chapter Two

Tips on Being Interviewed for Medical or Osteopathic School

The interview accounts for one-fourth to one-third of the selection value.

If your future depends on how much wood you can chop in one hour, you should spend the first ten minutes sharpening your ax.

(Based on a quote attributed to President Abraham Lincoln)

If you have a preferred school for your match, we recommend that you try not to do your first interview there. That means your first interview (at a different school) could amount to a practice run, but if there is any question, then go first with the school you want: *this relates to the importance of getting your application in early*. After every interview, go over what you learned from it. Ask other interviewees what they learned and what questions were asked of them. Some questions are very clever. You might use some of them when you conduct interviews in the future. Record this data.

Research each medical/osteopathic school as well as its locality. We suggest that you plan on visiting six to eight schools. You might live in a region of the country where you can drive to all of them. Do you know of any current medical students, e.g., high school and college friends, who you can contact? Their feedback can be invaluable. **Are they happy?** This is critical.

Can you find alumni from your preferred schools who practice in your area? Consider calling them to see if they might have thirty minutes to spend with you. This meeting also might result in your finding someone you can shadow.

Go to the town and school campus a day early to look around. You might get an offer to stay overnight with a medical student. While you are on campus, everyone you meet or encounter might be interviewing you in one way or another.

The multiple mini interview (MMI) is new and used in all the approximate twenty Canadian medical schools and a few dozen U.S. medical schools at the time of this writing (2017). During the MMI, the applicant reads a less-than-one-page situation, and then goes into a room with one or two interviewers for eight to ten minutes to discuss what was on the interview page. There may be seven to ten separate interviews. The applicant can prepare for this in several ways. A course in ethics would be of great value because the interview dialogue might include some medical ethics issues that usually don't have any straightforward answers. The interviewers want to see how you think about the dilemma. They are looking for poise, clear thinking, empathy, and being able to handle a difficult patient, which are all very important. You can't fake empathy; patients will detect it quickly if you try. You aren't expected to know the Science of Medicine. You can practice MMIs with your classmates.

There are several ways you can "prepare" to interview, such as by joining Toastmasters, taking speech courses in high school or college, acting in plays, and joining debate teams. These activities can benefit you for the rest of your life.

Some off-the-wall questions might include how you would solve the Middle East crisis, or poverty, or the health-care dilemma. During our interviews, we asked a number of students how they stay current on world and regional problems. It seemed that a majority had no answer to this because they didn't read newspapers or weekly news magazines or watch TV news. A few months before your first interview, we recommend that you at least start skimming some of these to get a feel for what is going on in the world. We "old folk" look to your generation to settle some of these crises.

Not all schools demand a personal interview. There might be financial reasons or travel limitations. Call the admissions office, and its personnel might arrange an interview with a physician in your town, especially if there is an alumnus. It might even be a phone interview.

Now For The Interview

• **Be yourself!** Don't try to be someone else. An experienced interviewer can tell the difference. And **relax**. If it is a morning interview, be cautious about eating too much sugar for breakfast—it is thought that it may dull your brain. Same for lunch for an afternoon meeting. *No chewing gum!*

• **Be on time always.** You only have one chance to make a good first impression, and this is it. It is also a sign of respect to be on time. How important is this interview? To many who are hiring (interviewing), being on time is a sign that you can be counted on. Have you taken into account that you might encounter a traffic jam, difficulty finding a parking place, or weather problems? We know of one physician who overslept for an oral medical exam and was a few minutes late. He flunked.

• Check in with the receptionist. And if he/she knows who is going to interview you, ask for the name and correct pronunciation (write it out phonetically).

• Always be kind and courteous to the receptionist, secretary, etc. When we were interviewing for residencies, we recall medical students who had great credentials and were very smart but were rude to the secretaries who arranged their visits. We didn't take them into our residencies. These employees (secretaries) have some input to admissions committees, and their input carries a lot of weight. Know the receptionist/secretary's name, and say it when you check in. But buttering up the secretary or receptionist can backfire. Act professional! You can't go wrong with that.

• Take something to read. If the interviewer is ready early, he/she will see your interest in what you are reading. It could be an icebreaker, as the interviewer might be interested in your reading material and ask about it. **Do not** work on your smartphone while you are waiting.

• Stand when someone comes in the room. Say not just "Hello," but "Good morning/Good afternoon, Dr./Mr./Mrs./Ms. his/her last name" (if you know it). Let the interviewer sit first unless he/she motions for you to do so. If you are in the examiner's office, there likely will be certificates of accomplishment on the wall—these might be a point of conversation to help you relax.

• Initially, sit with your feet flat on the floor. As you relax, you can cross your legs (ladies, not ankle over knee). Look and feel comfortable. Take a few slow, deep breaths, and then slowly let the air out. This will help you relieve some stress and relax. Avoid fidgeting. Don't sit on the edge of the chair.

• Don't apologize for being nervous; everyone interviewing is nervous.

Life is just one continuous interview—you just don't know it!

—Gina Vitali-Rasanen

• **Smile.** We can't stress the importance of this enough. *A genuine smile.* A phony smile doesn't involve the muscles around the eyes. There are many interviewers in different industries who, unbeknownst to you, count your smiles. The minimum is at least three, and maybe five, smiles in fifteen to thirty minutes; if you don't reach this, you may not be asked back for a follow-up interview! You can "see" and "hear" a smile in someone's voice on the phone. Just do it! It can become a habit and reflects your personality.

• Other things the interviewer might look for: Do you reflect a feeling of warmth? Do you have a capacity for hard work? Potential for leadership?

• **Poise.** Short of taking charisma lessons at a charm school, poise comes with maturity, good self-esteem, and self-confidence. Your **Body Language (BL)** is critical here *(see Chapter 3)*. Be aware of your BL during the interview.

• **Relax.** Smile when appropriate. Maintain eye contact. No slouching.

• When you meet someone, shake hands (BL again—this is **Touch**) using a *firm, but not strong,* grip. If your grip is too strong, it can work against you. A strong grip is not a sign that you are in control. Practice your grip with a friend. Men were taught in the "old days" to not shake a woman's hand unless she offered it first. Not anymore. We (authors) make a point of shaking a woman's hand before a man's as a courtesy. Say her name with "Good morning," etc. Don't believe that chivalry is a thing of the past; women still appreciate common courtesies from a man, such as holding the door open or helping with their coats. If in doubt, be chivalrous. A hug is good, but not everyone is comfortable with this, and it would be unusual after an interview.

• Establish **Eye Contact (BL).** *This is imperative, but don't stare.* "Touch" with your eyes. Smile when you look someone in the eye. Physicians must learn to be comfortable with eye contact. If eye contact is uncomfortable for you, practice it. Absence of this BL is commonly noted by an interviewer as well as by patients.

• Say hello (**BL: Voice**) to strangers. This attitude carries over to your interview and helps you relax and reduce stress. Do it every day! A monotone implies a lack of enthusiasm or being overly stressed.

• Hold the door open for people on your way to the interview (it might be the person interviewing you!). Women should go through the door and then turn to hold it open for the next person.

You may not really care for people—and you can't fake that you do!

• **Dress nicely (professionally).** If in doubt, overdress. Men, shine your shoes—it could make a difference! If you don't have leather shoes to shine, get some. Interviewers are looking for clues, and this is one of them: *Dress like you respect yourself.* Is your tie cinched up and the top button on your shirt buttoned? When traveling to an interview (mainly flying), be sure you don't pack your only suit in checked luggage. Learn to travel with only carry-on luggage for short trips. Women, no flip-flops or five-inch heels—wear sensible shoes. Do not wear too much makeup. No perfume; no chewing gum (we're saying this again). Cover obvious tattoos, if possible.

• Body piercings? It may be too late—depending on the position you are seeking and the kind of people you will be interacting with, body piercings can definitely work against you.

• **Attitude is everything.** Many people intuitively can judge someone's attitude and *passion* and make judgments on these alone. *You can't hide a negative attitude.* Experienced interviewers can judge from your attitude if you will be good with patients or customers. Some employers look for this first. Actually, passion and attitude are forms of the same thing. A friend who had uncomplicated total knee arthroplasty some years ago tells the story about a nurse who came into his room at two o'clock one morning. He was awake and facing away from the door but still knew immediately that she had a very caring attitude—even though he wasn't sure she had said anything. He just knew! To contrast this, he told the story of visiting a friend who was post-op shoulder surgery. The friend had his call light on, and when the nurse finally came to the doorway, she said in a rather gruff voice, "Well, what do you want?" There was no healing in her voice **or** her attitude! *What is your attitude?!*

• **Passion** is hard to define, but you know it when you see or feel it. It might be a quiet passion. It is showing up for work on time or even early and staying late, which shows that you truly love what you are doing.

• Be prepared to discuss your **Purpose** in life, but be realistic.

• **Hustle (BL).** What does hustle mean to you? What do you think it means to the interviewer? Or the selection committee? You can't chart or measure hustle! But you sure know it when you see it. A young man we interviewed was the captain of his college team but never played one down of football. In spite of that, he was always the first one at practice and the last one to leave. He had great leadership qualities, and he never complained. He had hustle. His coach recognized this and wrote this in his LOR. The admissions committee looked very favorably on this.

• **Listen (BL).** This accounts for at least two-thirds of communication in real life and is extremely important in medicine. Learn to never interrupt—especially during an interview—just to make a point.

• Be cautious about putting anything on Facebook, YouTube, and any other social network. Why put any pictures of you on them in the first place? They are there for perpetuity. Employers, including some in medical centers, are scanning these networks when assessing your qualifications (and **Maturity**). It is a well-known fact that many young people have not been hired or recruited because of what potential employers saw on one of these social networks. They probably will not tell you that they saw it. Skilled computer artists can use a picture of your face and attach any body to it. Cute!

• If you have a choice of being brilliant or being nice, pick **Nice (BL-Attitude)**. Of course, you can be both, but studies that show nice and kind people have a better chance of success in life than just brilliant people. Studies show that those who smile also have a better chance of success.

• Reminding you again, **do you know your body language?** There are experts in interpreting BL, but most of us have some intuition regarding this. A physician's BL can be healing or, worse, engender a lack of trust. Think about your BL. Can you improve it? The best way to improve your body language is to improve your attitude. Just being kind and smiling throughout the day improves your attitude.

• If possible, think out how you can turn a question(s) from the interviewer into describing your strengths, your passion for caring, an epiphany event that convinced you that you truly wanted to be a physician, and/or your ideal role model and how much value you hold in this person. Your strengths must include people. Quote the **Platinum Rule of Medicine**: *Treat every patient like you would want a member of your family treated.*

• Have questions in mind that you might be asked and some thought-out answers. One frequent question is "Why do you want to be a physician?" To say that you want to help mankind is pretty broad, perhaps "I find I'm happier with myself when I help others. An act of kindness for me is powerful." A common question is "What is your favorite book and why?" This could be an interview question for many types of education and work positions.

• Any physician role models? Consider emulating them. Do you have any family/relatives/friends who are physicians? Do you know any alumni of the institution?

More Possible Questions

• How would you describe your ideal physician role model? Immediately begin writing down the qualities of your ideal role model(s), and in a separate column, also describe the negative qualities you have witnessed by others and want to avoid. Many applicants have had family members who were either very sick or died and could describe their very competent, caring physicians who left lasting impressions. Be specific about how this affected you.

• What motivated you to go into medicine?

• Describe your strengths and weaknesses. You need to think about possible questions like this to formulate good answers. Don't stretch the truth; be humble. Avoid "ya knows."

- What would you do if you witnessed a classmate who appeared to be cheating on a written exam?
- Where do you envision yourself in ten years? Do you have a plan?
- What do you do for fun?
- What would you do to change our health-care system?
- What contributions do you think you could make to our medical school? To the field of medicine?
- Describe an interesting patient you saw when shadowing. What impressed you? You won't be expected to know medical details.
- An interviewer might ask how you would handle a hypothetical ethical problem. There usually are no good "yes" or "no" answers to ethical dilemmas. Your discussion can tell an interviewer a lot about you, including your poise, maturity, and passion, and how you handle pressure. You might consider taking a course on ethics in college—the information will last you a lifetime.
- Formulate your long-range goals before the interview, although we all know these can change. It's just the idea that you are thinking things out and looking ahead. Keep up with current events by reading either your tablet computer or daily newspaper and look for items on health-care delivery problems. How would you deal with some of these?! Your generation will need to solve these issues, like it or not. These are good items for discussion. Although the interviewer will ask definitive questions about you, it also would be common for him/her to ask questions that don't have specific answers. The interviewer wants to see how you think and reason.
- Say "yes" or "no," not "yeah" or "nope." Practice how to avoid these; it adds to your poise. This is something you could learn at Toastmasters.
- If you are comfortable with this, say, "Yes, sir" or "No, ma'am."
- Never look at your watch or stare out the window. Turn off your cell phone. If you forget to turn it off, don't answer it. When you are sitting in a lobby waiting for an interview, we suggest that you do not use your phone to talk or text.
- Never say anything negative about your last job, position, or college. If you are asked about your biggest weaknesses, don't admit to any, especially if they are related to the job you would like to get. Mention something like "I don't read as much as I would like," or "I easily get lost if driving through an unfamiliar town."
- If the interviewer asks you a question and you don't know the answer, say, "I don't know." A savvy person will know when you are faking an answer.
- Interviewers are looking for **maturity**, as well as attitude and passion. How would you rate your maturity on a scale of 1 to 10? (*See Chapter 11 on* Wisdom and Maturity.) Do you know where you are going? Or just waiting to be led?
- Have the latest copy of your curriculum vitae (CV) with you in case the interviewer asks for it. If you submitted your CV/résumé months earlier and updated it in the interval with new accomplishments—especially a published paper—this is an opportunity to hand the interviewer an updated copy and point out the major goal reached or recent award. Résumés aren't used much in pre-med interviews.
- Within a few days after the interview, **handwrite** a short note of thanks for the interviewer's time and interest. Don't go overboard on what else you might say. It's OK to write something like

"I'm very impressed with your program." **Never** just an email. If you don't get into the school but might reapply someday, then this handwritten note in your record will help the interviewer remember you. Your medical-school file might be reviewed if you eventually apply to a residency program at the same institution.

• Be cautious about using humor because it may not go over—the interviewer may not have a sense of humor, and you don't know his/her personality ahead of time. But you **must** have a sense of humor. Don't hold back a laugh.

• Be careful about what questions you ask regarding the interviewer's employer/company/medical center, especially at the first interview. Get some of your questions answered from the Internet before the interview, or if you have an opportunity to talk to the medical house staff, ask them. During interviews after medical school, don't inquire about salary, work hours, moonlighting, vacation, etc., which can easily be misinterpreted.

• At the end of the interview, say the interviewer's name when you again shake hands and thank him/her as you depart. And thank the receptionist.

• At a medical/osteopathic interview experience, you likely will have the opportunity to spend some time with medical students/residents/fellows. Use caution here as they may be asked what they think about you. Just be you!

• Finally, the admissions committee members most likely will complete summary forms outlining your qualities with a grade and then give you a bottom-line number. The summary will list things such as:

> *Passion*
> *Work ethic*
> *Leadership*
> *Capability to work as a team member*
> *Personal characteristics—would they like you as their physician?*
> *Communication skills*
> *Mutual respect*
> *Commitment to a career in medicine*

Questions You Can't Be Asked!

Are you ...

> Pregnant?
> Married?
> In debt?
> Disabled?

You also cannot be asked:

> What is your religious and/or political affiliation?
> How old are you?
> Do you have children or plan to?
> Do you drink or smoke?

Have fun! Nurture your sense of humor. It is **mandatory** for survival.

15

Chapter Three

So Now You Are Learning to Be a Doctor
or
The Making of the Ideal Physician

The Physician-Patient Interaction for the Medical Student and Young Physician

The very first time you see a patient **and all** subsequent encounters with patients are extremely important in the ongoing process of the making of the **PHYSICIAN throughout his/her entire career**. The encounters build on trust. As you will find out, this **trust** has great healing powers. The more trust there is, the more compliant your patients will be to your recommendations and, at the same time, allow them to maintain some autonomy over their own health. They will save a lot of health-care dollars and lessen the number of unnecessary return visits. They will sense that you care about them.

Unfortunately, the skills necessary for obtaining important information—from taking a thorough history to performing a complete physical examination—are going by the wayside. It is said that the diagnosis of an unexplained symptom(s) can be made in 80 percent of cases based on the patient's history and/or physical examination. If you listen carefully, the patient may tell you the diagnosis! It is not uncommon now for a skilled, master clinician to listen to a patient's heart and lungs through his/her clothes or gown! Patients know the difference. The current mind-think is to get imaging and laboratory studies first, and if that doesn't disclose an "answer," then do a history and exam! We sometimes hear now that a nurse will take a patient's history and do the physical examination and then have the physician sign the note. Cost control may not pay for the imaging or laboratory studies—you may have to! Practicing the Art of Medicine is one of the most important and enjoyable aspects of being a physician, but we are losing that skill and the patient knows it. It is up to you to maintain the practice of the Art of Medicine.

This chapter pertains primarily to your "first patient" and is a "how-to" regarding the physician-patient interaction. However, it applies not just to your very first patient encounter but also to the ongoing care of **all** your patients over your practicing lifetime. This interactive partnership relates strongly to the patient's well-being. There is one rule that you should keep in mind every time you encounter a patient—whether by phone or during his/her first visit or a subsequent one—and that is the Platinum Rule of Medicine:

> ### *Treat every patient like you would want a member of your family treated.*

Now Are You Ready for Your First Patient?

• Dress professionally. You only have one chance to make a good first impression. No chewing gum. You should have your medical center's identification badge on.

• **Be on time.** Of course, this is not always possible, but if you are running behind, have an office staff person tell your patient why you are late (every so often if need be). Or stick your head in the exam room, and let the patient know you are coming soon. And *apologize* for being late. Tell the patient you have been reviewing his/her record (with the attending physician if that is the situation) and haven't been on a coffee break. You must always remember that the patient's time also is important. Being on time is analogous to airline punctuality—if the plane is on time, no one complains about the service, the food, the baggage mishandling, etc. But when there are more delays, there will be complaints about everything.

> ### *Being on time enhances your bonding with the patient—you care!*

• Look over the record before you go into the room. Is there anything there that gives you an idea why he/she is here? If the patient has been to your office before but saw another doctor, know this. If the patient expected to see his/her previous doctor, apologize. Patients put a high priority on being able to have their own doctors. *This is continuity of care and demonstrates your professionalism.* If there are records from a referring physician, tell the patient that you have looked at them. This is very important. You should insert in your note that you have reviewed the outside records and images, as well as the internal record. You may need to do this to get paid!

> ### *There is a miraculous moment when the very presence of the physician is the most effective part of the treatment!*

• If the door is closed, knock **gently** before going in. Begin by saying the patient's name, and then offer a handshake while looking him/her in the eye. A warm smile is important. If you don't have the pronunciation correct, be sure you learn it; spell it out phonetically on the chart. Keep in mind that many patients intuitively judge whether or not they are going to like their doctors *within the first five seconds*—maybe even before the student or physician speaks. More on this under body language.

• If there are family members in the room, be sure to include them in the conversation. Shake their hands, look them in the eye, and get their names and relationships to the patient. Eventually, you may need to ask them to leave the room during a physical exam unless it is a very limited one. After you finish the exam and before you send the patient for further testing, call the family members back in, as appropriate, to explain your plans. Ask the patient and family members if they have any questions at this point. Always explain what tests you are going to schedule and why. Patients need to be involved with these decisions because this allows them to establish some autonomy.

• If you are a medical student, introduce yourself and explain that you are not yet a "doctor." Give the patient your professional card if you have one, or write out your name for him/her. Point to your name on your name badge. Young women in training, or even on staff, sometimes have a problem because patients intuitively insist on calling them by their first names. A woman should introduce herself as, "I'm Ms. Johnson, a medical student," and point to her name badge, which, ideally, should have the initial of her first name rather than her full name. But many physicians do prefer to be called by their first name.

• Remind patients that their medical records are very confidential to anyone not involved in their care.

• When you see children as patients, you usually can make them smile and relax by asking them how old they are—and then asking if they are married!

• If you are seeing patients as a medical student or resident, explain that you are going to find out what medical problems bring them to you, and then a staff physician will come in and go over your findings. It is uncommon for a patient to want to bypass the medical student; they seem to know that this is a part of his/her education. A male medical student must learn when it would be uncomfortable to examine a woman, as many ethnic groups allow only a woman to examine another woman. A female clinical assistant who roomed the patient can help you here. If there is any doubt, ask a female attendant to be present.

• As a student or resident/fellow, be very cautious when talking about the patient's possible condition or disease. Just say that there isn't enough information yet to speculate. This will save you a lot of embarrassment and backpedaling, as well as having to try to explain this to the staff. You will learn how and when to do this.

A patient new to a physician doesn't care about how much the physician knows until he/she knows how much the physician cares!

• Be cautious about using patients' first names. It is OK for patients younger than you, but until you establish a relationship, even a brief one, call them Mr., Ms., or Mrs. Last Name. If they insist that you call them by their first names, as many older patients will, then we always tell them to call us by our first names. Nursing home patients are a little different. Nursing home personnel commonly call patients by their first names. We disagree. These people, especially the elderly, have lost a lot of dignity by being in a nursing home, and we respect them by using Mr./Ms./Mrs. After you get to know a patient as a friend, using a first name is more natural. And never use terms like "dearie" or "honey," etc., which is what nursing home personnel are want to do.

> ### *... the average person is more interested in his or her own name than in all the other names on earth put together.*
> —Dale Carnegie

• The older we get, the more we appreciate the absolute importance of greeting all people we know by name, not just by "Hi" or "Hello." A person takes this as a very personal compliment—a form of bonding—that you cared enough to call him/her by name. It immediately enhances the power of your caring in the patient's eyes.

• With the physician-patient partnership, the physician tries to respect the patient's autonomy. But there may need to be a gentle push-pull between the patient and the doctor (often nonverbal) to allow the doctor to decide how much autonomy the patient really wants. The concept of loss of control on the part of some patients can't be underestimated. The struggle for control can be very stressful and is inversely proportional to the patient and the family's trust and comfort with the physician(s) and the health-care team.

• There is a relatively new approach referred to as *shared decision-making*. It is a form of a partnership (a dance) between you and the patient, which is critical when dealing with possible life-and-death decisions. This is more of a factor now than in decades past when patients almost always left all the decisions up to their physicians. Today's patient is much more informed, mostly because of the Internet. Physician empathy is critical here—as is trust. Some physicians are reluctant to give up their power of decision-making, and it becomes an unfriendly tussle—maybe to the point that the patient will seek care and another opinion elsewhere. Comparable terms to *shared decision-making* are *patient empowered, autonomy*, and *collaboration*. The decision often vacillates depending on input from family, friends, and physician-friends. The physician's ability to interpret the patient's body language can be a positive factor.

• Begin the dialogue with your patients by asking, "How can I help you?" rather than "Can I help you?" With the "how" question, you are more likely to get the information you need to help your patients. Ultimately, ask patients how their illnesses are affecting their *quality of life* and that of their families.

> ### *Research shows that the physician-patient relationship is the most consistently reported determinant of physician satisfaction!*
> #### *This statement is a great means of preventing the onset of apathy and burnout (see Chapter 12).*

• Being a patient in the best of hands and in the best of situations can still be a humiliating experience. We, the health-care team, must minimize this while, at the same time, be aware of this. Oftentimes, a physician doesn't appreciate the humility of being a patient until he/she becomes one. If a medical student has never been a hospital patient, he/she should arrange to be admitted overnight to experience what their patients do. Some medical schools do this routinely. Find out what it's like to be flat on your back in a hospital bed and pushed onto a crowded elevator with others, including your friends, "looking down" on you. You won't forget this!

• **Kindness/Being nice.** You don't need a definition of these terms because you know them when you experience them or, worse, when you don't. Body language expresses kindness. Similar human characteristics are "warmth," "respect," "caring with dignity," and "empathetic." These characteristics should be there for every patient every day, no matter how your day is going. Practice being a little kinder than necessary to everyone. Here is the Platinum Rule again. *And be kind and gentle with yourself.*

> ### *Three things in human life are important. The first is to be kind. The second is to be kind. And the third is to be kind.*
>
> —Henry James

• Appear relaxed. Sit down—we've heard of many physicians who stay standing in the exam room while they take a short history or give reports to the patient so they can get out of the room that much quicker! Some even stand at the door with their hand on the handle. This is rude and arrogant. Sit down! Do not lean back—the Mayo brothers (founders of Mayo Clinic) had office chairs built for their clinic that could not recline backward. And listen! *You will read about the importance of listening several times in this book.* You have limited time with most of your patients, so you need to pay strict attention—mindfulness—to them. Then they will feel like you have effectively communicated with them. As you sit before the patient, maintaining eye-to-eye contact, learn from him/her just by watching. There may be a mannerism or facial expression that is a tip-off to a clinical entity or his/her level of stress and how he/she is handling the illness.

• Don't look at your watch. If you need to know the time, place a clock behind the patient or on your desk between you and the patient. Or glance at the clock on the computer.

• A moment of small talk can be invaluable, e.g., "Tell me about yourself." If the patient bonds with you, he/she will want to know something about you, but keep this short. Ultimately, find a way to compliment the patient during a visit, and be empathetic by telling him/her that you know it must be hard to struggle with his/her disease. This is extremely important to the patient. Remember that two-thirds of patients over age sixty now have a chronic disease(s). We can summarize this by the motto of *Motivate, Educate, and Congratulate.* Do this with every patient when appropriate. It encourages compliance. It's possible that no one has ever done this before with your patient.

• If the caregiver is with the patient, compliment him/her. Studies show that nearly half of caregivers have chronic diseases themselves, which is twice the average for their age groups.

> ### *Wherever there is a human being, there is an opportunity for kindness!*

• Do you feel that the patient is comfortable with you? Never talk down to a patient. *And avoid medical jargon.*

• Studies have shown that a physician interrupts a patient after the *first eighteen seconds* and continues to do so. If you let the patient talk for up to three minutes, he/she will estimate that you spent twice as much time as you actually did with him/her and be much more satisfied. Similar studies have been done with surgeons, and it was found that if a surgeon allowed a patient to talk uninterrupted for two-plus minutes, the interview finished three minutes sooner. This included answering questions.

Be quiet! I'll do all the talking!

—From a physician to a patient

(This is an example of "awesome arrogance." We have many examples of similar comments.)

You can't heal if you are angry!

• **There is no such thing as an arrogant, compassionate physician.** Ask yourself, "Am I arrogant or perceived as being arrogant?" Arrogance is a weak man's imitation of strength.

• Ask patients what their expectations are for the visit.

• Never criticize another physician to the patient or the house staff, and never, never put this in writing. **Never.** If the patient hears this, he/she will almost certainly tell the physician you put down. This is not an uncommon factor in lawsuits. The patient's record is a legal document.

• Use great caution when criticizing or disagreeing with the diagnosis of another physician. You may be correct—remember, you probably have more up-to-date test results and a lapse of time since the patient last saw his/her physician—but it can really confuse the patient. Again, you can be sure the patient will tell the referring physician! Try to find a way to compliment the patient's physician (if you are not the primary physician). Criticizing a home physician is a good way to lose patient referrals.

• Never hesitate to say "I'm sorry"—two very powerful words—and look the patient in the eye. The arrogant physician can't do this.

• Why some patients are reluctant to disclose problems:
  ■ Distrust of the medical system
  ■ Embarrassed
  ■ Macho men
  ■ Belief that nothing can be done
  ■ Don't want family to find out
  ■ Worried that their fears about what is wrong will be confirmed
  ■ Blocking behaviors of the physician—switching the topic, explaining problems away by saying the distress is normal, attending to physical aspects only, offering advice and reassurance before the main problems have been identified, and telling patients that their problems are their fault!

Some patients are just really angry with physicians. They may want to talk about this, so give them a chance even if it takes a little more time. Until they deal with their anger, nothing good is going to happen.

• Never tell an off-color story in mixed company, and **never** use foul language. Show character and integrity. Patients, nurses, and other physicians will remember your good qualities, but they also will never forget your bad ones. Your "bad" character traits will be their first thoughts when they see you or hear your name. They will tell others that they wouldn't want that physician as their doctor!

• Avoid talking about patients in elevators, hallways, etc. This is a no-brainer, but it happens all the time. Some people's voices carry far. At the bedside, be cautious among yourselves when whispering. Don't think that the patient can't hear you. Wrong! When a patient is in a coma or semi-coma, it's known that hearing is the last sense to disappear; if a patient awakens, he/she may remember what he/she "overheard." Also, use caution about laughing in the hallways where very sick and even terminally ill patients and their families can hear. It is very inappropriate and reflects poorly on the institution. When you are in a group in a patient's room (most commonly a hospital room), never talk about another patient—your patient will assume you are talking about him/her. If this happens, explain to the patient and family, if present, that you were discussing another patient **and** apologize. If there is an urgent matter about another patient to discuss, step outside the room.

• Never use terms like "GOMER" (get out of my ER), a "hit," a "DUMP," or "PMS" (poor, miserable sap). It is disrespectful to refer to any patient as "impoverished"; a better term is "underserved." Never refer to a patient by a diagnosis, e.g., "the brain tumor down the hall." And don't tolerate anyone else using these terms **ever**. It undermines the culture of an institution and the reputation of the profession.

> *From a surgeon to his son going into surgical practice:*
> *Never operate on a stranger!*
>
> —Raymond A. Lee, MD

Communication

• Practice putting all your senses and expressions of caring together. The result will be a palpable empathy with a strong feeling of trust and bonding between you and your patient. *Listening* remains one of the most powerful forms of healing. *Suffering* is an affliction of the soul, not the body. It is separate from pain, shortness of breath, and any physical discomfort. *Do you think your senses are attuned to this?* Loneliness is another sensation that is hard to describe; men are often reluctant to admit to it, but it is one example of suffering. The extreme loner is frequently bullied and eventually, but rarely, may commit a serious crime. He's angry. Listening to a suffering person might be called *sympathetic listening.*

• Communicating is at the heart of the physician-patient encounter. Time constraints are making this a lost art, but it is the only way to establish trust. When patients are surveyed, "how my doctor talked to me" and "how my doctor listened to me" are very often listed as the most important characteristics of a physician.

Did my doctor listen to me or just hear me?

• You can get the diagnosis and treatment correct, but if you cannot communicate these to your patient and colleagues, you have failed your patient.

• We are communicating from the instant we meet a patient. Patients make judgments about physicians in a matter of seconds, although often they don't know that they are doing so. Most communication is nonverbal (see *Body Language* later in this chapter). If there is a lack of congruence between verbal and nonverbal communication, patients believe the nonverbal communication is more truthful and authentic.

• The foundation of our relationships with patients and colleagues is communicating with each other. Patient compliance is higher and symptom resolution is greater when physician-patient communication is satisfactory to the patient.

• Context and intonation in your voice are often paramount in medicine and difficult to communicate digitally. It is hard to go wrong with a phone call or face-to-face conversation. Patients appreciate physician-to-physician communication in their presence. It connotes transparency and honesty.

Successful communication is a combination of art, science, intuition, curiosity, and experience.

• Emotional intelligence—the ability to read and synthesize another's emotions—is the bedrock of good communication. Below are some characteristics of excellent physician communicators. Most patients intuitively recognize these qualities.

Empathy	Tolerance	Judgment
Inquisitiveness	Gratitude	Flexibility
Humor	Respect	Patience
Compassion	Passion	Engagement
Self-awareness	Self-discipline	
Temperance	Prudence	

• Some Barriers to Effective Communication:
   ■ Lack of training, including at home!
   ■ Lack of skills practice
   ■ Lack of observation and feedback by an experienced clinician
   ■ Lack of preparation before the patient encounter
   ■ Fear of upsetting the patient
   ■ Inability to read and respond to patient emotion
   ■ Paternalistic or arrogant mind-set
   ■ Fear of one's own emotions
   ■ Interruptions
   ■ Feeling rushed or harried
   ■ Insensitivity—doesn't really care! (apathy, burnout)

• Remember, you are always communicating, and communication begins the first time you meet a patient. A patient may assess you in seconds. First impressions tend to last.

• Here's something to mull over regarding a clinical trial reported in the surgical literature. In one trial group, anesthesiologists whispered calm and reassuring words in patients' ears shortly after they induced general anesthetic. Of course, the patients didn't remember hearing the words. A separate group of patients did not have anything whispered in their ears. Those who had the words whispered to them averaged one-day shorter hospital stays and less post-op complications. All the patients had surgical resection for chronic diverticulitis of the sigmoid colon.

• Dr. Hugh Butt, who was a Mayo Clinic physician for many years, described his experiences as a fellow with Dr. William J. "Dr. Will" Mayo, one of Mayo Clinic's founders, and Dr. Will's interactions with patients. According to Dr. Butt, Dr. Will always greeted every patient with a *smile*, usually a handshake or touch, got seated, and then made a nonmedical connection, e.g., asking the patient about his/her family or farm. Dr. Butt stated that Dr. Will could spend ten minutes with a patient, but the patient would feel that it had been forty-five. This method developed by Dr. Will has now been validated by scientific studies. Patients are more satisfied when their physicians smile, sit down, and conduct the interview using a biopsychosocial model.

• Generally, patients prefer some physical contact conducted in a professional manner. This could be a handshake, light touch on the shoulder, or an arm wrapped around the patient's shoulder as you walk down the hall. *Touch is a very important aspect of the physical exam.* Don't offer a hug unless you sense that the patient wants it. Respect for cultural differences should always be maintained.

Touch is a poorly understood method of communicating, but it can be powerful!

• When you sit, patients perceive that you are spending more time with them than when you stand. A large entourage in a hospital room standing near the door sends the wrong message to a patient.

Is there anything more doleful than the procession of four or five doctors into a sick man's room?
—Sir William Osler

• Your body language sends strong nonverbal signals to your patient. After being seated, assume a position close to the patient while giving him/her adequate personal space. Leaning in a bit toward the patient is generally preferable. Leaning back in the chair with your legs crossed, for example, is not a sign of caring and interest in the patient's needs.

• Eye contact is paramount and shows caring and concern, but avoid staring at the patient. Your facial expressions and small utterances ("Oh my!" said empathetically) can make a more lasting impression on the patient than any eloquent discussion of disease pathophysiology.

• Asking permission of the patient is almost never wrong and shows mutual respect. "May I sit down?" "Is it OK if I take notes?" "I need to look at the computer a few minutes; is that all right?"

"I need to call my colleague and ask her a couple of questions about your problem, OK?" Try to limit your time in front of the computer while with the patient. Never, ever spend the bulk of the interview looking at the computer and not having eye contact with the patient.

• Self-awareness (mindfulness; being in the moment) is key to effective communication. Be aware of your own emotions and body language, as well as those of your patient. This is more difficult than it sounds, especially when you are trying to juggle medical information in your mind. *It takes practice and intention to know yourself.*

The Patient Interview

• The first part of the patient interview deals primarily with information gathering. During this portion of the interview, questions should be open-ended and non-focused, e.g., "During the thirty minutes we have together today, what would you like to focus on?" As stated before, allow a patient to initially talk without interruption. Although it sounds a bit counterintuitive, this actually saves time as patients are allowed to express themselves, and most will not talk more than a couple of minutes.

Listen actively with the intent to learn.

• Use inviting language to be sure all their concerns are expressed: "Tell me more." "What else?"

• Summarize what you heard, and sketch a plan for the rest of the visit. For example, "So what I heard was that you would like to focus on your headaches, trouble sleeping, and concerns about your son's behavior. Let's talk about your headaches and sleep issues today. I understand the importance of your son's problems to you, and I will make sure we have plenty of time to talk about that when you return. This may be playing a significant role in how you are feeling."

• The next part of the interview should focus on the now-defined agenda with more close-ended questions. "Tell me about your headaches, when do they occur, what are they like, etc."

• After eliciting information about the patient's medical history using close-ended questions, turn your interview to understanding his/her perspective. Focus on the patient's expectations and how the illness is affecting his/her own life and that of his/her family. Try to gain insight into the patient's ideas and concerns about his/her health or illness.

• Acknowledge the patient's concerns or frustrations. "I don't know why I can't get my blood sugar under control." "My wife is really worried about me."

• Do a review of symptoms related to the chief complaints.

• Remember to speak plainly, give small pieces of information, and frequently check in. "Am I making sense?" "Do you have questions?" This also may be a time to respond to the patient's emotions, show empathy, and strengthen the physician-patient relationship.

Communication skills help with relationships, empathy, and emotions.

• To be an effective physician, you must not only be competent in your medical skills but also be able to have meaningful relationships with your patients. Physician-patient relationships are built on **trust**, which is the foundation of our profession. Patients must trust not only your medical knowledge and skills but also your integrity, compassion, and concern for their needs. By enhancing your communication skills for dealing with patient emotions and being able to convey empathy, you will go a long way toward building lasting relationships.

• To repeat again: During the course of your time with patients, find time to **motivate**, **educate**, and **congratulate** them for what they have done, e.g., quit smoking, lost weight, began exercising, etc. This is a powerful form of bonding and, in turn, healing. Remember to be empathetic by saying that you know how hard they have struggled with their conditions. All this can pay off with their compliance.

• **Ask-Tell-Ask.** This is a cornerstone of relationship-centered communication in health care. It sounds simple, but you might be surprised how many times physicians make *assumptions* about a patient's understanding of his/her health without taking time to clarify that knowledge. We think that is because we, as physicians, have been thorough in our explanations, and patients have insight into what they have been told. In fact, most of us can only remember a few facts of information even a few days after being told, much less synthesize and process them.

• **Ask-Tell-Ask** is simply what it says: "So I know you have seen several doctors lately, but just to be sure we are on the same page, can you tell me how you understand your medical condition?" "OK, great, would it now be all right if I told you how I understand your health-care issues?" Then, "What questions do you have?" "If you had to call your spouse now and summarize what we have just been over, what would you say?" If the spouse is there, ask what he/she understood. *Listen carefully—maybe you will learn more.*

Some Specific Communication Skills

Goals of Care, Recommendations, and Shared Decision-Making

• In an increasingly sophisticated and technological medical world, it is important to discern that patients get the kind of care they want and where they want it, and it should be congruent with their goals. And don't forget the **Platinum Rule of Medicine**.

• Understanding your patient's values, preferences, desires, hopes, and fears is key to providing the best and appropriate care. So it is helpful to make a nonmedical connection and use a biopsychosocial model of interviewing.

• To elicit goals of care, the **Ask-Tell-Ask** model should be the foundation of your discussion with a patient. However, before doing this, we suggest a rubric beginning with an understanding of your patient's "story." You might start the conversation something like this: "I am one of the doctors who will care for you in the ICU after your surgery if you go ahead with it, and I want to talk to you about your medical condition. Before we do that, tell me a little about you." Patients might tell you about where they were born and raised, their marriage and family, occupation, hobbies, and faith tradition. This helps the patient to relax.

   ■ Then continue with the question (**Ask**): "Thanks for sharing something about yourself; now can we talk about your health? So that we are on the same page, tell me how you understand your medical condition." Patient: "I had a heart attack and may need surgery."

■ **Tell:** "Would it be OK if I told you how I understand your medical condition? You did have a heart attack, so bypass surgery may be an option. However, there are risks involved for a person who is in his/her seventies and has diabetes and chronic kidney disease."

■ **Ask:** "Am I being clear? What questions do you have?" Patient: "I guess I am not sure what to do." At this juncture, a recommendation might be in order.

■ **Recommendation:** "Based on what we have talked about, you told me that remaining independent on the farm and not being in a nursing home are very important to you. It is hard for me to predict how you might do after heart surgery. Since your heart muscle is strong, I would suggest deferring surgery. Your new medicines we put you on also will help."

• **Shared decision-making:** Without knowing a patient's story, including his/her values, goals, and preferences, the above recommendation would not be possible. Remember, we each have our own unique narrative, yet you haven't taken away the patient's autonomy to make decisions. Shared decision-making keeps the patient central to the relationship and conversation. By presenting the clinical information in light of their values and preferences, we can help patients make decisions consistent with their goals. This allows the patient to maintain autonomy while looking to you for guidance and recommendations. This is extremely important in developing and maintaining trust.

• Another important communication skill—not only for attending physicians but also for surgeons—is "being there." After a surgeon performs an inpatient procedure, he/she should visit the patient and the family later that day for at least a few minutes to answer questions. The surgeon also should visit the patient for the next few days, assuming there are no complications. If there are complications, the surgeon should visit more often—this can't be delegated to the resident or nurse. The patient and the family deserve to have their questions answered.

Building Relationships and Responding to a Patient's Emotions

• Effective communication skills are the cornerstone of a meaningful physician-patient relationship and allow you to respond to a patient's emotions.

• The American Academy on Communication in Healthcare (AACHonline.org) uses the acronym **PEARLS**, which we find very helpful. Below are the acronym and some examples of helpful statements that correspond accordingly.

■ *Partnership.* "We are going to work on this problem together." "Together we can solve this." "I will give you information on how you can contact me."

■ *Empathy/Emotions.* Responding to a patient's emotions in an empathetic way can be challenging and requires learned skills and practice. If you know how to do this well, it also can be extremely fruitful and bond you with your patient. When a patient is upset, we sometimes find that a few seconds of silence can be helpful. A short time of quiet and reflection—not too long—rather than an immediate response can help tamp down tension and emotion. Another response that can be useful is simply naming what you see, e.g., "You appear very upset." Avoid saying how a patient feels—no one really knows how another person feels. But you can be sure that, at a minimum, most are apprehensive until they hear from you.

We have no idea what burdens many of our patients carry in their minds!

- **_Apology/Appreciation:_** "You have done a wonderful job caring for your mother." "I am sorry I am running late, but we are going to devote the next thirty minutes we have scheduled focusing on you."
- **_Respect:_** "I can't tell you how great it is to see that you have lost weight, and your blood sugars are much better." "Though we may have different opinions about that, I respect what you are telling me."
- **_Legitimation:_** "Anyone in your situation would be tearful." "It is normal to have the frustrations you are experiencing now."
- **Support autonomy and competence:** "I am going to call your doctor now so she knows we are all working together on this." "Here is my contact information. I am here to work with you."

• Other words we find helpful are "imagine" and "wish." "I _imagine_ the last few weeks have been very difficult for you." "I _wish_ I had different news for you." Also, "tell me more" can give you deeper insight into a patient's feelings when he/she is emotional: "You appear angry. Can you tell me more about that?"

"PEARLS" is a good summary of Motivate, Educate, and Congratulate.

Wrapping up the Interview

• At the end of the interview, we frequently ask one question that we have found enhances our communication with a patient: _So is there anything we did not talk about that we need to know in order to help us care for you?_ We are often surprised what patients will say and how much we can glean from that one question.

• It probably looks like following the outlined format adds more time to the patient's visit, but in the long run, it actually shortens it.

Body Language—Yours, Not the Patient's!

Studies show that 80 percent of person-to-person communication is _nonverbal_; some say it is closer to 90 percent. Nonverbal communication is a new science, and it is a powerful healer! It plays a significant role in effective communication. In addition to your voice and words, your body language (nonverbal) can express connection, complete attention, and engagement with your patient. Be aware of this—it is a very effective part of communication. Students in master's degree programs in body language interpretation learn more than 1,000 very, very subtle motions. Many people—like your patients—do this intuitively. They don't know what they are doing, but they are interpreting what you are "saying" with your body language and making judgments about you. We suggest that you learn to be an amateur interpreter of body language (a people watcher). The patient judges you constantly and makes decisions on this basis. As you become more experienced, you will intuitively learn how to interpret your patients' body language. During an interview, ask yourself, "Is this patient trying to tell me something through body language?" The following are some examples that are more important in you than in the patient.

• **Smile:** Absolutely powerful. Your smile raises good endorphins in you, as well as the recipient, and these may last for hours. It is the same in all languages. It is a form of bonding. Smiling boosts the immune systems of both you and the person receiving your smile and relieves stress. It disarms the angry patient. The oxytocin hormone, known as the "happy hormone," is released, just as it is by a mother and her newborn. Some businesses won't hire you if you don't smile during an interview. We now know your dog receives your smile with elevated oxytocin!

A smile is the shortest distance between two people.

We're emphasizing smiling here because it is so powerful, not just in a physician-patient relationship, but because it also works wonders in the real world! Here are more examples of what a smile can do:
- It changes our mood.
- It releases endorphins and oxytocin.
- It is contagious.
- It relieves stress.
- It helps you stay positive.
- It boosts your immune system.
- It makes you more attractive and lifts your face so you look younger. It makes you feel successful.

I have never seen anyone who was smiling who wasn't beautiful!

**It is OK to smile if you are with family members at the time of a death.
It is a smile of kindness and bonding if it is sincere. It warms the room.**

A smile is one of the most powerful weapons in healing we have!

• **Attitude:** A positive attitude can alter your life. You *cannot* hide your attitude. It really sends a message about you. Only **you** have control over this.

• **Facial expression:** The face can make *thousands* of microexpressions lasting only 0.1 second. The computer camera and some untrained people (including your patients) can read these. The face expresses five different emotions: (1) happiness, (2) concern, (3) sadness, (4) anger, and (5) surprise. Happiness communicates caring, sincerity, and compassion. Patients like to think their physician is happy.

• **Eye contact:** This is imperative when relating to another person because you are looking into his/her soul. About 75 percent of our interactions with a patient should involve eye contact. You can't be in tune with your patient without this—this is mindfulness. Don't stare. **Never** just concentrate on the computer—this is one of the most common patient complaints. *Smize is a new word that means smile with your eyes!*

- **Body position:** Crossed legs, twisting in your seat, and hands clasping and unclasping denote nervousness. This could relate to you or your patient. A reminder: Don't lean back in your chair because it can send the wrong message. In fact, lean forward every now and then.

- **Touch:** This is another powerful healer, but we don't understand it. A physician needs to learn the power of professional touching because it is a real act of bonding, especially when combined with a smile and caring words. You, the toucher, might get as much out of the touching as the person receiving it—not unlike a smile. There is a phenomenon in Eastern European countries related to newborns who are almost never held while waiting to be adopted, which sometimes takes many months and or even years. As these children get older, they are emotionless and "sterile." Their amygdala has atrophied. They are devoid of establishing interpersonal relationships and don't like to touch or be touched as adults.

- In another study of volunteers regarding the importance of touch, an electrical stimulus was perceived as less severe as measured by an fMRI when the person held hands with a friend. Americans are less "touchy" and less happy than those in South American countries and Western Europe, especially France, Italy, and Spain. Touching a pet also has been shown to have great healing power.

- **Olfactory:** Some dogs have a 10,000-fold ability to interpret odors. We think our olfactory centers have some ability to interpret extremely faint odors, but we never consciously appreciate it. This might explain the "chemistry" some people feel for others, or how patients can immediately and subconsciously judge a physician. What scent are you emanating? Maybe it is your attitude they "smell." It has been said that emotions are contagious; could this be what your patient is sensing?

- **Listen:** This can't be stressed enough. This is another sense that is extremely powerful as a healer and bonding agent and is essential for recognizing what is bothering your patient. Leaning in, nodding, and making a few expressions such as "go on," acknowledge that you want to help. Many patients just need someone to listen, no matter what they have to say.

A man can see further through a tear than a telescope.

—Lord Byron

- One of the biggest complaints patients have is "My doctor never seems to **listen** to me." *Listen with the intent to learn.* Nod every so often. Don't lean back in your chair. Maintain eye contact. *"It's not what's said; it's what's heard." Listen between the lines.* What is the patient trying to tell you? Hearing and listening are not the same things—remember this.

It's amazing how much you will hear when no one is talking!

- Most of us have no idea of the impact of the words we use, or don't use, when talking to a patient or of the patient's perception of us. You have to convey empathy, interest, and concern in your voice.

> ### *The most important thing in communication*
> ### *is to hear what isn't being said.*
> —Peter Drucker

- Negative behavior characteristics as judged by the patient are *angry, cold, callous, arrogant, hurried,* and more. Every so often, ask yourself if your patient might be observing these in your body language.
- **Voice:** Your voice and tone say much about you. Anger, caring, and happiness can all be picked up in your voice. Callers can detect if you smile when you answer the phone.

> ### *In life, you will have many opportunities to be quiet and not speak.*
> ### *Take advantage of every one of these.*
> —Raymond A. Lee, MD

Some Useful Phrases and Words
"Before we talk about your medical issues, tell me a little about yourself."
"What are your expectations for this visit?"
"I can only imagine."
"I wish."
"How can I help you?"
"Is there anything we have not talked about that I should know that would help me care for you?" This further closes the gap between you and the patient.
"Tell me more."
"I'm sorry."
"Anybody in your situation would feel this way."
"You have done a wonderful job caring for your (parent, spouse, etc.)."
"We are in this together."
"You appear (sad, upset, etc.)." *Never tell patients how they feel because you don't know and can't know.*
"Uh-huh" while nodding.
"So what I heard is ..."
"How do you understand the big picture of your health right now?"
"What other questions do you have?" This is better than "Do you have any questions?"
You also can be silent or pause. Sometimes a few seconds of silence when the patient is emotional can be therapeutic.

"Uh-oh" is an expression you should **not** use—it always has a negative connotation and frightens anyone who hears it.

• Remember that all the patients you encounter are worried about their health, although they'll say they aren't. Even in the absence of any symptoms, we call these patients "the worried well." Many patients have heard about the asymptomatic person who went to the physician to get a checkup and ended up being diagnosed with metastatic cancer.

The message your body language is sending would explain why the patient judges you within five seconds of your walking in the door without you having yet said one word!

More Words*

"Tell me about yourself."

"Do you have any ideas about what is causing your symptoms?"

"Go on."

"What else?" This encourages the patient to speak up if he/she is withholding some pertinent information.

"I think I'm beginning to understand how this is bothering you."

"I'm going to do everything I can to help you."

"What do you think is causing your symptoms?"

"How depressed are you over this?" This is more than "Are you depressed?"

"Everybody has stress in life; do you think you have an extra load of stress as a result of your problems?" "Might you have a form of post-traumatic stress disorder?" "How would you grade your stress on a scale of 1 to 10?"

"Let me see if I have this right."

"I share your sorrow. I consider your father a good friend."

*Be cautious about interrupting the patient inappropriately. Also be careful about using the word "closure" because it may sound too definitive to some family members.

• Don't hesitate to unmask a depression. About 25 percent to 50 percent of your patients may be depressed. Studies have shown that the patient with an undiagnosed mental problem (most often a depression) averages nearly a dozen office visits a year before diagnosis and treatment, which is a real burden to health-care costs and your time and frustration. After diagnosis, a patient averages only four visits the next year. The cost for hospitalized patients is even greater. If your time with a patient is too limited to get into the possibility of whether he/she is depressed, schedule another appointment soon. But tell the patient that you are going to help.

Above all things, let me urge upon you the absolute necessity of careful examinations for the purpose of diagnosis. My own experience has been that the public will forgive you an error in treatment more readily than one in diagnosis, and I fully believe that more than one-half of the failures in diagnosis are due to hasty and unmethodic examinations.

—**William J. Mayo, MD, 1895** *(The date is not a misprint.)*

• The next step is usually the physical exam. It is a very important part of the touch-communications. Touching throughout your exam is therapeutic and constitutes a form of bonding. Open this portion of your physician-patient interaction by asking, "Is it OK to examine you now?" And it should be unhurried, which takes a little skill. Don't forget that the physical exam can be a useful time to ask more questions if need be and also to listen. Be sure to explain any positive findings from the exam right then.

• How good are your exam skills? The best way to learn how to do a history and physical examination is to shadow an experienced clinician and get experience by practicing.

• Your examination of the patient should be appropriately thorough. "Appropriately," in this case, means that your exam generally is limited to the patient's symptoms and/or risk factors. But be prepared to answer why you aren't doing a "complete" exam.

• Wash your hands in front of the patient. Respect modesty with appropriate covering. Be gentle. Be sure your breath is fresh, and don't chew gum. Try to avoid words like "hurt" and "pain" as these lower the patient's pain threshold. "Discomfort" is more acceptable. This is especially true when doing a procedure on the patient. As you examine the patient, say what you are going to do next. Avoid using the expression "hmm," as it suggests something wrong or bad and is never used in a positive sense.

• Never listen to the heart and lungs through a patient's shirt or gown! Tell them that tenderness over the epigastrium (explain "epigastrium") is normal due to pressing on the abdominal aorta, which usually is mildly tender.

• Try not to answer the phone during an exam—you may end up in a long conversation while the patient is waiting on the exam table. And you don't want to be talking about personal things on the phone.

• After the exam, communication should include something on patient education, if appropriate, negotiating a plan, and summary/closure. This also is a good time to motivate and congratulate a patient on how he/she is handling medical problems. However, if your patient has an appreciable problem, he/she will want your thoughts now. Medical students aren't in a position to offer opinions so should defer to the senior resident or attending physician who sees the patient shortly after the student exam.

• After taking the history and performing the physical examination, if you are the responsible caregiver (this could be as a third-year resident in a position to order tests), keep in mind that the patient may have limited funds. The patient could end up paying $100 a month for a decade because you are curious about whether the spleen is enlarged, for example, or if he/she had a minor motorcycle accident and you want to be protected from a malpractice possibility. There would be no risk if you carefully follow up with the patient in a week or so. Put in the record why you are deferring more tests. You could offer your tentative impression with the proviso that you may need more information to give a more definitive differential diagnosis and plan of treatment. But you or the patient's primary care provider should see him/her back after an appropriate interval. This should be noted in the record. Better yet, call the patient in a few days to a week or so.

• If you are a first- or second-year medical student, excuse yourself after you have finished interviewing and examining the patient. Give the patient a gown and permission to move within the room. Tell him/her that it could be fifteen to thirty minutes or more before you are done presenting your findings and differential diagnosis to the attending primary caregiver who will come in after you. Presenting your findings to the resident on the service is good experience before presenting to the attending. When you return to the patient, knock gently on the door—the patient may have fallen asleep—and apologize for the delay. As a third-year resident, if you are in a position to order some tests, it could be the next morning before the findings are back.

You can't heal if you are angry!

• Never get angry with the patient or family (or the health-care personnel or anyone!). And never argue with the patient; disagreements should be handled in a calm, reassuring manner. With equanimity! *Never take your anger to work with you.* Deal with it! A psychiatrist will tell you that the inevitable result of not dealing with your anger is that you'll eventually have to deal with the source of the anger. Unresolved anger becomes "swallowed anger" and leads to more stress, a compromise of your values, and even physical ailments. We are impressed—in a negative way—with how much anger there is all around. Chronic anger leads to hatred. Can you afford this?! The angry person engenders very little respect. Most angry people are depressed.

• Always maintain tolerance for diversity because without it, you are, by definition, arrogant. It isn't so much a matter of tolerating differences in behaviors, race, religion, etc.; it's accepting that *it can't be any other way.* The opposite of intolerance is understanding. Tolerance also can have a negative impact if you accept someone's differences but still don't want any part of him/her because of those differences. This hurts almost as much as intolerance.

• Never talk down to the patient. Explain things in a language he/she can understand. Avoid medical jargon even if the patient uses medical terms. Write down the diagnoses for your patient, especially if they are brand new to him/her. If the patient wishes, include the family in the discussion, which may save you some time. In fact, it could very well prevent readmission to the hospital. Ask the patient or the family member to repeat the instructions you have given back to you. What may seem simple to you may be very complicated for him/her, especially if there is a language barrier or limited education.

• You might give the patient simple instructions, which you should write out on a prescription pad or a blank piece of paper. For example, if the patient is dealing with a nagging pain, such as acute low back pain, you might instruct him/her to use moist heat alternating with cool packs, use a cane, take one NSAID four times a day, go on bed rest, etc. In this example, tell the patient to show your instructions to a pharmacy technician who will help him/her understand how to implement them. Tell your patient to stay with the program for one to two weeks and not discontinue it just because he/she is much better in a day or so, or the symptoms will likely return.

• The patient may want an MRI "because my insurance will cover it." *Insurance may not cover it!* Tell him/her that you will consider ordering an imaging study if he/she is not better in a few weeks. Frequently, the symptoms regress in that interval.

Powerful Healing Actions

The mind (whatever that is) is more powerful than we can imagine. Physicians commonly take credit for what the mind really did. You must capitalize on this. Some examples:

- Empathy/caring
- Peace of mind
- The mind itself
- Use of a patient's name
- Role models
- Kindness
- Platinum Rule of Medicine
- Handwritten notes and phone calls
- Body language
- Two-way trust between the patient and primary care provider
- Not being arrogant
- A **SMILE**
- **Placebos**—these work even when a patient is told they are sugar pills; PET scans and fMRIs confirm this. The placebo response of "expectation" should be part of the healing process.
- *The very presence of the physician is when what we have most to offer is ourselves.*
- **Words**—these are in addition to the words mentioned previously. It's how they are delivered.
- **Reassuring words**—"*I'll be here to help you.*" Abandonment takes away all hope and is what many, many patients feel at the end of life.
- **Cringe words**, such as "If you weren't so fat, I could help you." This destroys all possible trust. Or, "That is the dumbest thing I ever heard!"

The good physician treats the disease; the great physician treats the patient who has the disease.

—Sir William Osler

Hope is a commonly used word by all, and patients, families, the clergy, and health-care personnel can offer **hope**—but only the physician can take it away. What the patient usually wants is not hope for a cure but *hope for a way through*—a way through to the end without being abandoned by the physician and the health-care system.

Wherever there is a human being, there is an opportunity for kindness!

If a physician practices at a medical center/hospital that has a reputation for excellence, this can help enhance a patient's confidence in the doctor.

- While evaluating a patient with unexplained symptom(s), ask yourself, "Am I missing something?" "What is the patient trying to tell me?" "Does it pass the 'sniff' test?" "Are the medications the patient is on contributing to the problem?" Be sure you know **all** the medications.

• Keep a tickler file of phone numbers and email addresses of all your active patients who are undergoing workups. You or a trusted office employee should check for test results at least twice each day. Email the normal or negative results, and personally call the patient with abnormal or sensitive test results. You care. It turns out that the results of some tests don't become available until after more than 40 percent of hospitalized patients are discharged. And a fair percent of these test results indicate the need for some urgent action—providing you are aware of the delayed results! Meanwhile, the patient sits at home and waits for the call with the results. Would you want a worried member of your family waiting for a delayed call?! **Remember the Platinum Rule of Medicine**.

• Guide the workup of the patient based on the potential seriousness of the problem and the patient's anxiety. The patient's time is important, too. Expedite the testing and then reporting the results to him/her. No woman should have to wait more than twenty-four hours for a mammogram result—she has a mammogram for one reason only: to rule out cancer. This emphasizes the value of a tickler file. Use it!

> *The convenience of the patient must take precedence over the convenience of the health-care team!*
>
> —Donald M. Berwick, MD

• After going over laboratory results with the patient, give him/her a copy that includes the normal values, and tell him/her to put it in a personal medical file. If the patient sees another physician for any reason, remind him/her to take along a copy (not the original).

> *A close relationship between the patient and you may not be valuable to you, but it can be absolutely priceless to the patient.*
>
> —Thomas J. Watson Jr., former IBM CEO and Mayo Clinic trustee

• If you are a medical student or resident on a hospital service, see your patients twice a day and more often if their illness requires it. If your patient goes to surgery or is admitted to an intensive care unit, visit every day and report back to the team the next time you are all together. The patient's family might ask you questions about the patient, but just tell them you are visiting out of concern and have no new information to pass on.

• Keep up with the science. Your patient may come back to you with the correct diagnosis after searching the Internet and know more about the disease than you do! Be tolerant of this.

• It is important that students and residents know how to present a patient workup to the team. This is especially important for undiagnosed, complicated problems. Observe other students and residents who know how to do this. A clean and succinct presentation, differential diagnosis, and plan of evaluation are the hallmarks of a very good physician or physician-to-be. This is done without resorting to your notes—we've seen residents present workups of six different patients without looking at their notes. On the following page, we've underlined what we think is the minimal information the attending needs to know without having to ask:

Example: *This is Mrs. XX, a 54-year-old woman, (name her occupation), and a farmer's wife from yyy, Wisconsin, referred by Dr. Olson from Eau Claire, with a chief complaint of two weeks of high fevers without an obvious explanation after a workup at home and empiric trials of antibiotics, namely zzz and sss. The fevers go as high as 39°C and are associated with chills and drenching sweats. She was well until all this began two weeks ago. She recently visited her daughter in Mexico. Her past history is negative except for minor indigestion problems. Her Review of Systems is pretty unremarkable except for generalized headaches for the last ten days. The only medications she is on are a statin and an antihypertensive. She denies taking any over-the-counter medications. Pertinent findings on the physical exam include ... The result of the admission blood work, chest x-ray, and urinalysis show ... Other tests I recommend are ... My differential diagnosis includes ...*

• There are two important physical exams that you take yourself: the weight of the patient in a gown and the blood pressure reading. Many patients are tagged with the diagnosis of "hypertension" on the basis of one reading. Hypertension is the single most common condition encountered in a medical practice—even more than obesity. It is a silent killer. If your patient's reading is even slightly high, wait a few minutes and repeat one or two more times, recording each one. Up to 50 percent of the time, the patient doesn't have hypertension but might carry this diagnosis through life. Don't start treatment on the basis of a few high readings. Have the patient return and take the reading again several times before you consider initiating therapy that includes weight reduction, exercise, and seeing a dietician regarding a low-salt diet. The patient should consider purchasing a sphygmomanometer for self-recording, and then bring that recorded information to your appointments. Many times, a clinical assistant or nurse will ask a patient for his/her blood pressure rather than actually taking it—but it should be taken during the appointment.

You may have seen hundreds of patients with breast cancer, but as far as I'm concerned, this is my first breast cancer!

Every patient is the only patient.

An unsolicited phone call from you, as the credit card ad goes, is "priceless." This is a tremendous act of bonding. The same goes for a house call. You care!

LEARN FROM YOUR ROLE MODELS—ALWAYS DO THE RIGHT THING!

Finally, as you are prepared to leave the room, ask, "What questions can I answer for you?" This is more open than "Do you have any questions?"

Buddhism teaches us to "think compassion." Don't wait until it comes to you!

What to Do Next When You Don't Know What to Do: A Very Common Problem

You have been seeing a patient for a few months and, as yet, have no established diagnosis. You have done a number of appropriate tests without an answer. Do not say, "There is nothing more I can do for you." Have you explained things in a way you would want a member of your family to hear (the **Platinum Rule of Medicine**)? Maybe you are the third or fourth doctor who has told the patient the same thing. Don't forget that he/she could be someone's mother or father. Have you ruled out depression? Have you asked the patient what he/she thinks might be wrong? On a scale of 1 to 10, what does the patient estimate as his/her level of stress? If it is high, why?

There are several alternatives:

1. First, reassure the patient that you have found no evidence of anything serious like a cancer, or you would have certainly relayed that information. This might be reassuring enough for the symptom to spontaneously improve.

2. Retake the history and redo an exam—maybe in a more complete fashion. "What am I missing?"

3. Order more tests? Probably not if a lot of tests have been done. Did you review the patient's images with a radiologist? This is like a free curbstone consultation.

4. **Think:** Could this be a Central Sensitization Syndrome? This is a newly appreciated condition in which peripheral pains, such as fibromyalgia, have their origin in various parts of the brain. This diagnosis includes other unexplained conditions, such as fatigue, irritable bowel syndrome, frailty, and even symptoms of post-traumatic stress disorder (PTSD). Consider referring these patients to a center that specializes in this condition; the treatment includes an intensive program of several months' duration.

5. Alternatively, if the patient is in no acute distress, suggest a follow-up appointment in four to eight weeks. Make the appointment now—this will show your commitment to the patient. But tell the patient to return sooner if needed or if new symptoms show up that might explain what is going on.

6. Before or after the period of observation, consider a trial of a pain medication, possibly along with a NSAID (avoid habit-forming drugs). If the patient has an aching or a poorly localized pain, tell him/her to call you before stopping the medication even if the symptoms greatly improve. If the pain is vague, consider a trial of something like amitriptyline. This helps central nervous system

pain and a depression, if present. You need to start with a low dose and gradually go higher. If a depression is improved, you will need to treat the patient for six to twelve months. Offer encouraging words (healing power) with the proviso, "Let's see how this works. I have used it in a number of patients, and it worked!"

7. Still no answer? Consider asking a partner for input or refer the patient to another physician for a consultation.

8. Plan a return visit: *"Maybe I'll think of something."* Stay with the patient; don't abandon him/her. Maybe the patient will consider a trial of a program for Central Sensitization Syndrome.

Working with Patients Who Do Not Speak English

Cross-cultural communication is necessary for all physicians in today's practice. It is always better if the physician speaks the patient's language, but when this isn't the situation, ideally you would have a professional interpreter available. (Health-care personnel, including physicians, overestimate their own second-language skills.) If your medical center does not have an interpreter for your patient's language, there are telephone services with interpreters of more than 100 languages. Your hospital telephone operators have this information.

Family members are notorious for not wanting to tell a patient the seriousness of a medical problem, including a pending death. When relating to your patient and the family, you may need a special sensitivity to the patient's culture and background. This enhances the clinical evaluation as well as the patient/family compliance and outcomes. All this may take extra time.

It is important that interpreters understand the nature of a patient's problem and, if possible, how much the patient and family understand the patient's health status. This requires a team visit with the interpreter before the visit with the patient. If you are using a telephone service, you will "meet" over the phone. If you meet the interpreter for the first time in the presence of the patient and family, it could confuse them because we may not understand how much English the interpreter comprehends; the family will pick up on scattered terms. The interpreter should minimize the use of medical terminology when interpreting to patients and their families.

You should look directly at the patient—not the interpreter—while the interpreter is talking. Do not look at the phone if you use a telephone service (the phone will be on speaker). Ask the interpreter if the patient has any questions. Avoid questions such as "Do you understand?" These are likely to be answered with a nod of "yes" or just a "yes." Ask the interpreter to have the patient say what he/she understands.

The Patient Bill of Rights*

The right to ...

+ respectful and compassionate care regardless of race, color, religion, sex, age, physical or mental impairment, or national origin.
+ pain and anguish management.
+ know the names of the physicians responsible for your care. You can have this in writing. You also can have the name(s) of other health-care providers, including nurses and those in supervised training (medical students, residents, and fellows) assisting with your treatment.
+ understand and agree to the treatment recommended by the physician most responsible for your care.
+ know the specifics and risks about your treatment or planned procedure.
+ complete information about your diagnosis, treatment, and prognosis.
+ have family members and surrogates be kept informed of your status, including the working diagnosis.
+ make decisions with your health-care team about your health care, which includes the right to accept or refuse medical or surgical treatment. Your physician will tell you your prognosis and consequences if you refuse treatment or a procedure, as permitted by law.
+ be told immediately of any medical mistake, including what has or hasn't been done and what is needed to correct it (your family members also have this right to be told).
+ prepare a Durable Power of Attorney or Living Will and to receive written information about these rights.
+ have your legally authorized representative make health-care decisions for you if you become incompetent according to the law or if your physician decides that you can't understand treatment(s) or procedure(s).
+ be provided with an interpreter—preferably not a family member or close friend—if you don't speak or understand English.
+ participate in discussions about any ethical issues affecting your care.
+ have all your medical records kept confidential and available only to those responsible for your medical care, as well as those authorized by law or those responsible for paying part of or all of your bill.
+ be informed of clinical research, which may provide you with an investigational drug, device, or other treatment available only through participation in an Institutional Review Board (IRB)-approved clinical research protocol.
+ express what you think your medical problem is.
+ examine and receive an explanation of your bill.
+ be free of restraints imposed for purposes of discipline or convenience and not required to treat medical symptoms.
+ express concerns about any aspect of your care without fear of retaliation.

* This is an incomplete listing of government-mandated rules for the patient's protection. Patients have access to the complete list from their hospital or physician.

You should attempt to be sure the patient gets a copy of his/her record, including consultations and laboratory results. Patients should keep these records in a secure place and give only a copy, never the originals, to their next physician, unless they are seen in the medical center where these records originated. The patient may have to pay to have copies made.

If you are working in an emergency room, by law (assuming your hospital accepts federal funds and most do), you must take care of the patient after he/she signs in. You must see that patient and evaluate him/her as to the urgency of the problem.

Chapter Four

Mentoring and Role Models

Background: *The assumption—false—that a student, resident, or young employee doesn't need further guidance/mentoring after he/she completes training. Mentoring has nothing to do with a person's knowledge, skills, age, or experience up to this point. Just ask someone who benefited from his/her association with a good mentor(s), formalized or not. Hopefully, this person is now actively mentoring others. Mentors and role models not only are important to physicians at academic medical centers but also to professionals at other medical and nonmedical organizations.*

The words "mentor," "mentoring," and "mentee" were never in our vocabularies or medical writings during the first two-thirds of our long medical careers. We think back to our years in college, medical school, and residencies, and as young staff members at our institutions, without any recollection of ever being formally mentored. During college, we usually had an "advisor" who guided us in selecting classes, but he/she was not someone we felt we could question about our futures.

Part of the problem was that physicians senior to physicians-to-be and young doctors frequently gave one impression—if not the actual verbiage: "I did it the hard way. Now you have to do it like I did." Or, in other words: "Find out yourself!" Fortunately, we never found this attitude as physicians at Mayo Clinic. Early on at Mayo, the vast majority of older residents/fellows and the staff were always open to questions and answered with some obvious pleasure. But this is not the same as sitting down over a cup of coffee or lunch and discussing in detail what we could expect during our lives, pitfalls to avoid, and, very importantly, the value of networking. It's kind of learning "the birds and the bees" of how to mature into a seasoned physician.

"He is a good resident but will never be outstanding!" This is a quote taken from a resident's record that awakened us to the importance of mentoring or—almost more importantly—to the lack of it. **Every student has the ability to be outstanding.** This can't be done without mentoring, nurturing, and maturing. Role modeling can only do so much. Role models, by definition, aren't usually asked for advice on a regular basis unless they also have agreed to be mentors. *But students should be told to look for good role models and emulate them.* Mentoring is a process of nurturing, not nature, unless you include the culture of the workplace as nature. *A very positive workplace **culture** can act as a **"giant role model,"** making the job for the mentor that much easier.* A negative culture, of course, has the opposite effect, which we would consider an awful trickle-down effect.

A definition of mentorship is the establishment of "a purposeful relationship between two individuals with the goal of furthering the less experienced participant's growth." (Another term for mentorship might be faculty development.) Keep in mind that the mentor will learn something from these interactions.

All staff members must consider themselves as mentors even if they don't actually have that assignment. They need to be available to answer questions on the spot if the mentee's mentor is not available.

It is difficult to formalize a mentorship program unless leadership and staff (potential mentors) strongly support it. Each division should have a mentoring committee with a chair; the chair asks for volunteers and should select highly respected persons with good track records for mentoring. The chair then shares the list with potential mentees. We suggest the institution involve recently retired physicians for mentoring. They have the time and some of the wisdom necessary to have most of the answers. These retirees/mentors would live in the same area, stay in touch with the division, still do some teaching, etc.

A good mentoring program will only enhance the quality of your training programs and the institution's reputation, which will help in your recruiting because these are very important to future staff. Leadership **must** repeatedly get this message to the staff. Two or more failed mentoring relationships reflect negatively on a division. Word gets around.

What I need is someone who will make me do what I can.

—Ralph Waldo Emerson

The Joint Commission (JC), formerly the Joint Commission on Accreditation of Healthcare Organizations (JCAHO), has standards that require leaders in medicine to develop programs for faculty development, recruitment, retention, and continuing education for all staff *with a key emphasis on mentoring.* **This all comes under the guise of *professionalism.***

Most students in graduate school or postdoctoral training have advisors who guide them in their research but, in actuality, are mentors. This often results in lifelong friendships and collaborations. The following are our thoughts on mentoring:

• Mentoring is the process of an association between a maturing individual and a more senior, mature professional who has "been there, done that" and knows most of the ropes and traps. The mentor also knows how to network for the mentee. Both the mentor and mentee should look at mentoring as part of a *continuous personal improvement program* and continuous orientation to the mission of the institution. Many institutions have faculty development committees. Mentoring must be dealt with in a positive fashion. Mayo Clinic inculcates in all staff the importance of its primary value: *The needs of the patient come first.* We will add to that the Platinum Rule of Medicine:

Treat every patient like you would want a member of your family treated. Of course, the Golden Rule also applies in any workplace. A good mentor will constantly be certain that the mentee is supporting these missions. As a reminder, many physicians have or will have children, grandchildren, nieces, or nephews interested in becoming physicians. You can only hope that these young people will be lucky enough to have some great mentors.

• The mentee must initiate the process of mentoring by selecting his/her mentor with input from the chair. It can't be done as an assignment. The two should decide on the frequency of meeting—certainly at least once a month at first and definitely more often if major decisions are pending. Some meetings might last only minutes, but this could be sufficient compared with the hours that the mentee might need otherwise without a mentor.

• Mentoring can be one of the greatest personal benefits an individual can offer to young people who might be struggling because of a lack of input from someone who, through experiences that may include making mistakes, knows the system and a lot about getting over the hurdles. The mentor has figured out faculty development, knows how to relate to peers, appreciates career satisfaction, and knows the proper responses to many different obstacles and many of life's ups and downs—*networking* at its greatest. It can make a huge difference in the mentee's success and especially in his/her happiness.

• A survey of college students listed *time management* and *mentoring* as what they thought most helped them get through college. We would add *networking*. A good mentor can be invaluable in facilitating networking. A phone call to a colleague—networking—can be a game changer for a mentee. In addition to the home institution, national meetings are great places for networking. The mentor and others in the division can introduce the mentee to some of their friends, as well as to the leadership of the organization. This leader can advise the mentee on how to work his/her way up the organization and maybe even introduce him/her to a mentor within it.

• The mentor should be a good role model who shows compassion, professionalism, and selflessness, and is not self-serving as it relates to the mentee, etc. The mentor also should be respected by members of his/her department/division, act as a career guide but remain flexible, and always be prompt for meetings with the mentee. The department/division must include the allied health members for mentoring—this is imperative.

• A mentor puts a high priority on establishing trust with the mentee so that he/she is able to successfully provide honest and pure feedback when necessary. The mentor also should be able to tell the mentee that everything will be OK.

• The mentor should concentrate on the following:
  - Effective communication, especially *listening*
  - Clinical skills, especially practicing the Art of Medicine
  - Knowledge and experience related to a mentee's research
  - Networking
  - Review of the mentee's grades and comments submitted to his/her record, with the division's education director or coordinator's approval
  - Supporting publications, but not expecting that his/her name will be on every paper *unless* he/she contributed to the project. By contributing to and preparing the potential publication, the mentor teaches the mentee the art of education via publishing.

- Work-life balance
- Polishing mentees' curricula vitae and making sure they are updated accordingly, again with the education coordinator's approval
- Educational skills
- Helping mentees rehearse upcoming presentations
- Academic appointments/promotions
- Career planning, e.g., five-year plans
- Interacting with other professionals, including referring physicians
- Relationships to allied health personnel
- The importance of going the extra mile—teamwork
- Other

• A mentor is **not** a psychotherapist.

• Mentoring is not limited to students. Just because a student has completed training and may have begun a career job, it doesn't mean that he/she knows all the answers. Mentees may think they do, but nothing short of experience will give them "all" the answers. A good mentor can fill in some of the gaps, and quickly. What we are saying is that all young people should maintain the mentoring relationship for a number of years or until they become mentors themselves. And even then, it doesn't mean they have to discontinue using a mentor.

• Less than half of white-collar workers, including professionals, can look back to someone they would call a mentor.

• Some years ago, the National Board of Medical Examiners (NBME) stated that professionalism is a competency that must be nurtured, monitored, and graded. The organization started with 150 positive behaviors and narrowed the list down to less than 20, including: *altruism, honesty, integrity, balance in life, absence of arrogance, committed to society and professionalism, caring and compassion, respect, responsibility, lifelong learning, communication, teamwork, teaching,* and **mentoring**. We add an appreciation of the altruistic value of practicing the **Platinum Rule of Medicine** and the Golden Rule, which should go without saying. A number of other educational organizations have bought into this. (*See Chapter 9 on* The Ideal Academic Medical Center and Private Practice Medical Center Professional.)

During the first visit with a potential mentor, the mentee needs to decide whether this is the right person to advise him/her over at least several years' time. The mentee should not be afraid to speak up because it is his/her decision. However, there should be no problem changing mentors, or, at least, there shouldn't be as this is part of the "rules." Women students/residents/young staff often prefer other women as their mentors. However, we (male authors) have mentored a number of women and felt very comfortable and think the mentees did also. The mentee could have more than one mentor, but the caution here is that getting mixed advice can be very confusing.

Medical students have reported in surveys that they felt they had been abused, bullied, belittled, and their coping skills chipped away during their medical-school years. Then they lose their confidence. As they advance in their training, they may then become the bullies—further perpetuating their own immaturity. We can say we never heard of any bullying at our institution. We were fortunate that all our role models were true gentlemen or ladies.

46

Leadership must make mentoring a high priority. We need to find ways of rewarding mentors for their time, wisdom, and motivation (more on this follows). Theoretically, students can gain the equivalent of a semester's training in the Art and Science of Medicine if they have a good mentoring relationship(s). What they are getting is the *wisdom of experience* from their mentor(s). You don't learn mentoring from reading a journal or textbook on this subject. It is very likely that a mature resident or trainee could be a good mentor, and maybe this should be included in the residents'/trainees' curricula. This experience may encourage them to continue mentoring when they become staff physicians or go into private practice. Our rewards for mentoring a number of pre-medical and medical students and physicians have been their appreciation, which they still have many decades later. It is likely that we mentors often gain more from this experience than the mentees do. The mentors should list their mentees in their CV, just like researchers list postdoctoral fellows.

The First Formal Encounter with Your Mentee

We usually start with lunch. If the institution isn't paying for it, we mentors pay out of our pockets. That is a small price to pay for the feeling that we may have really helped someone by providing insight that took us years (decades?) to acquire. *Remember that someday you hope your offspring will have mentors who care about them.*

We have a list of items to go over so that we don't forget the important things we want them to learn. We also may give them a few handouts pertinent to the encounter, including some history of the institution. We begin with reviewing his/her CV with a very critical eye *(see Chapter 5)*. The beauty of this, compared with only a few decades ago, is that the mentee can update the CV in minutes with his/her computer instead of having to retype the whole thing.

One "pearl" we emphasize to mentees is to keep a list of individuals encountered in their work, especially those they don't see regularly. This includes physicians outside of their subspecialty as well as surgeons, pathologists, radiologists, etc. Have them review the list before they go to regional and national meetings. Remind them to use these physicians' names when they talk to them because this is a very important means of bonding. Be sure they also keep a list of the allied health personnel they work with and are **always** nice and caring toward them. Always. They are not subordinates. They are partners in teamwork and delivering compassionate care to patients. They are one of the strengths of the culture of the institution.

Unfortunately, education/teaching is often a low priority, but mentoring (teaching) is the premise of the academic center. For mentees to advance academically, we point out that they should document **all** teaching activities, including preparation time for lectures; lectures prepared for and given to peers and medical students (even if they are only presented to two or three students during rounds); CME (continuing medical education) credits for the year; all publications, including the percentage of contribution to each; and on and on. Highlight (bold print) their names in bibliographies. Ultimately, most of this will be deleted as they move up the ladder, but we remind mentees "if it isn't documented, it didn't happen." We point out that Academic Promotion Committees (we called them Academic "Commotion" Committees) now, finally, promote on the grounds of education accomplishments, but this **must** be documented. If your institution doesn't already have them, establish awards to outstanding residents/fellows. These awards should not only be for internal medicine/subspecialty trainee residents but also for residents in surgery, radiology, anesthesia, pediatrics, etc.

> ### *The best way to attract excellent students and residents to your program—and then to your staff—is by having the best teaching reputation in the institution.*

The mentee should be urged to strive to become a **"Teacher of the Year."** This gives great credibility to his/her division and is a great attractant to younger physicians who will want to apply to its training program and, ultimately, a staff position. *While we teach, we learn* (Seneca). We always point out that teaching has been one of the greatest rewards of our careers. It is important to keep coming back to this throughout the hour or two you spend with a mentee. You can then go on with a number of other points about teaching, including the art of educating. Tell the mentee that he/she isn't going to be a full professor after two years; it usually takes five or so years between promotions assuming that he/she continues to publish and teach. After completion of training, he/she should be able to take the academic appointment with him/her. During a subspecialty fellow's early training, encourage him/her academically to become an instructor. Then he/she will hit the ground running upon completion.

> ### *We tell them that they are like the bamboo tree. During the first four years, they will be spreading their roots. During the fifth year, they will grow more than twenty feet.*

Urge the mentee to develop one-, five-, and ten-year plans. Write them out. At the end of every year, go over the plans and see where they stand. This is goal setting. But the plans also should be flexible.

Stress the importance of keeping up with health-care delivery and management issues through the media and other means. It will be up to them in the future to solve some of our problems.

Currently, most trainees and a number of residents do some research. The trainee may want to be a researcher (grants, etc.), but this may be beyond your expertise. If the chair hasn't already, he/she should talk to the trainee about visiting with a researcher. But you can network for the mentee if he/she doesn't have names. At this point, we can discuss the burdens and obligations of a researcher, especially with the changes that medicine is going through. A researcher eventually may end up a pure clinician because of limited dollars for grants. Knowing this will guide mentees in some decision-making over time. They can always fall back on being a master educator. Early on, they should start working toward becoming an educator and begin building a reputation.

The first meeting will conclude with a discussion on miscellaneous topics. The mentor could talk about the various people the mentee will encounter and how he/she can learn so much from really good role models. Another item to stress is the absolute importance of relationships to referring physicians. We all know of horror stories about complete rudeness to these physicians. Referrals are the lifeblood of subspecialties at academic centers. If the mentee is learning about the community, also talk about the area's social aspects, schools, etc. It is worth spending some time talking about what the area offers for the spouse and children.

Finally, remind them that maintaining a "Culture of Caring" to their patients is mandatory. Maybe there isn't a recognizable culture. The mentee should consider this as a challenge.

Occasionally, a good mentor is asked to take a potential staff candidate to lunch and spend up to two hours going over all the items we've mentioned, plus more. Much of this time will be spent answering questions and emphasizing the strengths of the division. We do this because we enjoy it. One recent experience was with a young man who was highly qualified in his prior training but wasn't sold on coming to our institution for a lot of reasons, but most were because of misunderstandings. After spending two hours with him, he signed on that afternoon. Within two years, he had two National Institutes of Health Research Project Grants (R01s).

Mentoring a young physician who has been asked to join a private practice group is just as rewarding as mentoring one interested in academic medicine. Most of what is written also applies.

Finally, remind all mentees of the most important rule in patient care: **the Platinum Rule of Medicine**—*Treat every patient like you would want a member of your family treated*.

Role Models

• Role models are very important in the health-care field, and we've learned how important they are in all walks of life. We hone our skills in empathy and equanimity from them, *but we have to want to*. We've learned from them since infancy (our family members are our first role models) and continue to do so regularly. For reasons unknown, many people beginning in their youth are attracted to negative role models, possibly because they never had positive ones. If they ever mature, they will realize the errors of their ways.

• The most important thing we can say about role models is to appreciate the good to excellent ones who are all around you. *This is a gift to you*, and you need to consciously take advantage of it.

• **Keep track of positive qualities you observe** on your smartphone or on four-by-six cards, and keep adding to them. Try to emulate these—your children will benefit from this. You also can learn from negative role models: "I would never want this physician to take care of my family." Role models are mentioned throughout this book because we believe they are so critical to your education and maturation.

The wise learn from fools, but fools seem to never learn from the wise.

The following are qualities to emulate. Note that **maturity** is necessary in all these. Go over this list occasionally and think about where you might need some areas of improvement, and add to the list when you think of more traits to emulate. These are characteristics of a person highly respected by all:

Humility	**Empathy**
Integrity	**Smiles easily**
Passion toward dreams	**Respect for others**
Good communication skills	**Knows how to listen**
Responsible/can be counted on	**Leadership abilities**
Acceptance of diversity	**Love of learning**
Absence of arrogance	**Resilience**
A warmth about you—you care	**Volunteers when needed**

Able to say: "I'm sorry," "How can I help you?" and "What am I missing?"

In Summary

- An effective, collegial working relationship in any medical group is an invaluable asset to the culture, reputation, and strength of an institution. Every member of the group should support this because they are all part of the "family." Professionalism permeates the culture of the institution.
- The mentee selects his/her mentor and should be able to change mentors to suit his/her goals.
- At the first meeting, the mentor should go over the mentee's CV, as well as talk about his/her one-, five-, and ten-year plans and goals.
- The mentor and mentee need to meet at regular intervals. There also will be interim meetings, depending on the needs of the mentee.
- The mentor can list his/her mentees on his/her CV, providing there have been at least six meetings. The mentor, as well as the chair of the mentors, keeps a record of the meetings.
- Role models are extremely important in any mentor-mentee program.

Keep in mind that the JC and the NBME accreditations of the institution could depend on the strength of the mentoring program. This is why it is important that the director of the mentoring program keep good records.

Chapter Five

The Making of the Ideal Resident

"XXXX is a good resident but will never be great!" We say, "Why not?"
By the time residents reach this level, they have shown significant
potential—they just need good nurturing and mentoring.

• Treat **every** patient like you would want a member of your family treated! Never forget this. This is the **Platinum Rule of Medicine**.

• Positive **attitude**. This is maturity. It will get you everywhere.

• Nurture your **passion** for medicine by improving the well-being of your patients, as well as for your own satisfaction. There is no other *calling* like the practice of medicine. This means demonstrating a *desire to learn* and to teach—a professional obligation.

• Always be on time for rounds. If you are going to be late, let someone know.

• Introduce yourself to the patient and the family. Write your name on a piece of paper, and give it or your card to the patient. *Wear your name tag. Explain your role.*

• **Common sense** is a real asset when **always doing the right thing**.

• Don't complain inappropriately. If you are concerned about something, discuss it with someone you trust.

• **Read, read, read.** Try to read at least a little bit on a disease or condition new to you every day.

• Develop a responsibility for self-discipline and self-improvement in continuing education by attending conferences, reading, and learning from your role models.

• We are repeating this: **Learn from your role models**.

• Ask questions. Educators appreciate questions because they mean that you are thinking. It is intellectual curiosity.

• Know your limitations. Never be afraid to say, "I don't know." Don't try to fake it; it will backfire.

51

• Always apologize when appropriate. "I'm sorry," says a lot about you. Remember, you can't say this if you are arrogant!

• Always use eye contact to earn the patient's trust.

• Be pleasant to *all* support personnel. They may have some input regarding your grades. This includes the custodians, kitchen personnel, and others. They are part of the team and contribute to the culture of the institution. Mutual respect is imperative. Know their names. *Thank and praise them when appropriate.*

• Balance your life. Work at being happy. Don't take yourself too seriously. **Have fun!** A good sense of humor is imperative in life.

• Develop **patience**. You will be less stressed and less likely of becoming angry. Plus, you will be more effective, calmer, and relaxed. Remember counting to ten? Ten slow, deep breaths are even more effective. *(See Chapter 12, which focuses on stress.)*

• **Never get angry.** This is **equanimity**, which Osler said could be one of a physician's greatest virtues. You can tell a lot about a person by knowing what makes him/her angry. You will quickly lose respect for angry people, no matter what their accomplishments.

• Seek maturity: emotional stability, equanimity, flexibility, compassion, self-confidence, humility, and the ability to "roll with the punches." *(See Chapter 11 on* Wisdom and Maturity.)

• **Listen.** Listen to the patient, to the family, and to the nurse. *It's not what's said; it's what's heard.* They may be trying to tell you something very important, but it doesn't come out very clear.

• Develop tolerance. Accept diversity.

• **Think.** This requires mindfulness, but thinking is the hallmark of the excellent physician, especially when combined with caring and empathy. It is estimated that the average adult spends less than ten minutes a day actually thinking!

• **Never** say anything disparaging about the referring physician; if possible, find something positive to say. If you say something disparaging, it will almost certainly get back to him/her.

• Maintain a professional attitude at all times. Don't tell off-color stories during professional activities (anytime?). Never use offensive four-letter words.

• If you become aware that a fellow resident or student, or even a staff physician, is depressed or acting inappropriately, deal with it. Tell someone, such as your program director or chair of the division/department.

• Learn how to interact with other physicians. This is one of Mayo Clinic's strengths. In some cases, it is imperative that you call the home physician. Tell the patient you are going to do so, and then put this in the record. If a physician calls to tell you about a patient, you—not a nurse or clinical assistant—return the call. This leads to teamwork, continuity of care, and, in turn, improved quality of care. Patients notice this. Don't forget that you represent your institution.

• **Never** discuss a patient's case in the elevators, hallways, etc., where you could be overheard. Know the institution's policy on patient confidentiality. You could lose your job in a breach of this policy *(see page 57).*

• **Document! Document! Document!** Remember, if you don't document it, it didn't happen! The patient's record is a legal document. If you have to improve something in the record, be sure your signature is readable, and then print your name below it. If you write something and then cross it off for any reason, initial what you crossed off.

• If your patient goes to surgery, consider visiting him/her postoperatively alone or with your team.

• There is no room for arrogance in the medical profession. Every now and then, ask yourself, "Could I be perceived as arrogant?" *Success can be more dangerous than an occasional failure.* The arrogant physician never says, "I'm sorry." *Humility* remains one of the major virtues of a caring physician.

• Keep a tickler file on index cards or on your smartphone with patients' names and test results that need follow-up. Check it daily.

• **Keep your promises!**

While on the Hospital Service

• Always be neat and professional in your appearance. You only have one chance to make a good first impression. Minimize the need to wear scrubs on morning rounds. Patients and visiting physicians have told us many times how impressed they are to see professionals, including residents and medical students, in business attire.

• Again: Be on time to start rounds.

• Keep the family informed after making sure you have the patient's permission to do so. Be sure the team is all on the same page.

• Encourage the patient's primary nurse to accompany you while on rounds.

• See new admissions as soon as possible if only to say hello and that you will return soon. Quickly prioritize the urgency of each new patient's situation. Call the responsible staff after you've worked up the patient if there is some urgency. And if you are the responsible staff, encourage residents to call you at home if there is a problem or concern. Never discourage this. This is professionalism.

• If a staff physician admits a patient to the hospital, call or electronically communicate your findings, etc., to him/her.

• When you are on rounds, don't take personal calls or read text messages on your cell phone. You may find that many attendings are intolerant of this.

• Know the patients who are being treated by other residents on your service. Never tell another physician who inquires about a patient on your service, "I don't know anything about that individual—he's not my patient!" Some physicians don't forget this.

• Round on all patients when other residents on the service are not available to round on their own patients.

• Don't try to one-up fellow residents, and always be considerate of everyone—especially fellow residents of the opposite sex. Include them when meeting for hospital coffees, meals, and social occasions. One of them may be your primary physician someday! It happens!

• Quietly assist other residents who are not quite up to par.

• Stay in the room with the consultant when you are both with a patient; don't drift out into the hallway unless an issue related to the care of another patient needs to be handled immediately.

• Some residents are offended if the responsible staff physician seems to be too involved. On the contrary, how will you know what you missed? This is part of your education.

• Difficulty with an attending happens! Don't overreact. Is it just you or are all the residents on the service having problems? How much longer do you have the service with him (this rarely occurs with a woman attending)? If it is only a week, ride it out. The next step would be to talk to a chief resident for his/her input. If you are still uncomfortable, talk to your program director and ask to present your interpretation of events if the attending submits a negative grade with comments. If this problem also is with other residents, the program director should talk to all of them.

• Never argue about the appropriateness of an admission.

• If you are a student or first- or second-year resident who is seeing a patient and will be followed by the staff physician, be cautious about discussing diseases, physical findings, etc., so the patient doesn't think the worst. You may mention that lupus can do this or that but fail to tell the patient that he/she doesn't have it; more commonly, the patient isn't listening closely and only thinks about the worst possibility. Or you can feel the liver on deep inspiration, but this can be normal in some people. And you don't right away need an imaging study, which can cost thousands of dollars. A faint murmur is not uncommon in many people, and the attending thinks it is of no consequence, so the patient needs to be told this with an explanation. The patient may have a relative or friend with a murmur who died or someone with liver disease and an enlarged liver. Again, the patient always thinks the worst until you explain things. **Be sure you answer all the patient's questions!** The point is that if you are inexperienced, don't discuss your thoughts with the patient until after the staff physician explains the findings to him/her, the family, and you.

• Arrange with the institution, if it has not already been done, to get a report of all the costs of your patient's hospital stay. It shouldn't include anything that will identify the patient, but you will know because you recognize the pattern of the testing. It will amaze, astound, and floor you! It is truly educational.

As a Senior/Chief Resident

• By definition, you now have significant responsibilities for patient care, but don't forget your attending is ultimately responsible. Make sure the attending is aware of what is going on with your patients.

• Return phone calls promptly and with a smile. This is **integrity** and **professionalism**. If an email relates to a patient, answer it quickly. If you have reliable clinical assistants, trust them to make sure you stay informed about patients in your care and that your instructions are carried out.

• Discuss options. Allow patients to be involved in decision-making. Empowering patients to partner with you in their care is very important. However, many patients will have established great **trust** in you to the point that they want you to make all the decisions. Even so, you need to get their input and approval of your decisions, and make sure they understand them. This is shared decision-making. At this point, it may be necessary to bring in a member of the family, if the patient approves. After the staff has seen the patient, you can ask if he/she has any other questions. Again, be cautious about getting beyond your range of knowledge.

• **Never** tell a patient there is nothing more you can do. ***Do something!*** This might be as simple as saying, "Let's sit tight, and I'll plan to see you again in a few weeks or few months and recheck, or call me in a few weeks to update me." "I'm pretty sure I know that you do **not** have anything serious, but we'll stay on top of this until you are feeling better." Your tickler file will have the date when your patient is to call you; if he/she doesn't call, then you make the call! A good clinical assistant will help you stay in touch with your patients. This enhances tremendous *trust*. Another option is to have the patient try a medication that you know is harmless and see what happens. *Placebos are powerful.* If the patient is depressed, this could be a cause of his/her unexplained symptoms. Tricyclic antidepressants work on some symptoms in nondepressed patients with peripheral neuropathies and many other conditions, but these aren't without some side effects. Behavior modification also works. So might a pet.

• Ask for the patient's permission to speak to the referring physician and to the family, which may include members of the extended family (this can be difficult if they disagree with the patient's care). Then make a note in the record that you have these permissions. Be cautious when someone calls and claims to be a family member. If you are in doubt, tell the caller you need to call him/her back, and then check with the patient. In the past, this kind of thing was never a problem, but now with patient confidentiality laws *(the Health Insurance Portability and Accountability Act; see later in the chapter)*, you can't be too cautious.

• Finally, if a patient dies, send a sympathy card to the family. If the funeral is local, attend it or the visitation if it feels congruent with your sense of propriety. The family will never forget you and your institution *(see Chapter 14)*.

Prewriting Conundrums

Young physicians should be aware that academic medicine requires publishing. What follows are some things we have learned—sometimes the hard way—that will prevent you from wasting a considerable amount of time. As soon as the idea of a paper is conceived, ask yourself the questions that follow to save yourself a great deal of frustration and regrets.

• What is the subject? Who is the audience?

• Who suggested the topic for the paper?

• What is your role? Are you the first author, i.e., the one expected to do most of the work?

• If you are in training, do you have a choice about whether to write a paper if you are asked to do so by one of your attendings? If you are concerned, check with your mentor.

• What do you know about the paper's subject? Did one of the senior authors sit with everyone involved to discuss the merits of the subject? If not, ask for a meeting with those involved unless it is a simple case report. Even then, be sure the subject is worthy of your time.

• What is the message of the paper? Is it worth your time? Is the message something you might regret later on? You can't very well retract your name from the paper after it is published.

• Is the information new, original, and contributing to new knowledge?

• Have you reviewed the literature and abstracts from recent meetings to be certain someone else hasn't already done the work?

• It takes an average of about four years, or longer, from the conception to the publication. It may be old data by then, or someone else could have published on the subject in the interval.

• Are there ethical issues? If so, be cautious unless you are experienced in the field and an experienced writer. Get outside help on this before embarking on the paper.

• If you agree to be the first author, do you have the time? Researching the literature and writing the first draft always takes longer than you or the attending physician who suggested the paper thinks it will. If you are going into private practice soon, you may not have time for writing.

• Authorship: How many? Who? Is one of the coauthors an expert on the subject? This helps.

• What is the role of each coauthor, and can everyone be counted on?

• Will the coauthors help, or is this just a paper that will have their names on it? Get this in writing as you will find that sometimes the "authors" will disappear for a long time and then appear out of nowhere the closer you get to completion. Too many authors on a paper create a loss of credibility with the editors and dilute your contribution.

• Is there a conflict of interest? A turf issue? If this isn't clarified ahead of time, you could get caught in the middle and the paper may never get completed, or it could be completed but never submitted, or it could be submitted and rejected by peer reviewers because of turf issues. Does your institution distribute a registration of subject so that no one can say they were unaware of the project? Ask to have conflicts of interest with industry, etc., clarified by the coauthors early on.

• Remember, most editors expect that all authors will be actively involved in writing the paper, proofreading it as often as necessary, and be willing to critique it for scientific validity and ethical issues. The authors may have to testify to this in writing and sign a statement to that effect.

• Some people fight to get their name as the last author because it makes them look like the "senior expert." You might do most of the work but be the second or third author.

• **Never plagiarize!**

• Do you have a mentor who isn't an author to help you with issues that could arise?

• Is there a time line? If you are writing a book chapter or an article for a quarterly journal by invitation that is covering one subject in detail, there always is a deadline. It is flattering to be asked to write in this situation, but you might consider gracefully declining if you are stretched. But if you were asked because of your expertise, consider asking a resident/fellow to help and start working on the project immediately.

• Patient record review? Will it be necessary? This will require Institutional Review Board (IRB) approval. If so, how many charts? Some charts might take a minimum of thirty to sixty minutes to extract the data. Will any of the other authors help?

• IRB approval is not an automatic thing. If you are going to need IRB approval, begin with this very early.

• Statistical analysis? Extensive? Could your paper be rejected because of your statistical interpretation? Will the statistician be an author? Is there financial support to "hire" statistical analysis?

• Is imaging needed? If so, is it of good quality? If pathologists and/or radiologists are serving as coauthors, be sure they agree with the case material available.

• Tables and charts must be of good, easily interpretable quality.

Remember, a paper isn't worth doing unless it is of good quality and makes a contribution to medicine. It has your name on it and will be in print forever. Can you defend your message in a "letter to the editor" after the paper is published?

PATIENT PRIVACY

Patient privacy also is known as patient confidentiality via the **Health Insurance Portability and Accountability Act (HIPAA)**. Know your institution's policy—to the word. Privacy policies are pretty much the same everywhere, but your medical center may have a few additional recommendations and warnings. A breach of your policy could cause you to lose your job without the need for due process. This is happening more and more nationally. The federal government could fine your institution tens of thousands of dollars and even put it on probation.

Remember that if you are affiliated with an institution, you represent it. If it receives federal dollars (all academic centers do), government officials can put the institution on probation for violating anything they think is inappropriate.

Follow the guidelines of "Need to Know" for medical purposes and "For Your Eyes Only." If you are in doubt about something, contact your compliance officers. Document in the record that the patient has given you (the primary care provider[s]) permission to share his/her record with anyone involved in his/her care. We're repeating this, but if you don't follow the law, it could lead to a lot of problems.

After you look at a patient's electronic medical record (EMR), be sure to log off. If you don't, anyone who opens the computer after that will encounter the last patient's EMR.

Repeating this: Never, never discuss a patient's case in the hallways, cafeteria, elevators, or any place where there is even a remote chance you will be overheard—even if you don't mention the patient's name, room number, or diagnoses. You'd be surprised how a voice carries. If your patient happens to be in a double-bed room or a ward, find a way to talk to your patient in private.

After a patient is discharged, give him/her a summary copy of all their EMRs, including dismissal summaries from the hospital, clinic, or emergency room. When these EMRs are given to patients or mailed to them within twenty-four hours, it can abrogate some of physicians' responsibilities about patients' wishes to look at their records (this is done often online). *(See Chapter 3 or 17 for the Patient Bill of Rights.)*

Tell your patients to keep these records and give the next health-care center a *copy* (unless they are returning to the same institution). Remember the Platinum Rule of Medicine.

We're repeating this: A disclaimer somewhere on the record and a list of who the patient permits to see his/her records will lessen the risk of uncertainty. Ask the responsible staff if it is OK to call the patient at home to check on him/her, and then note that in the record.

Most medical centers don't have a formal method of teaching how to handle death, especially when it is unexpected. As a resident, a patient's death can weigh heavily on you—and result in significant stress—if you blame yourself. Talk to your attending—the sooner, the better. Ideally, you would learn from your attendings, but they aren't always available when this occurs. Ask for some lectures from physicians and clergy. Remember to deal with the death of a patient like you would want it managed for a member of your family. There are no magic words to say. In many cases, the best thing you can do is just listen; silence can say a lot. Stay in the room for a while. If the family members weren't available at the time of their loved one's death, be sure to come back to the room when they arrive. Use some of your instincts. Men, it is OK to cry.

Accepting a Position of Practice

This relates primarily to a position in an academic medical center because it is more complicated than going into private practice. What follows are certain things you should know before you "sign on."

1. What are the expectations for you? Get them in writing.
2. Type of assignments:
   - Hospital (number of hospitals covered)
   - All consultations? Of some primary care? Work with hospitalists?
   - Outpatient only? Primary care? Consults only?
3. Time for administration? For research? For balance in life? For attending regional and/or national meetings?
4. Number in the medical group of:
   - Physician assistants and nurse practitioners?
   - RNs?
   - Patient care assistants (PCAs)?
   - Clinical assistants?
   - Scribes?
   - Pharmacy technicians?
   - Secretaries?
5. How many medical students, residents, and fellows would you be responsible for?
6. What is the center's approach to recruiting new staff?
7. Describe typical rotations: One week? Two weeks? Other?
8. What are the teaching obligations? Opportunities?
9. Any hidden agendas? Any pending lawsuits?
10. What kind of support is there from leadership?
11. What about my research? Get the details.
12. What are my obligations regarding committees?
13. What are my leadership duties?

****

As a resident or subspecialty fellow, you will need a curriculum vitae (CV). It is time to bring it up to date. The division/department secretaries will know how to do this. There is a sample on the opposite page. This should be updated with every milestone in your career from now on. We point out that this is your "obituary," which has information about everything that is important to you professionally. Your family may not know everything on your CV. The CV has some components that aren't in REAIMS (Research and Education Academic Information Management System), such as date and place of birth and marital status. REAIMS is a database of the scholarly activities of participating staff members that includes articles published, classes taught, presentations, active grants, and applications for academic appointments and promotions. Some academicians prefer to have a second CV of their own making. Any upgrade of a CV by a staff member should be forwarded to the secretary so it also can be entered into the REAIMS.

Sample Curriculum Vitae

NAME Include MD, MS, PhD, FACP, etc. Include academic appointment.

Division of Primary Care Internal Medicine
ABC Medical Center
Address
City, State, Zip
Phone #; Fax #
Cell phone# if you wish; Email address

Date and place of birth: xxxxx xxxxxxx
Marital Status: Optional

EDUCATION:

1994–1998	BS	College/University	City/State
1998–2002	MD	College/University	City/State
2002–2006	PhD (pharmacology)	College/University	City/State

POSTGRADUATE TRAINING:

2006–2009	ABC Medical Center, City, State
	Resident in Internal Medicine
2009–2012	ABC Medical Center, City, State
	Fellow in Cardiology

BOARD CERTIFICATION:

2009   Diplomat in Internal Medicine, American Board of Internal Medicine

APPOINTMENTS AND PROFESSIONAL EXPERIENCE:

2012–   Consultant in Internal Medicine, Division of Cardiology, ABC Medical Center, City, State
2012–   Instructor in Medicine, ABC Medical Center, City, State
2013–   American College of Physicians, member

HONORS AND AWARDS:

1997   Outstanding Science student, College/University, City, State
1998   Phi Beta Kappa honor society, College/University, City, State
2012   Sir William Osler Award for Outstanding Teacher, ABC Medical Center, City, State

BIBLIOGRAPHY:

Peer Reviewed*

Invited Articles*

Chapters*

Books*

(Insert date of last CV update here, e.g., February 23, 2017.)

*Print your name in bold. Print title of article/chapter in italics.

As your career progresses, some of the items listed in your CV will be less important, and you will delete them. This is your decision. Ask your mentor or your division's director of education to review your CV with you. After you make any updates, send a copy to the secretaries of your division chair and director of education.

Since your CV is on your computer, there is no excuse for any misspellings, grammatical errors, etc. Your CV represents you and is something you can be proud of. Many people will read it over your lifetime.

Always put the date of the newest addition on the bottom of the first page.

Chapter Six

The Art of Educating

I desire no other epitaph ... than the statement that
I taught medical students in the wards ...

—Sir William Osler

- A professional never stops learning and never wants to stop learning. To teach is to learn again.
- We have learned a tremendous amount about medicine from those we were supposed to be teaching. It is a remarkable two-way street.
- Educating others is an obligation and a privilege for a professional. It is passing on not only what you know but also how you do things—and with a passion. This is an art. It is sharing your knowledge of how to think your way through to an answer. This is one of the traits of the ideal role model.
- Teaching is one of the most rewarding aspects of being a physician. You don't have to be in an academic center to teach. Unfortunately, teaching is often a low priority because of external time pressures on physicians; plus, how do they get paid for it? The government pays out billions of dollars for medical education—is the government getting its money's worth at your institution? We have to remember that **learning** is the reason that students are in medical school and residents and fellows are in training at our institutions.
- The successful educator is able to instill in students the passion to learn, teach, and develop a curiosity about all aspects of medicine.
- While you are teaching, you are a role model to your audience. Your body language is closely observed. How you talk about a patient is analyzed. Anything said in a disparaging way is a sign of a lack of respect. You can assess this in the bedside-teaching physician even when he/she is not saying anything. (*See Chapter 13 on* The Art of Medicine.)

61

Never forget the Platinum Rule of Medicine: Treat every patient like you would want a member of your family treated.

• Even when you become an educator, your role models are still your most important teachers of the Art of Medicine. Role models may be younger than you and may be nurses or other non-physicians. Never turn down an opportunity to learn from these health professionals. Keep your eyes and ears open to this.

• As a teacher, you will witness negativity many times, and you should consider these incidents to be learning experiences just as much as positive ones. After observing a negative incident, tell yourself that you don't want to treat any patient that way. Again, the Platinum Rule.

• Three words to remember when interacting with a student: **Respect**, **Respect**, and **Respect**! Learners respond to the same values that patients do: caring, empathy, and respect.

• The educator is a coach as well as a teacher. A coach takes raw material and hones, shapes, and molds it into a nearly finished product. The students will respond depending on how much they respect you **and** how much you respect them.

As an educator, you have to appreciate, unfortunately, that students have learned multitasking, which is a great hindrance to learning. Their brains can only process one fact at a time in spite of what they think.

• In the 1980s, the *Journal of the American Medical Association (JAMA)* published a scathing statement from a student (more than a letter to the editor) about his/her negative experiences. The school was named! This could happen anywhere. Just don't let it happen at your institution.

• Medical literature states that the vast majority of medical students report being abused during their schooling. Isn't this bullying?! This is intolerable and must be dealt with. We thought this was limited to K-12 education. Residents and nurses were common sources of the abuse. After going through this, medical students become the abusers when they get to their residencies! These abusers are negative role models. It may be that some of the students who feel they are being abused are overly sensitive or even depressed. Maybe they received constructive criticism. You, the educator, must keep this in mind. The students will recognize before you do that another student is depressed or burned out. You may need to act on this.

You <u>must</u> become the person you see as the ideal role model!

• The Platinum Rule of the Art of Educating might be: ***Treat every student like you would want your child treated if he/she were in medical training***. Many students are the children of physicians. I (author ECR) am a third-generation physician, but I never was bullied at any level.

• How well you teach, relate to, and respect a student could have a downstream effect—someday a member of your family or even you could be admitted to his/her service! It happens. Now you are thinking, "Was I kind to this student? Did I teach him/her good medicine?"

• Remind students to never use their cell phones for personal calls or texts during learning time. You might ask them to leave the room.

• Encourage your residents and fellows to begin developing lecture series to be used during their training and post-training periods. Have them continually build on them and change accordingly with new information. House staff love handouts. A repertoire of fifteen or so topics gives them plenty to work with. Carry them on a memory stick.

• Faculty should earn the privilege of being on a teaching service. A nonteaching or a subpar-teaching faculty member should not be given the responsibility to work with students. The students must have the opportunity to grade the teacher.

• How can you expect students to be on time for rounds if you aren't?

• Have **fun** on rounds. The students should look forward to this time.

• In addition to bedside teaching, try to teach every day even if it is only for fifteen to twenty minutes. There are significant time constraints on students now. If you have to start rounds thirty or more minutes early, then do it. Remember, they are there to learn.

• Students always appreciate coffee breaks, which are great opportunities for you to teach. Consider asking a student who worked up one of the patients to review the literature related to the patient's problems. The student should present his/her findings during the group coffee break the next day or shortly after that.

• When you entertain a medical student/applicant for a matching program, have him/her join morning rounds to witness your teaching and talk to the residents. This could make a difference in how high the applicant ranks your program. Even if the applicant doesn't come to your institution, he/she will tell a lot of others about what was observed. Overall, this can significantly affect the reputation of your academic medical center.

• Show images, and question the students about them. "What are you thinking?" "What is your differential?" "What do you see on the image?" "What is your differential of the abnormality on the image?" "What would you do next?" Add pearls in between. Always praise them when they answer correctly. **Never** degrade them. Remember, someday one of your children or grandchildren might be a medical student or resident—how do you want them treated? We keep repeating this because it is a common scenario. And have **fun**!

• Spoon-feeding doesn't work anymore. Teach them to **think**!

The great contribution we can make is to prepare the oncoming generations to think that they can and will think for themselves.

—Charles H. Mayo, MD

Instruction from teachers and books teaches a man what to think, but the great need is that he should learn how to think.

—William J. Mayo, MD

• Call a resident by his/her name (usually the first name), but if you are with a patient, you should refer to him/her as "Dr. (or Mr./Ms. for a student) Last Name." Discourage the patient/family from calling women physicians by their first names. Some patients tend to call young women by their first names, but this is not necessarily the case with young men. A female student or resident shouldn't have her first name on her badge, just "Dr./Ms. First Initial and Last Name."

• At the bedside, call the patient "Mr./Ms./Mrs. Last Name"—never use the first name unless he/she is under twenty-five or so. Introduce the students if this is their first visit. Touch the patient. Explain to the patient that you are teaching future physicians. Then ask the patient for permission to demonstrate physical findings. Be sure the patient remains appropriately draped. Keep explaining things to the patient as you do the examination.

• When discussing the problem and/or the physical findings, be sure to use terms the patient will understand. Before leaving, ask the patient and/or the family what questions they might have. How you handle this will tell the students and residents a lot. If this person is your patient, you should plan to return after teaching rounds to discuss things with him/her.

• Never hesitate to admit that you don't know something or that the student was right and you were wrong.

• Teach cost constraints. Show the costs of tests that the student wanted as well as the tests that were done.

• "I'm sorry" are powerful words.

• **Never** complain in front of the students about the following:
  ■ The patient—Never!
  ■ Another physician—Never!
  ■ The system
  ■ The nursing care
  ■ The institution
  ■ The leadership
  ■ Problems with the practice of medicine; this doesn't preclude an honest discussion of the situation over coffee

• Instead of complaining, try to be upbeat. Medicine is still the greatest profession.

• Treat all support personnel with respect. Know their names. Expect the students also to know their names if they are working in the area.

• **Never** criticize a student in front of anyone. If there is a need for criticism, make it in the form of a constructive suggestion and always treat the student like you would want a member of your family treated if he/she was training at your institution.

• Encourage students to teach while you observe and critique their presentations. Always tell them ahead of time that you are going to do this.

• When you are on hospital service, never discourage students/residents from calling you at home. This is a learning experience for them that will engender a great deal of respect for you.

• You may be asked to write a letter supporting a student for a residency, fellowship, or job. If it is a good letter, send the student a copy, along with a personal note. Always send a copy to his/her file in the education office. If one of the student's parents is a physician, send a copy to him/her. This will be appreciated more than you can imagine.

• Never whisper with another physician or nurse in the presence of a patient. The patient will assume the worst. But if you forget and do this, explain to the patient that you weren't whispering about him/her.

• Use great caution about disagreeing with the diagnosis of other physicians, including colleagues and referring physicians. If you criticize the referring physician to the patient, you can be sure the patient will tell this physician! But it is a good way to cut down on referrals if this is your goal.

• At the end of a rotation, take the students to lunch. Invite them to your home.

Learning is not compulsory ... neither is survival.
—W. Edwards Deming

Follow the guidelines listed in this chapter and any other positive ones not mentioned here. Be a role model, always respect the student, and the student **WILL NEVER FORGET YOU**. This is your reward.

Chapter Seven

Preparing and Giving a Medical Talk

Formal Presentation: This chapter relates to a presentation you give as a guest to a group of physicians, most of whom you don't know, versus one you give at your home institution to your colleagues.

1. Be sure you understand what your host expects from you. Who suggested the topic(s)—you or your host? Make sure that the exact topic is established, and affirm it in the letter of acceptance. What will the title be? Avoid changing the title after your host has advertised your presentation.

2. Know who will be in the audience—MDs, PhDs, RNs, others, etc.? What is the breakdown of the specialties of the physicians? Who do you aim your presentation to?

3. Don't overestimate or underestimate the level of understanding of your topic. Think about this. Never talk down to your audience. If you have a mixed audience of internists, subspecialists, family physicians, and radiologists, for example, define the topics that might be confusing to some of them during your presentation. But only allow a minute or so for this.

4. Your PowerPoint slides should not have any misspellings or errors (more later in the chapter).

5. Always carry a backup of your talk(s) on a flash drive or disk.

6. If your host requests handouts, your PowerPoint slides probably are sufficient. Use six slides per page, back-to-back, so you can get thirty-six slides on three sheets of paper. Email the presentation with your latest changes to the host's secretary several days before your arrival, so he/she has time to print copies. Don't wait until you are on the airplane to make significant changes.

7. Practice your talk, especially if it is brand new, you've made some changes, or added to your slides/images. When you are before an audience, it takes approximately 20 percent longer to give a presentation than when you practice it alone. Your introduction, which includes a "thank you" for the invitation, recognition of a few friends in the audience, and a vignette, clean joke, or short story if appropriate, always takes more time than you estimated.

8. If you can handle criticism (self-criticism!), videotape your practice presentation and then critique it, maybe with a colleague. This can be enlightening.

9. Familiarize yourself with the podium, microphone, laser pointer, etc., a few minutes ahead of time. If there is a media-support person there, know his/her name in case you need help in the middle of your talk. Let him/her set up your first slide, and then be sure you are able to open it if someone introducing you has some slides. If you are short, ask for a step stool.

10. While acquainting yourself with the podium and before the audience comes in, you can put the first slide up on the screen and hit "B" on the computer to blank it. When you are ready to begin your talk, hit "B" again to put the first slide back on the screen. You can do this anytime during your presentation if you temporarily have no need for slides. This makes it look like you know what you are doing!

11. Find a clock on the wall or podium, and watch it.

12. Use a lavalier microphone, and be sure it is turned on so you can wander from the podium. Most experienced speakers do this because it helps keep the audience interested, which means you will convey your message more effectively. Have the remote slide changer with you, preferably one with a laser pointer. Ask the media-support person for a pointer if there is not one on the podium (pointers are easily stolen, so they may not be kept with the podium equipment), or bring your own laser pointer.

13. Lights should be turned down (not off) over the screen if you are projecting images or histology.

14. Be prepared if the computer projector goes down. It happens. Can you wing it alone?

15. You will learn the right and wrong ways to give presentations after listening to speakers at every conference/event you attend. Each is a free lesson. *Don't think that just because you are an expert on a subject that you automatically know how to give a masterful presentation.*

At the Podium

• Relax. Take a few deep breaths. Look over your audience. Stand tall. Act poised and confident. Look like you know what you are talking about.

• Do not drink any carbonated beverages in the last hour before your talk. You could be eructating every several seconds.

• If you tell an anecdote or a clean joke (think about what you are doing here; some people can't tell a joke), keep it brief. The clock is running.

• Don't lean on the podium. Don't shuffle from one foot to the other. This is distracting.

• We prefer that the speaker work from the slide on the screen rather than from the laptop computer on the podium. This way, he/she is likely to look at the audience more often. Use **eye contact** when looking at the audience. Look at all parts of the seated auditorium, not just the first few rows, even though it might be dark in the back and you can't see anybody.

• If you are not using slides, then you had better be a good extemporaneous speaker. When you don't use slides, such as during a graduation speech, write down **topic** words on three-by-five-inch cards and have these cards on the podium to guide you.

• When using a laser pointer, never zigzag the laser light back and forth across the screen. Point to what you are emphasizing but for no more than three to four seconds. If you have a slight tremor, rest the pointer on the edge of the podium or on your hip. This is especially important if you are a long way from the screen, which would exaggerate any tremor.

• **Talk slowly!** Rushing a talk is not natural.

• Think about your mannerisms—you may not even know that you have any until you review a video of yourself. These can ruin an otherwise good lecture. One senior speaker we observed bobbed up and down three or four inches every fifteen seconds. After a while, audience members were counting to themselves the number of seconds between bobs! It turned out that he was as accurate as an atomic clock. Distracting! *Don't become part of the show!*

• All mannerisms are distracting. Using your hands is a common one—fidgety. A nervous facial twitch is another one. **Try not to say, "Ya Know"!** *Never* allow yourself to get into this habit—you don't even know you are doing it. Again, the audience might be counting how many "ya knows" you use in sixty seconds. There have been a few indoor records set and broken with this. Same with "Uh" and "Ah." Distracting. Your talk should flow smoothly. If you need professional help to learn how to give a presentation, get it.

• Never just discuss the first two or three bullets or skip a few bullets. The audience may still be reading the third or fourth of five bullets while you are on to the next slide. So when they look at your next slide, they try to quickly read all the bullets because they think you are going to cut them off again. If you have shortened your talk to pertain to just some of the bullets, make new slides with only those you want.

• Most audiences like human-interest stories (interesting patient problems). It keeps their attention.

• **Never read your slides word for word** unless you've spotted someone in the audience with sunglasses, a white cane, and a dog. The audience will have read everything before you are halfway through. In fact, full sentences on a slide are no-nos.

• If you say during your talk that you will come back to a point "in a little while" or "later," the audience will think you plan to talk for a few hours. Instead, say that you'll come back to this point "in a few moments."

• Never put someone down—i.e., don't criticize someone who can't defend himself/herself. This is arrogance and quickly recognized. Someone in the audience will tell that person.

• Use great caution when talking about yourself. Don't be a name-dropper.

• When you have finished your presentation and are beginning the question and answer (Q and A) session, hit the "B" rather than leave your last irrelevant slide on the screen, unless it is a beautiful scene. Otherwise, it is distracting.

• Again, thank your host(s) and make any comments you wish about the hospitality, etc.

• Stay within the time limit given to you. *There never has been a documented peer-reviewed report of complaints about a speaker ending his/her talk before the time was up.* Many speakers have ruined good presentations by talking too long. ("What I have to say is too important to leave anything out.")

Q and A

• Check with your host ahead of time to see if a Q and A session is usual. If there are less than twenty people in the audience, you can announce at the beginning of your presentation that it is OK to interrupt with questions but to keep them short.

• Before the Q and A session begins, think about whether you stuck to the content anticipated based on the title of your presentation. If not, make a few points in this regard.

• **Always repeat a question.** This gives you a few extra seconds to think about the question and if you understand it.

• Don't let a questioner get you into an argument. Cut off the conversation, and don't promise a discussion afterward.

• If you don't know the answer to any question, say, "I don't know." This might be humbling, but it is better than faking it. Trying to fake it takes longer than if you had the answer because you will be hemming and hawing while you try to think of something to say. Maybe someone in the audience knows the answer.

PowerPoint Slides

• The quality of these slides reflects the time you put in to create them. They speak for themselves. They aren't your message—they just enhance it.

• Use the same background color on each slide in a presentation. Never use a black background, and never use white print on any color.

• If your institution has a media-support service, ask for that department's help to polish your slides. Why not have them done right the first time? And you'll learn something. Or you could go to a local grade school—third graders know how to make PowerPoint slides!

• Don't apologize for the slides. You made them (or had them made).

• Always crop your image slides. If you don't, you now have a reason to apologize for *your* slides. We can't tell you how many slides of images we've seen that were not cropped. For example, some included all the data from the radiology department, while others showed large areas outside the thorax on Computed Tomography (CT). Both of these left little space for the part of the image that the speaker wanted to show. Poor and distracting. This affects the quality of your talk. Again, get help from your media-support service.

• Avoid unknown abbreviations.

• Limit the number of words used per bullet.

• No more than five or six lines per slide.

• Forty slides should be the maximum for a thirty-minute talk. *Remember, you must stick to your time limit.*

• If you have a reference citation, reduce this font size by two and use italics. Put the author's name first, followed by the journal, year, volume, and beginning page number. If it is important to your message, give the audience time to write this down. If the citation is in your handout, point that out and move on.

• Always credit a reference source if you used a chart or image to make a slide.

• If your slide looks too busy to you, it **is** too busy. What can you do to fix this? Make a duplicate of this slide, and then crop it down to highlight the area you want to discuss.

• Too many slides will fatigue your audience.

• Avoid gimmicky fade-ins and fade-outs. Use the same fades throughout your talk. One lecturer used a different fade for each bullet. Pretty soon, the audience was waiting to see the next fade and not concentrating on the slide materials. Entertaining, but distracting.

• If you anticipate questions about something you didn't cover, have the pertinent slides available to use after the last slide (but you may not need them). Remember that additional slide's number, and then you can type the number on the computer and hit "Enter."

For the last slide (before the Q and A), close with a pretty scene with a graphic *THANK YOU*. But don't leave this slide on for more than a few minutes; hit the "B" key to blank the slide.

A special thanks to Dr. Udaya Prakash for the use of some of his teaching materials on this subject and especially for his expertise as an excellent speaker.

Chapter Eight

Entertaining Visiting Faculty

A visiting faculty member is your guest. Most likely, this will be the faculty member's first visit to your institution as an invited guest. Ideally, the host should be someone who has been a visiting professor a number of times, as he/she will know and appreciate the little amenities that can make the visit memorable. *The results of this visit will affect your institution's reputation.*

The invitation should be initiated with a phone call, followed by a letter. **The call and subsequent letter should contain most of the information that follows, which the visitor needs to know:**

• The date of the talk—make this clear. And the town. For example, there are many anecdotal stories of Mayo Clinic guests coming on the wrong day and even to the wrong Rochester.

• The exact time of the talk(s) and the maximum length. Are there any special audiovisual needs?

• The letter should include a discussion of the possible topic(s) with the final topic(s) to be determined at least three weeks in advance, so the visit can be properly publicized.

• The visitor needs to know who will be in the audience and how much time is allotted for the talk. Point out the option to leave time for Q and A.

• If a handout is needed, the guest must be told this in the letter. After you receive the handout from your guest, email it to your secretary to make copies.

• If this is an invitation for speaking at a course, send at least a rough draft of the program that includes the names and titles of the other speakers. Be sure to include the length of the recipient's talk and whether to leave time for questions. Urge the speaker to keep his/her talk to the allotted time.

• Mention the honorarium in the initial letter.

• Your visitor should be given your secretary's contact information in the initial letter.

• Is the speaker expected to make rounds and visit with residents? If so, when?

• Is it anticipated that the visitor should meet with the division/department chair? The dean? Others? If so, plan ahead. There should be no surprises. Get the visit on everyone's schedules. Be

TIMELINE FOR VISITING PROFESSOR

Initial phone call and follow-up letter:

1. **Topic(s) of the talk(s)** _____

2. **Date(s)** _____ **Day(s) of the week** _____

3. **Time(s) of the talk(s)** _____

4. **Honorarium amount** *(optional to mention)* $ _____

5. **Dinner the night before?** _____**Where?** _____

6. **Day and time the guest can plan to leave** _____

7. **Host** _____ **Cell** _____

8. **Host secretary** _____

    A. Phone numbers: Office _____ **Cell** _____

    B. Email address _____

9. **Guest secretary** _____

    A. Phone numbers: Office _____ **Cell** _____

    B. Email address _____

    C. Request for the guest's latest CV _____ **Bibliography?** _____

    D. Mention if a handout will be needed

10. **Expected to make rounds? Yes_____ No_____**

11. **To meet with leadership? _____ Who?_____ When?_____**

12. **Arrival date _____ Time_____ Airline _____ Flight # _____**

13. **Pickup arrangements: Cab** _____

    Limo _____ **Phone #** _____ **Code** _____

    Host _____ **Who will pick up the guest?** _____

14. **Hotel**_____ **Conf. #**_____ **Phone #** _____

    Address _____

(Host secretary makes the hotel and restaurant reservations.)

15. **Host secretary responsibilities:**

    A. Fills in all of the above

    B. Makes sure there is appropriate publicity for the presentation

    C. Receives the CV (or searches for it on the Internet, if needed) _____ Handout? _____

    D. Emails the guest one week before arrival. Confirms flight specifics and who will pick him/her up and where, or arranges for a limo or cab with the guest's name at the airport.

    E. Emails this sheet to the guest

    F. Reminds the guest to announce any conflict of interest at the start of the lecture

    G. Emails information from numbers 1 to 8 above to everyone involved

    H. Gives the guest an envelope with his/her address on it so the guest can mail back all expense receipts; the check should be mailed within ten days.

sure that someone is available to escort the guest around, and that escort must be on time. Use caution when assigning this responsibility to junior residents.

• Ask your guest for his/her secretary's name, phone number, and email address. As soon as you get this, ask this secretary to email the speaker's most recent CV to you. Follow up on this if it is forgotten.

• Indicate when the guest should arrive (in time for dinner the night before?) and when he/she can plan to leave. Most guests will want to make their own plane reservations. Offer your guest different options for travel, such as an express or limousine from the airport or renting a car rather than taking a second or third flight. These little things can be "crowd-pleasers" to a guest new to your institution. Minimize the hassles!

• Do not invite the guest to stay in your home unless he/she is a good friend and knows your spouse. Many professional visitors don't like to stay in someone's house and prefer some privacy. He/she needs a place to relax, go over the presentation, etc.

• Two weeks before the guest's arrival, fax or email the full visit agenda. This should include the reservation confirmation number for the hotel where he/she will stay, along with the hotel's location information and phone number. Your email should be copied to everyone involved with the visit; put these names at the bottom of the email so the guest will have this before arriving. In this email, ask the guest to confirm that he/she received the information and for his/her travel plans, including flight numbers and arrival time.

• In the above fax/email, remind the guest of your secretary's phone number and email address, and your cell and home phone numbers. (Did you get his/her CV?)

• The host should call or email the visitor about a week ahead of time to make sure there are no unanswered questions on either side. At a minimum, leave a message with the secretary.

During the Visit to Your City

A designated, experienced secretary is the best person to make sure that all the arrangements are made so you can take care of your guest when he/she is at your institution.

• Meeting the visitor at the airport is a good job for a resident/trainee, who would then have the opportunity to talk privately with him/her. Go over these plans with the resident/trainee.

• If your guest is not being met by someone from your institution, how will he/she get from the airport to the hotel? Will the speaker be picked up by a limo?

• After the guest gets to the hotel, give him/her some time there to clean up, make calls, etc. What time will you pick him/her up at the hotel?

• After dinner, return to the hotel at a reasonable time; remember that the guest may have traveled from a different time zone.

• If you are not taking the guest to breakfast the next day, tell him/her so he/she can make other plans at the hotel.

• During the day, be sure to offer your guest some time for finalizing his/her talk, bathroom breaks, coffee, and some rest. These days can be very tiring.

• Don't expect him/her to eat in a rush fifteen minutes before the lecture is to start.

• Try to include at least one resident or fellow at any lunch or dinner.

• You should know your guest's departure time, so you can get him/her to the airport in plenty of time with no last-minute rushing to the gate.

Secretary's Duties

• Ideally, one secretary should be in charge of each visit, although every division and/or department involved will probably have its own secretary working on it to some degree. Secretaries who have experience in planning events—making hotel reservations, reserving limo service, following up on publicity, etc.—can prevent some major oversights.

• Send an email to the guest one week before arrival to confirm flight specifics and how he/she will get from the airport to the hotel.

• Make sure the talks are publicized well ahead of time.

• Make sure the host has the CV.

• Expedite the reimbursement of expenses. These should be paid by the institution within seven to ten working days after receiving the list of expenses with appropriate receipts.

Remember, a smoothly run visit reinforces a positive impression of your institution. Almost all your guests will have visited other institutions that they can compare with yours.

Chapter Nine

The Ideal Academic Medical Center and Private Practice Medical Center Professional

Professionalism Criteria

The ideal professional is **respected by all**. This professional is the ultimate **role model** because he/she always does the right thing and cares about people. Achieving respect should be one of your primary goals. This includes being respected by professionals from other institutions. How many full professors or chairs of large group practices do you know who are jerks? Do you still respect them?

This *ideal physician* always practices the **Platinum Rule of Medicine**:

> *Treat every patient like you would want*
> *a member of your family treated.*

- Does this individual represent your group?
- Would you want him/her as your physician?
- Is the physician a team player? Teamwork imbues loyalty and **pride** in your institution. Those who lack pride and dedication will become apathetic, lose their work ethic, and do the least amount of work and social interaction possible. This is contagious.
- If you work in an academic medical center, your ultimate career goal should be to become a full professor. Seeing patients may be your primary interest, but there's no reason why you also can't write papers and teach to work toward qualifying for academic promotion. If you write two peer-reviewed papers a year, this would result in sixty papers in thirty years. You should work with a resident or two on most papers.
- If you are the attending on hospital service, you are the physician of record. You must be sure that the patient is getting the best possible care. After rounds are completed, consider going back

to the patient without the house staff (or with just one resident) to clarify some matters. This is extremely important if things are not going as well as expected. It is just not right to make the patient wait twenty-four more hours for your next visit. This doesn't undermine the experience of the residents; on the contrary, it will teach them a lot. You are the role model! Be sure the patient has the written names of all the physicians who are taking care of him/her.

These are some traits of the ideal professional:
- Trustworthy and demonstrates high integrity.
- Known for having **common sense**.
- Has a passion for **mentoring** and considers mentoring a professional obligation.
- Has no hidden agendas, is not self-serving, and is transparent in his/her professionalism.
- Sees patients and enjoys this part of the job, even if he/she also is a researcher. Goes the extra mile, e.g., sees patients not on the schedule. This also would include taking a call from a referring physician and working a patient in within a day or two when appropriate.

> *The good physician treats the disease; the great physician treats the patient who has the disease.*
>
> —Sir William Osler

- Keeps a tickler file of patients with undiagnosed problems or who are due back at a definitive time while awaiting test results. The physician's clinical assistant will check this file daily. A call from you is immensely valuable and will help your patient while he/she is healing. The ideal physician never leaves a voice mail or sends an email when he/she has to tell a patient about abnormal test results. This physician will try again to reach the patient or take the patient's return call right away.
- Relates well to referring physicians (*see Chapter 10 on* Qualities of a Chairperson in an Academic Medical Center or Private Practice Medical Center).
- Is very appreciative of the value of teaching—sees it as an obligation and makes it a high priority.
- Is **always** a gentleman or lady.

> *It is the patient who carries the burden of illness, but the compassionate physician shares that burden, lifting it when possible and lightening it when that is all that can be done. This sharing of the burden has always been the hallmark of the medical profession.*
>
> —Richard S. Hollis, MD

Virtuous Qualities of the Ideal Physician

• **Character** is what you are—it is your *reputation*, which takes years to build but can be lost in minutes. Building your reputation is a continuous journey, not a destination. It's always doing the right thing. It's looking in the mirror in the morning and asking, "Is the image I'm seeing someone I can greatly respect at the end of the day?" The ideal physician never gossips. The physician with character always remembers who he/she is working for—*the patient!*

• **Integrity** is a firm adherence to a code of moral values. It is an implicit obedience to the dictates of your conscience. Integrity is what you do every day, whereas character is a long-term quality—your reputation. An example of integrity is doing something good while knowing that no one will ever know that you did it.

• **Humility** is the ability to see yourself, including your faults, from a distance. The ideal physician is confident (but not cocky), self-effacing, grateful, and able to respect himself/herself.

• **Lack of arrogance (humility).** There is no such thing as an arrogant, compassionate physician. The arrogant physician is easily angered and brings this to work with him (we see arrogant women much less often). The arrogant physician exudes a professional detachment.

• **Trustworthiness.** Honesty. To many patients, trust is more important than compassion, integrity, and other virtues. Trust is sacred to our profession, but we are rapidly losing the public's trust, mostly as a result of the commercialization of medicine. The patient's trust in his/her physician is an unquestioning **belief** that the physician will do what is best for him/her without compromise. The ideal physician is a partner with his/her patients. This physician practices the Platinum Rule of Medicine.

Trust is a two-way street. The physician trusts the patient to be compliant. The satisfaction that the physician and the patient have in each other greatly relates to their mutual trust. Satisfaction is an outcome measure of mutual trust: a perception that represents past experiences and fulfillment of a patient's expectations. *This is recognized as good continuity of care*, which is highly valued by the patient.

Trust itself is a powerful healer.

• **A Positive Attitude** is everything. It is the intent to be happy and optimistic. It is the first thing anyone notices about you and is the result of the power of positive thinking. You reflect your attitude in your body language. You can't hide it.

• **Empathy** is demonstrated by **caring**, **compassion**, and **kindness**. It is **humanism**. Empathy is the capacity to put yourself in the patient's world and understand what he/she is experiencing. It is a feeling while *sympathy* is an emotion. *Compassion* is a feeling of deep sympathy for someone who is suffering, which is accompanied by a strong desire to alleviate the pain.

Empathy cannot be taught through reading or playacting. It has to be learned, preferably at home first and later through effective *role models*. Charisma lessons have been shown to have little effect! You must **want** to care for the patient. You can't fake this!

... For the secret of the care of the patient is in caring for the patient.

—Francis W. Peabody, MD

You can demonstrate your empathy with acts of kindness. You may think that you don't have time for empathy, but in the long run, you will find that it takes less—not more—time to take care of a patient when you are empathetic. Reassurance is not the same as empathy, especially if there are no diagnostic grounds for confidence if the problem remains undiagnosed. *But never take away hope.* Remember, more and more often, patients see a different practitioner (MD, DO, PA, NP, RN) every visit! Continuity of care is one of patients' greatest desires. How can a practitioner and patient develop a good relationship knowing that they probably will not see each other again? *The only way is for every practitioner to deliver the Art of Medicine by* **caring** *for the patient.* It can take a patient several subsequent visits to overcome one negative experience—if he/she ever does.

• **It is fun to be kind.** If you smile, you are more likely to be kind. If the patient senses empathy, he/she is more likely to comply with your recommendations. When a patient doesn't trust his/her physician, the patient often is less compliant with the physician's recommendations, which becomes a big, expensive problem. By the end of a visit with a patient, you can probably tell by his/her body language if he/she is receptive of your empathy and your trust.

• **Tolerance** for diversity/tolerance for people who want to be what they are. You can't have it any other way because *this is the way it is*! Another term for tolerance is *acceptance*.

• **Intuition**—and acting on it.

• Portraying a sense of **purpose**—this is *passion*.

• **Resiliency:** the process of adapting well in the face of tragedy, serious illness, and other adversities. Resilience requires good coping skills, and these strongly correlate with social connections. A sense of humor and having hobbies that are enjoyed are invaluable.

• **Equanimity:** maturity. Osler said that one of the greatest virtues a physician can have is equanimity. It is calm patience, inner strength, and imperturbability. Learn to forget. **Let. It. Go!**

A physician's *passion* is the deep feeling of obligation to serve others.

The person with passion gets things done!

• Every employer seeks people who have **passion**. A person's passion may not be outwardly obvious, but employers can sense passion through body language and by learning about an applicant's accomplishments.

• **Communication skills** and the desire to use them (*see Chapter 13 on* The Art of Medicine).

• **Consistency, reliability, dependability,** and **punctuality.** Always being on time is one of the most underappreciated virtues you can have; this defines your reliability and dependability.

• Self-recognition as a positive role model. Good self-esteem. The ideal physician is confident and proud of his/her accomplishments.

• **Spiritual acceptance.**

• **Collegiality**—the ideal physician is nice, composed, mature, sociable, and friendly.

- Knowing what you don't know shows wisdom and maturity *(see Chapter 11)*.
- **Emotional intelligence.** Social skills.
- **Respect** for yourself.
- **Loyalty.** This person is dedicated, proud, and supports the mission and vision of the institution.
- **Balanced life**. Remember that you can never get time "back." Enjoy every moment with your family and your professional life as well!

For the most part, these virtues are self-explanatory. These are virtues that you hope your children will acquire from you.

Professionalism

Professionalism is a mind-think. It is an attitude of upholding what the public thinks those in a profession should be doing to advance the well-being of society, and doing it without compromise or self-serving financial gain. Ask yourself, "Would I want my family (or myself—it happens) cared for in a less-than-professional culture/institution by less-than-professional people?"

Professionalism is the foundation of the social contract we maintain with the public and our patients. But as the practice of medicine becomes more corporate, the physician becomes an employee with less commitment and loyalty to the institution and to the patient! What was once a covenant of trust between the patient and the physician has become more of a contractual relationship based on mistrust. We must do everything we can to reverse this trend.

Professionalism can be looked at as another name for ***trust***.

There are a number of criteria for professionalism, but you really don't need to know each one. You will know when you see (or don't see) them in your ideal role model.

Some expectations of a professional are as follows:
- Ideal role model and mentor
- Supports the mission of his/her department and the institution
- Adheres to high ethical and moral standards
- Demonstrates a continued commitment to excellence
- A patient advocate who never takes away hope
- Promotes a Culture of Caring
- Accountable
- Compassionate
- No conflict of interest
- A constant learner who feels an obligation to teach others
- Makes sacrifices for the betterment of patient care and the institution
- Never arrogant or greedy
- Highly respectful of referring physicians
- Never makes derogatory comments and never uses foul language

The qualities listed above include most of the basic tenants of professionalism.

There is a great overlap between *bioethics* and professionalism. The physician must realize that every interaction between the patient and the physician has a moral component.

Institutional professionalism is the totality of actions by all your medical center's employees. In one study of employees, two-thirds of respondents reported that they had never received recognition or praise for the quality of their work.

Deprofessionalism is the long-term erosion of the public's trust because of the impairment of the qualities listed above. Financial interests take precedence, followed by maintaining the bureaucracy. The patient's needs become a lower priority.

Ten percent of overall mortality is related to poor medical care.

The Accreditation Council for Graduate Medical Education (ACGME) and the American Board of Medical Specialties (ABMS) listed the following six competencies of internal medicine and medical subspecialty residents/fellows that must be evaluated and documented:
- Patient Care and Procedural Skills
- Medical Knowledge
- Practice-based Learning and Improvement
- Interpersonal and Communication Skills
- Professionalism
- Systems-based Practice

There are six **"Cs"** that are **imperative** to the ideal physician-patient relationship:

1. **Communication.** This is one of the most important skills needed for any relationship in life, not just the physician-patient relationship. Remember that 80 percent of communication is nonverbal. Good interpersonal communication skills include the ability to break bad news, along with being able to effectively deal with the difficult patient, unusual patient expectations, refusal of recommended care, end-of-life care, management of medical errors, impaired colleagues, and any situation that seems futile. Communication also includes the ability to *listen*!

2. **Competence.** The competent physician always seeks new knowledge and stays current with medical news. This physician knows what he/she doesn't know. The patient can look up a physician's credentials, including his/her last Maintenance of Certification (MOC) score.

3. **Compassion.** Would you send your family members to a physician who was not empathetic? The **Platinum Rule of Medicine** again!

4. **(No) Conflict of interest.** *Greed* for money and power is becoming more and more pervasive, and physicians are not immune. Once greed is hardwired in someone's brain, it is very hard to reverse. These "sins" easily override integrity. This can ruin the reputation that you have worked so hard to build.

5. **Choice.** Patients relate that choice is one of the most important components of a positive physician-patient relationship. If a patient likes his/her current caregiver and is moved to someone else (including MDs, DOs, PAs, NPs, RNs, etc.), he/she loses trust in the system. The patient won't know which caregiver to expect at the next visit. An absence of trust will lead to noncompliance, demand for more testing, mistrust of caregiver recommendations, doctor shopping, etc.—all of which leads to more expensive health care. And the patient will be more likely to sue.

6. **Continuity of care.** With the depersonalization and industrialization of the physician-patient relationship, everyone has to work harder to maintain continuity. Some physicians discourage continuity because they don't like people. If the staff recognizes this in a physician, action needs to be taken. Maybe this physician shouldn't be seeing patients! These physicians are without remorse—a form of abandonment. It's possible for a patient to never see the same person again in spite of many visits. *This is a form of abandonment—a loss of **hope**.*

We would add the following to the 6 "Cs":
   • **Autonomy for patients.** They must be given the choice of having autonomy versus turning over their care completely to the physician. Autonomy includes establishing trust, maintaining confidentiality, encouraging advance planning, always telling the truth, and allowing the patient complete access to his/her records. After the completion of a visit or hospitalization, send a copy of the summary with lab results to the patient (or make sure the patient knows how to find this online, if this option is available).
   • **Beneficence.** Improving the patient's quality of life.
   • **Nonmaleficence.** Above all, *do no harm. And never take away **hope***.
   • **Fairness to all.**
   • **Good coping skills.**
Most of the above cannot be tested for on a written exam. It is very likely that a physician's compensation will depend on patient evaluations in the near future.

All boards have established their own set of competencies. Can professionalism be taught out of books and in medical schools? Maybe, but only the *ideal role model* and the *culture* of the institution can truly teach it by example.

Avoiding Malpractice and Traits of the Nonideal Physician

The following are all unprofessional through and through *(see also Chapter 10)*:
   • **Poor communication/miscommunication** is the single-most common cause of malpractice. Although patient dissatisfaction with his/her health care may be another factor, a patient is unlikely to initiate a malpractice claim based solely on dissatisfaction.
   • It may not be just verbal communication that is at fault but also body language. A patient intuitively can "see" that a physician is uninterested and maybe even angry with him/her. The physician's body language may be evident in his/her facial expressions and if he/she is not listening, making eye contact, smiling, and/or touching.
   • There could be another reason that patients sue for malpractice found in a letter that the physician writes to the referring physician (with a copy sent to the patient) or if there is a delay of more than a month before it is mailed. The physician may even refuse to send the letter to the patient, but this is contrary to the Patient Bill of Rights *(see Chapter 3 or 17)*.
   • Delays in getting significant abnormal results reported to the patient.
   • Failure to discuss alternatives, goals, and risks of any planned procedure, and making a record of these discussions. Good records are the first line of a malpractice defense.
   • Criticizing another physician's care.

• About 1 percent of hospitalized patients suffer a significant injury due to negligence, but less than 3 percent of these patients will sue.

• Be sure that team members always are on the same page.

• Patients who sue have stated that their physicians always **seemed rushed, tended to ignore them, didn't return phone calls, spent too much time on the phone while with them**, and **gave inadequate explanations (or no explanations) about diagnoses and plans for treatments**. These physicians also were described as **arrogant, callous, insensitive**, and/or **disrespectful**. *These descriptions (listed in bold) could be part of a textbook on true unprofessionalism on the part of the physician and are a setup for a malpractice lawsuit!* At a minimum, these physicians are burned out and stressed. They should be given a reprieve from the practice of medicine until they have received some sort of therapy—otherwise, they should remove themselves from patient care.

There are more!

There are several types of communication problems:

1. Deserting the patient! This is *abandonment*, an increasingly common problem that causes much frustration for patients and their families.
2. Delivering information poorly; this demonstrates an anxiousness to get out of the room.
3. Devaluing the patient's views.
4. Not really knowing the patient's perspectives and, at the end of life, not knowing his/her end-of-life wishes—and not caring!
5. Using only medical jargon.
6. Just not listening.
7. Avoiding/ignoring family members who have questions.
8. Not admitting that a medical error has been committed.
9. The patient's inability to choose his/her physician or not getting the same physician whom he/she likes.
10. Not returning phone calls.

These problems are present in the majority of malpractice dispositions. It may be the family members—because of their anger—who urge the patient to see a lawyer. It is not uncommon for a patient to be concerned that he/she will not be allowed to return to a medical center if he/she files a complaint.

See the sample "Commitment Contract" that follows. Some of the information is geared toward physicians in academic medical centers, so the contract may need to be adjusted to reflect this. Mayo Clinic is referenced as the institution in this example contract. However, note that the contract is an example only and not used by Mayo Clinic. (The Mayo Clinic professional staff is salaried.)

The Ideal Academic Medical Center And Private Practice Medical Center Professional

COMMITMENT CONTRACT* **

By reading and initialing each underlined item (and then having this in our files), you cannot come back to the chair and say, "You never told me this before!"

**This is a memorandum of understanding, not a formal contract.*

In the process of finalizing your appointment to the staff in the_____ division, I, _____, the division chair, am asking you to read each item word-for-word and initial each item regarding your commitment to the institution. This is not legally binding (with a few exceptions), but it does serve as a reminder that you are committing yourself to associate with a large group of people and many, many patients who have put their trust, as well as their lives, in our hands. Every action, good and bad, reflects on our institution as well as on the medical profession.

> *The best interest of the patient is the only interest to be considered, and in order that the sick may have the benefit of advancing knowledge, union of forces is necessary.*
>
> **—William J. Mayo, MD, in a commencement address at Rush Medical College, 1910**

This led to Mayo Clinic's primary value: "The needs of the patient come first," which must take precedence over all other missions you/we might have! It has brought us this far.

Some of our **strengths**:
- Quality and quantity of *role models*
- Allied health personnel (AHP) with their strong *work ethic* and genuine kindness to all
- No prima donnas here—those who feel they aren't getting the recognition they expected do not stay

Institutional Guidelines
Mission and Vision Statements
Bylaws
Employee Handbook

History of the Organization
(Add historical reference books and notes about the institution here.)

Institution's Expectations of You:
excellent patient care—our highest priority!

Treat every patient like you would want a member of your family treated.

The Platinum Rule of Medicine

Support the institution's **Culture of Caring**.

Never be angry. If you have a problem with this, deal with it, or we will.

Treat *all* allied health personnel with kindness and like a member of your family. Our concept of *family* has been one of the major reasons for our success. Rudeness of any kind toward AHP puts you at risk of dismissal. Because of their very strong work ethic, they expect as much from the professional staff.

Nurses, just like all other health-care providers, are invaluable to the mission of health-care centers. Studies have shown that nurses are more likely to quit their jobs because they feel a lack of respect as opposed to feeling dissatisfied with their salaries and perks. Find a way to recognize their accomplishments.

Patients commonly tell us that they are so impressed that physicians talk to each other here. This adds up to teamwork at its greatest.

Relate well to *referring physicians*. Keep a list of "active" referring physicians with their patients' names, and keep in contact with them. We could not exist without them.

Maintain a professional demeanor, including in your appearance and clothing, at all times. Everything you do reflects on the institution.

Follow the rules of *common sense*. ***Always do the right thing***. There are no instruction books for these.

Be an **Ideal Role Model**. This is one of an institution's absolute strengths because of the quality and quantity of superb individuals who are teaching a great deal about the *Art and Science of Medicine* and the *Art of Living*. Are you the kind of role model others can look up to while enhancing both your own and the institution's reputation? You can go to these role models for advice at almost any time. Remember, too, that not all role models are positive, but you can still learn from them.

What does hustle mean to you?

All new Mayo Clinic staff members are appointed as Senior Associate Consultants (SAC). During an initial period of "engagement," the new SAC and the current staff evaluate each other. Toward the end of the third year, the division decides if the SAC will be offered a permanent staff position; 10 percent are not.

Mentoring: Not all role models are good mentors, but all mentors should be good role models. You have to want to mentor to be a good mentor. (*See Chapter 4 on* Mentoring and Role Models.)

If there are certain patients you don't like to see (e.g., those with mental disorders), forget it. They have to be taken care of if they are in the system, and you are obligated to provide your best care if you are scheduled to see them. Don't pass the buck or treat them indifferently.

Volunteering: List previous and current experiences. You are encouraged to continue.

How would you handle *medical mistakes*? You made? Someone else made?

Maintain your CV and your Research and Education Academic Information Management System (REAIMS). Update it appropriately, and put the date somewhere on the first page. After each update, send an electronic copy to the chair's secretary and your own secretary.

Education

• All staff members are expected to teach, especially to the students, residents, and fellows. The quality of our students and our eventual professional staff depends on the education we give them. Teaching every day during hospital rounds is imperative.

• Strive for the "Teacher of the Year" and other education awards. They are among the most rewarding achievements.

• Attend all education conferences and social functions.

• Publish two to four papers a year. Involve students. Practicing physicians in academia have access to an extensive record system. Physicians in the real world of practice rely on us to relate our vast experiences with conditions that they seldom encounter. They value our knowledge about these conditions.

• Become an "expert" in a few narrowed areas. Publish on these.

• Know the institution's academic promotion guidelines. Set your goal at becoming a full professor.

• Join national education organizations (if you haven't done so), and get involved in their committee systems.

• You must have certification in your specialty(s). Recertify on schedule.

• If you have just started a one-hour experiment in the lab and get a call that you have a patient waiting to be seen, what would you do?

Your Goals and Expectations

(Attach a list that includes volunteer activities.)

Do you have a five-year plan?

Do you have a Living Will or a Durable Power of Attorney? Are you an organ donor?

Risks for Dismissal*

• Breach of patient confidentiality—could be immediate.

• Sexual harassment, which would be immediate.

• Unacceptance of diversity—could be immediate.

• Poorly controlled anger.

• Difficulty with alcoholism and/or drugs.

• Unprofessional behavior and improprieties (unacceptable act, remark, and/or language).

• Repeated complaints by patients and AHP; three or more complaints could result in probation.

• Refractory mediocrity.

• Not being a team player.

• Not taking or failing certifying/recertifying examinations.

• Conflicts of interest, as well as any financial improprieties, must have been previously disclosed. If in doubt, ask ahead of time.

• A lapse of integrity—any impairment of integrity reflects negatively on the institution.

• Any fraudulent act.

Likely preceded by due process and probation.

Attention: Chairperson—Is there any reason you should call this physician's previous employers, letter writers, and/or education program director? This would be your opportunity to ask how this physician treated patients and AHP. It could save you grief.

Signed _____ Date _____

Printed name_____

Chair signature _____Date_____

Vice Chair signature *(optional)* _____Date_____

Chapter Ten

Qualities of a Chairperson in an Academic Medical Center or Private Practice Medical Center

Make your division the BEST at your institution—right from the start. We think this should be the single most important goal for a new leader in any capacity—and especially for a chair in an academic medical center or large group practice. It begins with your passion and is followed by a collegial group of dedicated caregivers (family) with the same attitude. The trickle-down effect has significant benefits. The result of reaching this goal will be your division's accomplishments. Everyone's pride will be obvious; it will permeate the institution.

Everything else—including national recognition—can follow. This reflects on your reputation. Set goals, and celebrate when you achieve them. Some ideas on how to achieve professionalism in your department follow (also see Chapter 9).

Leadership

There are numerous books, magazines, articles, courses, and on and on about how to become a leader. But you only can learn so much from these. Essentially, no one comes out of a residency or fellowship and suddenly becomes a division chair. Throwing you in the water to teach you how to swim doesn't work here—you'll drown first.

As an aside, I (author ECR) didn't become a division chair until I was on the Mayo Clinic staff nearly twenty years. No one had talked to me about the possibility of someday becoming a chair—in fact, I was more interested in patient care and education. As a result, I didn't really know what it took to be a chair, and there was no break-in period because my predecessor left for Mayo Clinic Scottsdale shortly after my appointment.

I didn't receive any manuals that might have helped me. There was no orientation of any kind. I hadn't made any mental notes from my observations of previous chairs. My only real exposure was sitting in on division committee meetings.

When I agreed to be the chair, my ascension began immediately. I had a full 7:30 a.m. to 6:00 p.m. schedule of patients for the next six weeks. I couldn't cancel them. And my first problem was dealing with a staff member's personal issue not at all related to work! I didn't know of any books that dealt with medical personnel issues since no two problems are alike. Back then, the Mayo departments didn't have vice chairs, so there was no "passing the buck." I was in this alone.

The chair of any division/department or of any business must exhibit qualities that exceed those outlined in Chapter 9 *(The Ideal Academic Medical Center and Private Practice Medical Center Professional)*. As a chair, you have the opportunity to positively impact the lives of everyone you are responsible for. You can best assess the status of those in your division by monitoring their morale.

Being a leader is a *mind-think*. The leader/chair assumes *responsibility* for the well-being of all the personnel—professionals (physicians and scientists) as well as the allied health personnel (AHP)—in his/her section/division/department. This is your new family. This concept of family has been a very important element of the Mayo Clinic success story. Leadership is a people business. *You must be visible!* Encouraging the family concept in your division greatly contributes to **teamwork**. *The priorities of the institution/division and the people in it must supersede those of the leaders.*

Ideally, you would learn leadership qualities before you assume the role of the chair, but there is no substitute for on-the-job training—provided you are willing to learn! If your institution offers leadership courses, take them even if your future goals don't necessarily include a leadership role or it would be many years away. *But if you don't truly care for people, then you shouldn't accept a leadership position!*

Are you going places? Or just being led?

The following ideas are based on what we learned during our years on the job and also from very closely observing role model leaders, reading extensively, and talking to people about leadership. We've put in boldface what we think are the qualities necessary to become an effective leader. One of those important qualities is a **sense of humor**. If you don't have one, get one—you'll need it!

• Remind yourself frequently that you have a mission and a dream, and follow them. *Be the best you can be.* Remind all the members of your team, including the

AHP, of your division's mission/goal to be the best at your institution. Everyone shares a **sense of purpose**. Outline the specifics of how to best reach that goal. Be cautious when delegating certain obligations too quickly; some of these responsibilities will need to be nurtured at a slower pace. Consider listing milestones on a common wall. And have fun doing this. Celebrate when a goal is reached.

• Review the institutional staff manual. Talk to the chairperson you are responsible to about his/her expectations of you, and write these down. Know the institution's mission, goals, and rules. Be aware of the guidelines of the Joint Commission (JC), Residency Review Committee (RRC), Association of American Medical Colleges (AAMC), Maintenance of Certification (MOC), and all specialty boards. Is there a job description?

• Tell everyone in your division what you expect of them and the resulting rewards. Put these in writing so they can't come back later and say, "You never told us!" (This works with your kids as well.)

> *You need to be the role model for the whole division that you lead. Are you? And you must work harder than anyone else. Don't accept an appointment to chair your division just to pad your CV.*

• Do you consider an appointment to division chair to be a stepping-stone to a similar position at a larger institution in the not-too-distant future? This should not be your hidden agenda, so if this is the case, make this known before accepting the appointment. This is **integrity**, which could be the most important quality you bring to this position.

• Chairing a division/department is not a lifetime job. At Mayo Clinic, it is an unwritten rule that most chairs will serve about seven to eight years. At that point, another qualified person will provide new blood and ideas to the division.

• As a chair, you must be **fair** and **transparent**. This means **no favoritism** and **no hidden agendas**. Remember, you are responsible for dozens of people.

• As the leader, one of your most important priorities will be to continue as, or create, a patient-centered division. This is a priority, and you must continue to see patients. This means that you most likely will be working on some of your administrative duties at night and on the weekends.

• You must be willing to **accept change**, which is inevitable. This is critical to effective leadership and especially important when a change isn't your idea. Give credit where it is due.

> *If you are the leader and you stop rowing, you shouldn't be surprised if everyone else slows down.*

• Two of us (authors) learned a lot from our experiences as chairs of large divisions and from chairs of other divisions. First, you must be visible at least two to three times a week in the "work area." Talk to the desk attendants—they know a lot about what is going on as they have their fingers on the division's overall morale. Make time for one-on-one communication with your personnel. See patients who have been overbooked, are waiting to be worked in with at least a semi-urgent problem, and/or referred by a physician. See disgruntled patients who want to see the chair. Be the last one to leave for the day. Not following these suggestions could lead to apathy within your division *(see Chapter 12)*.

• Instill **pride** in your group (your family). You can't do this if you don't have pride in yourself. We don't think you can be a leader if you don't have it. Some might suggest you aren't supposed to be in a leadership position.

• **Listening** is another one of the most important qualities of a leader. Listen with the intent to learn. You'll read this again. This engenders **trust** and **humility**.

• **Smile.** Make this a habit. It is infectious. Give an award to the best smiler(s). Smiling begets kindness and a positive attitude. At some major medical centers, employees are reminded to smile and greet everyone they see. Make a mental note of those who never seem to smile.

• There is a lot more to leadership than overseeing a group of people—a leader has to be an **outstanding role model/mentor** *(see Chapter 4)*. You already must have the respect of the people in your division. If you aren't already an outstanding role model, it might not be too late to become an "effective" leader. Strive for this. Learn all you can from the role models you respect. Make a list of their qualities and review them frequently. This is something you can pass along to your kids and grandkids.

• The division leader's goal is to bring **reputation** to the top of everyone's mind when they think about your division. Your reputation is based on providing the best possible medical care for your patients, recognition of outstanding educational endeavors with awards, significant cooperation among all members of the institution, respect for throughput, obtainment of research grants, and collegiality. Surprisingly, division collegiality is one of the qualities that is most respected by those not in your division. It reflects teamwork and that you are having fun. All this is important to the **morale** of the division.

• The AHP are among an institution's most important assets. They are significant to the institution's core culture. The leader is responsible for their need for recognition ("what I *do* is important to others") and need for acceptance ("what I *am* is important to others"). This is **respect**, which is imperative. Without this respect, the morale of your people will decline, and apathy will set in. Keep in mind that it is not uncommon for this to be the supervisor's fault. The leader is ultimately responsible. And you must respect yourself! Could you be at fault for the division's low morale? Many studies have shown that leadership qualities likely affect the satisfaction of physicians who work in health-care organizations.

> ### *Employees say the number one reason that they leave a workplace is because they don't feel appreciated. The main reason is not pay, position, or perks.*

• Find ways to **compliment your AHP and professional staff** whenever you can. The Mayo Clinic Karis (caring) Award and other similar awards of excellence (best role model, best smiler, etc.) are superb ways of recognizing members of your division. Post these awards in your work area.

A handwritten note, a cake, or cookies go a long way, and you also might consider sending a letter to the family. Your employee will never forget this.

> ***We wildly underestimate the power of the tiniest personal touch.***
> ***And of all personal touches, I find the short, handwritten***
> ***"nice job" note to have the greatest impact.***
>
> —Tom Peters

• If you receive a letter from a patient in gratitude for the care given by one of your division members, read it at a division (department) meeting.

• Post a copy of the first page of any recently published article written by one of your staff members, and list it in your meeting minutes.

• Be aware that 15 percent of your patients will leave your practice because of the rudeness of your receptionist or another AHP. Examples of this could include ignoring patients, long holds on the phone, negative body language (obviously an unhappy person), and office chitchat while the patient waits. You could learn about this through exit questionnaires. Your administrative assistant and supervisor should be on top of this. You should appoint a chair for practice.

• Learn a lot about your division by conducting nonjudgmental exit interviews with the professionals. The administrator/supervisor should do the same with the allied health personnel, and you need to see these summaries.

• **No favoritism.** Repeating this. This is divisive and counterproductive. Don't allow cliques.

• Begin grooming a vice chair. This person should know that this doesn't mean that he/she automatically will be appointed the division chair someday. Since your vice chair may not be ready to serve as the chair when your appointment ends, be sure to also identify two to four other physicians whom you can groom as your replacement.

• You will need an administrator (depending on the size of your division). This person would, preferably, have some finance experience. You should learn finances. Go over the division's accounting status every month with your administrator.

• In addition to your administrator's responsibilities for finance, if you have a physician staff member who has an MBA and/or is interested in accounting, appoint him/her to be your finance chair. But keep track of the finances as if they are your responsibility—because they are. Maintain and teach cost containment. Make this part of your education program. Where can you save dollars without affecting the quality of your practice?

• The finance chair should make available the costs of patient care, which should be shared with the medical students, residents, and fellows.

• It is very important that you appoint an education chair. This person will oversee the quality of the seminars in the division and make sure the staff is maintaining certification. The education chair will work closely with the fellows and young staff to make sure they have the correct mentors. This chair also should work with the fellows and staff to make sure their CVs are up to date.

• The supervisors of your allied health personnel can be a great asset to you—trust them. Extend that trust to the receptionists because they will know a lot about how patients relate to your division and the professional staff.

• If you work in an academic center, you should not recruit anyone who isn't interested in **teaching** and **publishing**. Imagine a division in an academic medical center that doesn't publish. What if this were the case in every division? The practicing physician wants to know how your specialty cares for the person with a condition that your academic center has seen in hundreds of patients, but he/she is seeing for the first time.

• A paper's senior author (resident/fellow) can become a world authority on a medical subject as a result of recording the division's experiences. This begets referrals. We rate this as a high priority for a division and its reputation.

• If your people don't go all out and have a **passion** for teaching, how can you expect to attract medical students, residents/fellows, and staff to your program? Your division's reputation for teaching—good or bad—is known throughout the institution. In order to be the best division, you have to be known for your teaching. The students will pass this around. Teach the students to be good teachers. You also must have a way of rewarding good teachers. If there isn't a "Teacher of the Year" award or something similar, start one. Encourage your staff to give grand rounds and arrange to give lectures at local/regional hospitals.

Ha! Ha! Your end of the boat is sinking!

• Recognize that teaching may be more important than publishing. Motivate your students, residents, and fellows to strive to win your division's teaching awards. The payoff will include attracting the best students to your program and, eventually, to your staff. Always teach with respect (*see Chapter 6 on* The Art of Educating). It is easier now to get an academic promotion with educational accomplishments because only publishing counted in the past.

• You should have a chair of mentoring (*see Chapter 4*). All mentors are good role models, but not all good role models are good mentors. Mentoring is absolutely imperative unless you are in business for yourself. As a young staff physician, you should pick the mentor best suited to you (provided the person is willing). The value of a good mentor is priceless, especially if you need advice regarding your potential as a leader. As you move along in your career, you should open yourself up to mentoring students, residents, and young staff. This can result in lifelong rewards for both the mentor and mentee, and it is priceless to the young staff member. Mentors can prepare young staff members for future leadership roles, including that of division chair. This is an obligation of the more senior staff.

Some leaders consider "passing the buck" the same as delegating authority!

• Be sure that you and your staff introduce your new staff and fellows to physicians from other academic medical centers during national meetings. Nurture this.

• Carefully vet anyone you are considering for recruitment; it can take almost a hundredfold more time to get rid of someone than it did to recruit him/her.

• **Never get angry.** If you are angry about something, never take it to work. Those who witness it will consider it part of your reputation, and they will make it a topic of conversation with anyone who will listen. Your temper—not your accomplishments and good qualities—will be the first thing that people remember about you. *You can measure the size of a person by what makes him/her angry.*

• **Never tolerate arrogance**, which is a lack of humility and empathy. There are so many other descriptions of arrogance, but you need to know that one person can adversely influence the reputation of your division. Some descriptions of an arrogant person include: doesn't know what he/she doesn't know (this is an arrogance of ignorance), blames the patient for not getting better, disregards the value of maturity and wisdom, doesn't recognize that others consider him/her arrogant, doesn't appreciate that he/she will be remembered as arrogant over his/her good qualities or accomplishments, and is generally unfriendly to anyone he/she considers inferior or of no value to him/her. Arrogance begets arrogance. Arrogant people tend to be greedy—they are so good that they become entitled to wealth!

• Bullying is prevalent in industry, and this includes medical centers. Bullying not only is painful for its victims but also creates a huge cost burden to the economy. Never tolerate it.

• Never criticize someone in front of others, and criticism should always be constructive. When you are ready to voice a concern to someone, first compliment the person about something he/she has done positively. End the conversation with an upbeat attitude. Do this with empathy.

• Have a great imagination and stimulate it in others. Develop a long-range plan and write it down. Set goals with input from all your division members, including key allied health personnel. **Recognize and give credit** to people with good ideas (innovation). Share the ideas with others who may be able to add to them. Go over ideas every quarter at division meetings.

• During division meetings, ask the members to list what they consider to be the *qualities of a leader*. Write them on a whiteboard and record them. The members also can submit ideas anonymously later on. Compile and add to these ideas over time. Ask the residents, fellows, and even some AHP to contribute. Where do you, the leader, fit in? It is imperative that you conduct 360-degree reviews on your physicians and scientists on a regular basis.

• Compile also a list of goals and a five-year plan. These are always works in progress, so keep adding ideas as they are received.

• You must have **loyalty** to your employees and to the institution by supporting its mission, vision, and culture. This is *pride*. Don't knock it. If you can't do this, maybe you don't belong at this institution as a leader or even an employee. If you or members of your staff have concerns, deal with them with the right people. Do not complain to all who will listen—this is demoralizing.

• When you need to make major decisions that affect the division, do so only after input from all the members.

• **Recognize apathy, stress, mediocrity**, and **burnout** in your staff and allied health personnel and deal with them *(see Chapter 12)*. Depressed? Interpersonal relationship problems may consume more of your time than you can imagine. The problems won't go away by not dealing with them either. The sooner you deal with these matters, the better the chance of satisfactory resolutions. You may not be able to delegate these issues.

• *I'm sorry* is a powerful phrase. The arrogant person can't say this. He/she is never wrong and will blame others. Swallow your pride. Arrogance is easily recognized in a person's body language. This doesn't reflect well on your division.

• Saying *"I don't know"* engenders **trust**. It imbues self-integrity. Make sure your staff knows the importance of this phrase and uses it.

• Staff members should document their teaching efforts, including preparation time.

• Give compassionate care to your patients and don't tolerate any employee who doesn't. Deal with this! You certainly should not hire anyone who can't deliver care with empathy. This is the Art of Medicine *(see Chapter 13)*. The data from patient-satisfaction surveys should be used appropriately, including to recognize or award ideal role models. Strongly support and reward the good role models in your division.

• Never tolerate any lack of kindness toward the allied health personnel. Never. Again, never tolerate arrogance.

• **Maturity** and good leadership are synonymous *(see Chapter 11 on* Wisdom and Maturity*)*. Osler said that equanimity could be one of a physician's greatest virtues.

• If research is your forte, you may have to give up some of it to maintain your visibility in the practice and education areas. Sacrifice is a prerequisite for a leader. Do your share of seeing patients and taking the hospital service.

• Attend every educational conference you can, and make sure your staff does the same. Encourage your nurses also to do so.

Responsibilities of the Chairperson

There will be some responsibilities that you may not have appreciated when you accepted the position as chair. Early in your experience, you should be involved in all of them—they are your responsibility. Eventually, you can delegate some of these to your vice chair or someone of maturity. But you will still need to stay in touch as they can reflect on your division's reputation.

1. *Develop a Culture of Caring* within your division *(see Chapter 13 on* The Art of Medicine*)*. This is a function of practicing the **Platinum Rule of Medicine**; this culture is a learned behavior from ideal role models. Honor your division's ideal role models, which could include AHP, nurses, and even the custodians, at a recognition event. Awards should recognize what your division's members consider to be ideal qualities. Your allied health personnel are major contributors to a positive culture, and many are great role models. So award those great role models, and put up plaques on the walls. Even the division members who don't earn these awards will notice that good qualities are recognized and rewarded.

Nurses should be members of some of your committees. Recognize your nurses during National Nurses Day/National Nurses Week. It's amazing what some special desserts and coffee can do!

Be as nice to the custodian as you are to the top guy!

Be aware that a compliment resides in a person's mind for only about two weeks, but inappropriate criticism could be remembered at every encounter for months or longer. Nonconstructive criticism will destroy almost any incentive for improvement. This is why you (the leader) need to maintain a positive air about your workplace—a workplace with an attitude! Exit surveys are an excellent way to find out what employees are thinking.

> ### *If you take good care of your employees,*
> ### *they will take good care of your customers.*

2. *Divisions within a department.* If you are the department chair, the divisions and sections within your department are your responsibility. You might ask the vice chair to oversee them, but they are still **your** responsibility. A lot could happen before you know it if they go unmonitored, and then you have to fix any problems and answer to your boss. You need to meet with the division chairs and other members of your department at least every two weeks; if things are going smoothly, then meeting every four weeks is appropriate. Always have an agenda sent out at least twenty-four hours in advance.

3. *Problem physician or employee.* This requires due process and the sooner, the better. After you have discussed a problem one-on-one with the involved staff (medical or paramedical), immediately handwrite a note with the date and time on it and then file it away. Any witnesses also should complete a note. *Document! If it isn't documented, it didn't happen, but be careful what you put on your computer. Do not write anything damning.* And do not forward anything. Print it out (put a copy in a folder in your locked files), and handwrite anything necessary, such as a note to the personnel committee, a colleague, etc. All this could be retrievable and discoverable. In your documentation, state that the employee received a full explanation of the allegations, the recommendations that you had given previously regarding correcting the problem, and the written reprimand that makes clear the reason that he/she is being fired. If the firing is due to an issue, such as a sexual indiscretion, be sure to get assistance from the institution's lawyer. The personnel committee, which needs to be involved from the beginning, will help with this.

Your AHP supervisor can be a great help to you, even with a problem physician. If a physician has a problem, first rule out any medical issues, including alcoholism and drug use. This may be an *impaired physician.* If this physician doesn't have any medical issues, the state board of medical examiners needs to be involved. Every state has policies regarding the incompetent/impaired physician, who is defined as a physician unable to practice medicine for any reason. Discuss this with your human resources department liaison. You can insist on a medical evaluation, including a psychiatric evaluation. Don't try to settle everything at once if the situation is complicated (*see Chapter 12 on* Apathy, Mediocrity, Burnout, and the Consequences of Stress and Depression on Health-Care Professionals). If you must dismiss someone from his/her position, do this with class, not anger. *We have no idea what burdens some people carry in their minds.* This will impact many lives. Are you sure the person is not suicidal?

4. *Conflicts of interest* are best handled by the chair. This requires a sense of calmness. You must be nonjudgmental during deliberations. Get both sides of the issue from each person separately and then with both of them in the room. Ask the vice chair and administrative assistant to sit in and record the deliberations. Give both parties some time to think about what transpired at the meeting. Then make a decision or meet again if you need more details. *Decisiveness* and *fairness* are the keys. This leads to *transparency*.

It's been said that the sign of a good leader is that his/her employees always knew where they stood.

5. *Difficult patients*. Studies show that 10 percent to 30 percent of patients in group practices and academic medical centers are unhappy and want to complain to someone. They may vote with their feet and never return, but they will tell ten to fifty people at home, including friends, family, and neighbors—really anybody who will listen—and always will tell the referring physician. We define the difficult patient as someone who isn't psychotic or who doesn't have a severe personality disorder. Many are just unhappy people who are looking to take out their anger on someone. But they could have a legitimate complaint. So before you (as the chair) see this patient for the first time, it may help to see the patient's medical record but remember that you must get written permission first. The **ideal physician** *(see Chapter 9)* intuitively knows how to handle them.

Difficult patients make up a high percentage of those who sue physicians. If more than 10 percent of your division's patients register complaints, then you, the leader, should look for the source. Many complaints are due to long waits. Are the same few physicians the target of these complaints? Beware of the patient who also criticizes other physicians who are caring for him/her; tread lightly as the complaints may be valid. The patient may be referred to a patient affairs office to determine if he/she should talk to a physician. This is often **you**, the leader. Knowing how to handle this may stave off a malpractice suit. We think that up to 90 percent of difficult patient problems can be assuaged, but it takes an emotionally mature physician—one who is practicing the Art of Medicine. Or you could do what a number of other physicians have done—escort the difficult patient from the clinic or shuttle him/her to another physician. Keep in mind that a small—but definite—number of these patients will have a significant disease that remains undiagnosed. Ask yourself, "Are we missing something?"

There are ways of dealing with difficult patients as many—most—have legitimate complaints. Many have been difficult before; some might have a less severe personality disorder or depression, but they still need their concerns heard. They drive up appreciable health-care costs. Those patients with psychiatric problems who agree to receive psychiatric care will cut their visits to primary care providers from approximately twelve per year to three or four. You may not be able to talk about a patient's mental problems until the second or third visit. The incidence of depression in difficult patients is about twice that of the overall population.

You should check with your patient affairs personnel to see what complaints have been lodged against any of your division members.

Who is the patient angry at or what is he/she angry about?

- His/her primary physician.
- You, because you represent the "enemy" (the opposition).
- Another physician not in your division.
- The health-care system after being told there is nothing wrong with him/her: "It's all in your head."
- An incomplete physical exam (something missed) is the most common complaint about an "improperly performed procedure."
- The physician who refused to write a prescription or authorize a surgical procedure that the patient insists is needed.
- Costs of medical care
- Life in general.
- Medical error (see the next section).
- All of the above!

Above all things, let me urge upon you the absolute necessity of careful examinations for the purpose of diagnosis. My own experience has been that the public will forgive you an error in treatment more readily than one in diagnosis, and I fully believe that more than one-half of the failures in diagnosis are due to hasty and unmethodic examinations.

—William J. Mayo, MD, 1895 *(Yes, that is the correct date!)*

Four Imperatives When Dealing with a Difficult Patient

Communicate

Listen. Let the patient know how much time you have to listen and that you can reschedule for another time if needed. Let the patient talk for several minutes without interruption. Nod or frown. If the complaint is unreasonable, just let him/her keep talking. Listening and hearing are not the same things—which are you practicing? Listen to learn. Remember, the complaint may be very legitimate. What you learn from these complaints may improve your practice.

Use the patient's name frequently. Find out exactly what the patient wants that would make him/her less unhappy. If he/she is right about something, say, "You're right." Avoid blame on both sides. Don't try to get the person to see your point of view—it usually doesn't work and could make things worse.

Empathize

"I'm sorry you're angry/unhappy"—but don't say this until you have the full picture. Don't escalate the problem by arguing against what he/she is saying. Don't apologize too quickly if you are so inclined. The patient may think you are trying to end the conversation and get him/her out of the office. Don't keep looking at your watch.

Empathy turns defensiveness around.

"I think I understand your anger." *Do not get upset with the patient.* "Funny, a friend of mine had the same complaint here two weeks ago, and we are working on the problem."

Ask the patient if it is OK for you to take some notes. This demonstrates your interest. Talk to the spouse and/or the grown children if they are present; they are often the unhappy ones about the situation.

Body Language—Yours!

Eye contact. Don't look at your watch or computer. Sit at or below the patient's eye level. He/she doesn't want to lose any more control.

Smile appropriately. The patient can usually sense your arrogance (if you have it).

What Can You Offer?

Assume the primary care of this patient if he/she is willing to stay with the system. You've won! You are busy, but you also are responsible for the care delivered by your division. If you didn't solve the problem, you should see the patient again. The importance of the care delivered by your division/institution supersedes your research time. You may end up saying, "I'm sorry. I really don't think we can satisfy you here. We'll give you your laboratory and imaging test results."

If you think these recommendations will take too much of your time, wait until you are involved in a malpractice lawsuit!

Managing the Violent or Potentially Violent Patient

Managing the violent or potentially violent patient is another matter, and it usually happens unexpectedly. Don't ignore the patient or any threats. Be vigilant and closely observe his/her body language while encouraging him/her to talk. Don't lean back in your chair. Listen! Don't allow a lull in the conversation. Your body language must be calm and reassuring to show that you are interested in helping, but keep your distance. Don't encroach on his/her personal space! Never turn your back on this patient, and if possible, get between him/her and the door. Document everything. Your goal? Reassure the patient that you will help, and maybe prescribe a short supply of tranquilizers until he/she can see a psychiatrist (if he/she agrees to see one).

The Joint Commission estimates that there are more than 20,000 assaults in health-care settings every year in the United States! Many assaults occur in nursing homes and in the ER. Some are fatal. You must know your institution's plans for minimizing this number and what action to take if there is an incident. Share this with the members of your division including the AHP.

The Leader's Role in a Division's Legal Issues and Conflict Resolutions

1. *Medical error.* It is estimated that 100,000 deaths occur every year in this country due to medical errors. Medical errors have been estimated to be one of the leading causes of death behind heart disease and cancer! Even if this is only partly true, it is a horrendous number of preventable deaths. All medical centers now have safety teams that work hard to prevent these mistakes, e.g., putting a large **"X"** on the joint to be operated on, etc. Not too many years ago, these errors were swept under the rug.

The protocol for handling errors is pretty standardized; your institution almost certainly has a written policy. Read it. Don't wait until there is a problem. Be sure all your division members do the same.

A. The patient is told right away of an error even if there was no harm. Patients are aware that mistakes do happen and want to know the details. The division chair should determine who should tell the patient—in person—about the mistake. In most cases, the person who made the mistake will tell the patient and must do so promptly.

B. No room for arrogance here!

C. Most patients don't automatically expect to be compensated unless there is pain and suffering. They do want the medical fees related to the error to be waived.

D. They want the doctor to say, "I'm sorry." Apologies or statements of regret are inadmissible in court in many states. However, when the fault is clear, "partial" apologies may be worse than none at all. Rehearse what you plan to say.

E. Record this interaction right away.

F. Placing **blame** is almost unique to the medical error. This is most common in intensive care units and usually aimed at the nurses and residents. This can be devastating and even result in suicide for the person who is blamed. At a minimum, it can result in depression, guilt, post-traumatic stress disorder, thoughts of inadequacy, and thoughts of leaving the job. The blamed person will be ashamed and may be shunned by others in the institution.

You should tell your staff to never blame anyone—even the person who caused the error (especially a death)—and avoid using the word "blame." After every unexpected event, there should be a debriefing with you (the chair) and the people involved, always including the allied health staff. What did you learn from the event? The AHP may be taking the error harder than you appreciate; ask the person's supervisor to monitor this closely.

2. *Malpractice.* There is nothing that can prepare a person in any division for being sued. Dr. Sara C. Charles has published extensively on this. Remember that the challenge against the staff person, fellow, resident, or AHP is not so much about his/her competence but for his/her pocketbook. About 1 percent of hospital patients suffer a preventable medical injury, but only 3 percent of those initiate a malpractice claim. Less than 15 percent of those who do go against the physician.

A number of lawsuits are settled out of court per the input of insurance companies. Miscommunication between the patient and the physician is the primary determinant—the physician wasn't practicing the **Platinum Rule of Medicine**. Arrogance is almost always a factor when a patient decides to sue, but quality of care, surprisingly, is not (*see Chapter 9 on* The Ideal Academic Medical Center and Private Practice Medical Center Professional).

You, the chair, must reaffirm the trust you have in your sued staff person because he/she is suffering. As the chair, you also might be brought into the lawsuit. In the meantime, the sued physician must deal with the case head-on. Talk to your lawyer and get the options. The lawyer will likely tell the defendant(s) not to talk to **anyone** about the case, but anyone being sued needs to ventilate. Those named in the lawsuit can't live with the stress alone; they could seek out support groups of previously sued physicians for help (*see Chapter 12*). More than 90 percent of physicians named in a lawsuit end up with a form of post-traumatic stress disorder even when the matter clearly wasn't their fault. If you are being sued, your integrity is challenged, and you are sure your name will be splashed all over the newspapers, but this rarely happens. It could take two years before the suit comes to trial if it isn't settled out of court earlier.

The best way to prevent litigation is to practice the Platinum Rule of Medicine. Keep in mind that you will be remembered for what you do and have done for probably hundreds or even thousands of patients. Finally, record your thoughts in "write therapy" (*see Chapter 12*). Then **Let. It. Go!**

3. *Sexual harassment.* This can be worse than medical malpractice. Any harassment, sexual and otherwise, is intolerable. Urge division employees who experience harassment to come to you, as the leader. If there is a problem, don't delegate it to someone else in the division (your institution's legal office ultimately will be responsible). Most institutions provide courses on avoiding sexual harassment, which all employees must take. Ask that someone from your human resources department give a presentation on this subject at least annually during a division meeting. It is a **legal** offense. It reflects on your whole division and adversely affects its reputation. This reckless behavior warrants almost immediate dismissal.

Here are several more suggestions on how to prevent any litigation:
A. Good records are the first line of defense.
B. Never argue in the patient's record over the appropriateness of care, and never criticize another physician in front of a patient.
C. There should be a statement in the record of goals, risks, and alternatives of any planned procedure.
D. Never admit to negligence verbally and/or in writing.
E. Avoid making statements to the patient that conflict with the record. *All team members should be on the same page.*
F. Arrogance and anger are major factors in the majority of lawsuits.
G. Minimize any delays in getting test results, especially biopsy results, to the patient.
H. Admit to medical mistakes right away; the person primarily responsible for the mistake would be the best person to deliver this information. However, the physician responsible for the division will decide who will tell the patient. The attending physician, if different, also should talk to the patient.

I. Keep the CVs of all staff members up-to-date and never falsely enhance them. The lawyers would attack this.

J. Maintain good working order of equipment.

K. Keep the allied health personnel in the loop.

You, the chair, should review and go over these guidelines and your medical center's own policies once a year with your entire division, including the AHP, residents, and fellows.

4. *Conflict resolution.* Jealousies (differences) are facts of life that suddenly can become conflicts, and you, the chair, must deal with them so they don't become divisive. The best way of managing these is by prevention. You need to find out if there are hidden agendas driving these differences. Don't get caught being dragged into one side. You must hear both sides without prejudice (listen with the intent to learn), and then meet with the parties. Just getting the issue off their chests may be sufficient. But some differences are irreconcilable to the point that one or both sides won't compromise. How does this affect the people involved? The division? The institution? If there seems to be no satisfactory resolution, consider suggesting that one or both parties go elsewhere, especially if the person(s) is having problems following the mission of the institution and/or is not carrying his/her load. If you think one of the parties just needs to be in a different place and your institution has affiliated practices outside your city, a transfer might be an option.

Working with the People in Your Division

The deepest principle in human nature is the craving to be appreciated!

1. *Your relationships with coworkers* affect the morale/happiness of everyone in your division, including your allied health personnel *(see Chapters 9 and 12)*. Like it or not, this is your responsibility. Surveys show that people quit their jobs because they don't feel appreciated—not because they are dissatisfied with their pay and/or benefits. Ask a third party to assess the reasons that people leave your division—perhaps with an anonymous questionnaire. Poor morale leads to apathy, reduced productivity, and an increased dropout (transfer; quit) rate. This reflects on your division's reputation as well as on your recruitment of trainees and staff, including good AHP. Remember that your single most important goal is to make your division the **best** in your institution. If word gets around that you have a happy, functioning division, good people will want to come and work in it.

They may forget what you said, but they will never forget how you made them feel!

2. *Academic promotion.* Every academic medical center has its own guidelines for academic appointment and promotion. Be sure you are aware of these. Essentially, all centers use the Research and Education Academic Information Management System (REAIMS), a database of the scholarly activities of physicians and scientists (this is in addition to having a CV). It documents their efforts in areas such as teaching activities, presentations, mentorships, curriculum development, visiting professorships, publications, citations, and funded research. There is limited access to REAIMS, but most medical secretaries are familiar with its workings and usually are responsible for maintaining the necessary information on it. Additional information is manually entered from your personal CV. Remind your staff to keep good records of their accomplishments, including educational endeavors, in their CVs. Ask all the members and fellows to forward their updated CVs to you, their mentors, and your education chair. The CVs should be reviewed with a staff member twice a year, and the education chair should help them polish their CVs accordingly. When you write a letter supporting an academic appointment/promotion for a staff person, allow the person you are supporting to give input. (You can delegate your education chair to write these letters of support.) Your subspecialty fellows may easily qualify as instructors in their first year, and some will make it to assistant professor during their training.

3. *Committees—they're everywhere!* Beware of committees, frequently referred to as "black holes." You can get caught up in these and waste a tremendous amount of time. Committees are well-known for diffusing responsibility and delaying decisions—or killing them! Try to attend some of your division subspecialty meetings for education, practice, and research. Always read the minutes, and talk to the person (administrator?) who wrote them to be sure nothing was left out.

Do not allow a committee to become any one person's turf, but committees are good places to develop your replacement. Urge committee chairs to cancel meetings when there isn't any agenda item that can't wait. If a committee-meeting attendee has something to say, his/her topic should be placed on the agenda, and he/she should be heard. Meeting agendas should always be published beforehand. The most important items should be first on the agenda. Use the KISS—Keep It Simple, Stupid—process. If a committee meeting is scheduled for an hour, then it will take two-plus hours; if it is scheduled for thirty minutes, then it will take thirty minutes.

You, the chair, and some of your subcommittee chairs should get on institutional committees, but don't let that overwhelm you. Learn to say "no" appropriately.

How do you know if you have a loose cannon on one or more of your committees? It is usually obvious, but some of the characteristics are (1) always speaking up first; (2) frequently interrupting; (3) insisting that he/she is always right and not being interested in others' ideas; (4) doesn't have the institution's or department's mission in mind, which borders on disloyalty; (5) use of vulgarity; (6) doesn't carry out an assignment; (7) doesn't know how to listen; and more that you can fill in with experience!

No park has a statue dedicated to a committee.

Immature committees spend too much time exploring all possibilities and then do nothing!

No good ideas are born in a committee, but many are destroyed there.

Committees are

- a practice of playing it safe … involve excessive copying … formed to "share responsibility," according to Thomas J. Watson Jr.
- a theme park for workaholics.
- a way of getting out of work, which is not a good morale booster for those working.
- ten people doing the work of one.
- a place where people go who like to hear themselves talk.
- a group of people who meet to sit and think, but mostly to sit.

4. *Collegiality.* Not too many decades ago, it was common for physicians on the hospital service to stop for fifteen minutes or so in the "doctors' lounge" for a cup of coffee, to relax for a bit, and to "chew the fat." The physicians would meet in the cafeteria during or after rounds, and if there were residents in the group, the staff always bought the coffee and snacks. The conversation might be strictly social, e.g., sports, or about specific patients—"curbstone consultations." The talk could be focused on getting to know the residents better (invaluable) or didactic with the staff ("professors") discussing specifics about a disease, maybe showing some slides, and/or allowing a resident the opportunity to give a short prepared presentation about a patient. These breaks were always self-rewarding as the doctors shared experiences, bonded with one another, and became friends. The physicians looked forward to this.

These sessions were always *fun*. We encouraged a sense of humor. Collegiality! Some of these conversations resulted in lifelong friendships, either from working together or by staying in touch at national meetings after a resident had left the institution. Many times, this camaraderie also resulted in referrals after the resident went into practice elsewhere. Time constraints have taken much of this away. We encourage you to fight to reestablish these sessions or strengthen what you have because a continuing disconnect from the "family" of physicians will lead to a decline in the quality of medical practice.

This personal disconnect is not limited to physicians, but that doesn't mean we need to accept it. If we do, the result could be a decline in the quality of medical care, an erosion of public trust, and apathy/burnout of the health-care team. A suggestion we have is to establish a competitive incentive system based on patient satisfaction surveys. Physicians thrive on competition.

Note that congeniality is not the same as collegiality; a culture of congeniality is a culture that cannot achieve greatness or success.

5. *The referring physician.* Every member of your division, including your secretaries, the nurses, and the residents who take or make phone calls to referring physicians, must relate well to them. This is another imperative. You are responsible to maintain or build a good referral center. This is one area where you can enhance your regional reputation.

Return all phone calls as soon as possible. This is **professionalism**. Be cautious when you delegate this responsibility. If the referring physician detects **any arrogance**, you will likely hear about it because he/she will not send you any more referrals. **Apologize.** You know those phone calls where you hear "This call may be recorded to maintain a high quality of service." If your institution makes these recordings, find out what is done with the information.

Compliment the referring physician. Never put down the referring physician (or a fellow colleague) to the house staff, and use great discretion if you tell a patient that you disagree with his/her physician's diagnosis. The patient will almost always tell that physician what was said! It takes months—and sometimes years—to develop a good referring-physician relationship but only a few seconds to lose it! Nurture these relationships by phone consultations as appropriate, one-day education programs, etc. All this will result in more kudos for your division's reputation.

Make sure that appropriate correspondence is sent to the patient's physician within three working days or sooner—the same day if the home physician "needs to know." Don't delegate this if it is a serious issue. The same goes for the hospital service. Get a note in the record that you called the physician.

If the referring physician is in your specialty, he/she expects you, not a resident, to see the patient. Always have the patient return to the referring physician. It is not uncommon, though, for the patient to want to stay with your division physician(s); this can be uncomfortable. A good compromise is to ask the patient to talk to the referring physician and arrange for visits to your division two or three times a year for the subspecialty problem. Be sure this is clarified first.

If a patient is referred to anyone in your division and then has surgery or an invasive procedure in another area, the physician performing the procedure ideally should contact your division's physician that day or the day after if he/she is awaiting biopsy results. If the other physician doesn't contact your division, then your people should make the contact. The referring physician will be getting calls from the patient's relatives and has to be able to tell them something. *This is important!* Patients love it when you contact their physicians—especially in their presence.

6. *Expert witness.* A member of your division may be asked to be an expert witness by the press or in a trial. You need to know about this in advance because it will reflect on your division. Go over what the "expert" plans to say. Be aware that the media can distort the facts to its own conclusions!

7. *The physical and mental health of the people in your division* isn't your direct responsibility, but this subject should be brought up during annual reviews.

Events You May Not Be Prepared For
- Unethical acts: falsifying data, plagiarism
- Suicide
- A cover-up of a medical mistake
- Deaths in your division's "family" (including AHP)

Specific Areas of Concern
- Communicate well; never underestimate this because this is transparency. If you are the leader, you have to be available. Be cautious about delegating this.
- Listen well! It is one of the most important things you can do. Always have an "open door"—and truly have an open-door policy.
- Motivate. Nurture.
- Create an atmosphere of collegiality. Avoid turf wars. Compromise.

- Celebrate the little things—birthdays, promotions, births, etc.—with your staff and the AHP.
- Document significant achievements on the department/division's award wall.
- If there is a death in a division member's family, at a minimum send a sympathy card and maybe send flowers. A visit to the funeral home or service is appropriate.
- If a patient dies while on your division's hospital service, or shortly after, send a sympathy card. All your division members who cared for the patient, including the nurses, should sign the card. Your staff may take the death of a patient especially hard; be aware of this.
- Be tolerant of diversity. Respect all.
- No favoritism.
- Don't tolerate cliques.
- Be fair.
- Keep promises.
- Keep your CV up to date. Be sure that all your staff and trainees do the same.
- You must maintain the highest integrity. How can you expect others to do this if you don't? What kind of role model are you?
- Learn time management.
- **Never** burn your bridges.

Have *fun*!

Attention, all personnel:
The firings will continue until morale improves!

Chapter Eleven

Wisdom and Maturity

eek Wisdom and Maturity. It will save you an immense amount of time and even some grief. Ideally, we would inherit some wisdom and then acquire more during our youth while also developing maturity. We would gain both wisdom and maturity through experiences and *role models*. We have to work on acquiring them through forethought, common sense, learning from our role models' experiences, our own mistakes, and always doing the right thing. Wisdom and maturity have nothing to do with IQ, but a great deal to do with emotional and social intelligence and integrity. A great source of education can be other people's mistakes—and then knowing not to repeat them. An act of stupidity may require weeks to overcome. **Learn to think!**

> *When knowledge is translated into proper action, we speak of it as wisdom.*
>
> —William J. Mayo, MD

We think that mature people have an above-average level of wisdom, but we don't think that a wise person automatically is a mature person.

Some Thoughts About Wisdom
- The first step to wisdom is silence/quiet solitude, the second step is listening, and then the third step is practicing how to think.
- **Think.** The best place for thinking is a favorite place of peace—a place where you can practice meditation.
- Knowledge comes and goes, but wisdom lingers.
- A wise person knows how to avoid saying and doing **stupid things**. Every day we hear and read about celebrities, athletes, politicians, and prominent, intelligent people doing stupid things.

- Good judgment; **common sense**. You can't buy these. Count your blessings if you have them.
- Ethical; follows the mores of society.
- A good comprehension of mastering the Art of Living.
- Wisdom is the application of knowledge using an instinctive adaptation.
- Knowing how to take a hint.

> ### *God, grant me the serenity to accept the things I cannot change, the courage to change the things I can, and the wisdom to know the difference.*
> —The Serenity Prayer

- It is enlightenment and comes from humility.

> ### *Education is when you read the fine print. Experience is what you get if you don't.*
> —Pete Seeger

- The proper handling of failure leads to greater wisdom.
- Wisdom is the quality that keeps you from getting into situations where you need it.
- Wisdom is insight—seeing only the facts and not seeing what isn't there.
- Hearing the unspoken.

> ### *Intelligent people believe only half of what they hear. Wise people know which half.*
> —Harvey Mackay

> ### *Honesty is the first chapter in the book of wisdom.*
> —President Thomas Jefferson

- Waiting and knowing when to wait—this sometimes is the only way a problem can resolve itself.
- You can't develop wisdom without thinking—and thinking about just one thing at a time. This is *mindfulness*.
- Knowing what you don't know. Assumptions are not facts. The wise wait until they have all the facts and weigh them before making decisions.
- It's paying less attention to what others say and, instead, watching what they do.
- Suffering brings wisdom.
- **Learning from mistakes—preferably made by others.** You'll never live long enough to make every possible mistake—just read the daily newspapers! Stupidity plays a big role here. Yet failure is part of life. Every successful person could tell you about several personal failures and how these struggles strengthened him/her.

The two most common substances in the world are hydrogen and STUPIDITY!

- Knowing that others might be right.
- Insight: an ability to discern.
- *"I don't know"* are powerful words together.

Kindness is more important than wisdom, and the recognition of this is the beginning of wisdom.

—Theodore Isaac Rubin

- The price of greatness is responsibility.
- We are drowning in information and starving for wisdom.

Maturity

As you read the following list of examples of maturity, mentally check off your strengths. Most of these attributes can be learned.

- **Equanimity:** a calm patience; an inner strength. Contentment. Imperturbability; an absence of anger. Serenity.
- **Always doing the right thing**—even when there is no possibility that someone is watching.
- A philosophy of life; **a purpose in life**.
- **Resilience** gives you strength to cope with the adverse events that everyone will experience. This would include the deaths of people close to you, bad luck, missed opportunities, accidents, illnesses, thefts, disappointments, destruction of property, financial misfortunes, and other setbacks.
- Knowing and accepting that life isn't always fair. This is the way it is. You will appreciate this all the more when life does seem fair and things are going your way. It more than evens out. When life isn't fair, calling on the ability to **persevere** is maturity.
- The ability to see things as they are and not as we wish them to be.
- Following the **Golden Rule** is a religion.
- An awareness of the feelings of others: **Empathy**.
- Grace under pressure; being **humble**.
- **Decisiveness**; making a decision and not looking back (unless new facts surface).
- Willing to change your mind in the presence of new or different information.
- The ability to laugh at yourself.

The art of being wise is the art of knowing what to overlook.

—William James

- Always using good manners. Acting professional.
- **You can't please everyone.**
- Appreciating the value of education.
- Never showing arrogance. Every now and then, reflecting on whether people might think that you are arrogant (or greedy).
- Knowing the value of a role model and appreciating your own role models. Thinking about whether you are an ideal role model. What kind of role model are you?
- Knowing when to keep your mouth shut. *No one knows how dumb you are until you open your mouth.*
- Always keeping your word. Can be counted on. **Integrity**.
- **Dependability:** On time always (integrity again).
- **Honest.** Plagiarism is out of the question; would never fudge data. This also is integrity.
- Thoughtful. Knows how to be tactful.
- Willing to **forgive** and then **forget**.
- Doesn't let criticism be a worry. Will it make any difference in five years? Or even one year?
- Ability to tolerate an injustice without wanting to get even. Road rage!
- Accepting the inevitable.
- Appreciating that **hustle** doesn't take talent—it takes work. And you have to show up.

Nothing great was ever achieved without enthusiasm.

—Ralph Waldo Emerson

- Not trying to be someone you are not.
- The ability to gracefully accept a compliment. This is underappreciated!
- Accepting responsibility for all actions and not looking to blame anyone else.
- The capacity to face unpleasantness, frustration, and defeat without complaint, and not attempt to find someone to blame.
- The ability to face adversity and defeat without complaint or collapse.
- **Humility:** "I was wrong"—three more powerful words when put together.
- Tolerates delayed gratification.
- **Disciplined**. **Perseveres**. Always completes projects. Doesn't alibi.
- *"I'm sorry!"* are very powerful words together. The mature individual never hesitates to use them when appropriate. The arrogant person won't—can't—use them.
- Learning to want what you have.
- Making haste slowly. Think!
- Ability gets you there; enthusiasm keeps you there. This is **passion**.
- The price of greatness is **responsibility**. Your level of maturity will determine how you handle your greatness.
- Preparing for the worst. How you handle adverse events also is determined by your maturity.
- Caring about the less fortunate; valuing human dignity.
- Always being grateful. You can't be happy without **gratitude**.

- Doing more than expected.
- Refusing to accept mediocrity or laziness.
- Able to live one day at a time.
- Taking pride and pleasure in the accomplishments of others.

Have patience! In time, even grass becomes milk.
—Charan Singh

- A good interpreter of other people's body language—and your own. Do you know what your body language is saying? How is it being interpreted?
- **Diversity-tolerant.** It is this way because that is the way it is.
- Realizing that you alone are responsible for your own happiness.
- Always being a **nice** person.
- Accepting weather conditions as they are—no matter how much they might interfere with your plans.

When you get to the end zone, act like you've been there before!

Traits of the Immature

You can't legislate stupidity!

- Immature people spend too much time exploring all possibilities and then do nothing. Immature people **procrastinate**! Beware if two or more get on a committee—they can kill progress.
- **Inconsiderate** of others.
- **Entitlement** is a constant mind-think and becomes a way of life.
- Self-centered, narcissistic, and rude.
- Have low self-esteem and negative attitudes.
- **Greedy**. They always need immediate gratification and are possession-obsessed (the pleasure of acquisition).
- Lack emotional and social intelligence.
- Empathy-challenged.
- Tend to be arrogant as a poor coping skill.
- See themselves as victims; self-pity becomes addicting.
- They don't hesitate to lie without guilt and are prone to making excuses (alibis).
- **Blame** is a way of life. When you blame others, you give up your power to change.
- They are constant negative thinkers.
- They accept **mediocrity**.
- They rarely complete a project.

- Immaturity begets immaturity through self-pity, anger, and more blame. This becomes hardwired in a person's brain.
- The world is full of stupid idiots who fit in this class. Alcohol can easily push people, at least temporarily, into this group.
- Unfortunately, society tends to reward immaturity. Here is an example of a poster child of immaturity:

In 2004, Latrell Sprewell of the Minnesota Timberwolves NBA team was "insulted" when he was offered "only" $30 million for a three-year contract extension (he was getting $14.6 million per season). "Why would I want to help them win a title? They're not doing anything for me ... I got my family to feed."

Chapter Twelve

Apathy, Mediocrity, Burnout, and the Consequences of Stress and Depression on Health-Care Professionals

Remember the Platinum Rule of Medicine:
Treat every patient like you would want a
member of your family treated.

Authors' Note: We include apathy, mediocrity, burnout, depression, alcoholism, suppressed anger, and the impaired physician on the list of disorders and problems that may affect health-care professionals. Later in the chapter, the focus is on stress, including how it affects all these disorders. In any business, including professions, the presence of personality disorders in employees, professionals, or students can be tremendously destructive and demoralizing to the morale within that work group, as well as to customers, colleagues, and patients. We have witnessed and dealt with these. If they aren't recognized, they won't be treated. When they are recognized, the sooner they are dealt with, the better the chance of response. If these disorders become institution-wide, there will be a significant breakdown in morale and in the quality of patient care. Studies show that at least one of these conditions is present in up to 50 percent of physicians at some time during their careers. It seems the more mature people have learned to adjust and cope, and so are less afflicted. This is another reason to maintain a mentoring program within an institution. Tait Shanafelt, MD, et al., have published extensively on the topics of this chapter.

Some of the attributes of a physician who needs help are listed below. These are self-descriptive terms that, in some ways, overlap with all the disorders discussed in this chapter.

- No recognition from leadership
- Work ethic has been challenged
- Depersonalization
- Exhaustion because of excessive demands on energy, strength, resources, and reserves
- Loss of feelings for people
- Loss of self-esteem
- Doesn't feel like part of the team
- Withdrawn
- Lonely
- Loss of control over his/her calendar
- Disinterested/no longer motivated
- Feels like he/she has too many bureaucratic tasks
- Worries about technology taking over the practice of medicine
- Stressed out
- Feels sorry for himself/herself
- Unmanageable problems at home (or too much time away from home)
- Bored
- Feels that expectations are unachievable
- And on and on

The physician also might feel that the mission statements have become rearranged with the economic bottom line ahead of everything.

We have to remember that alcoholism is prevalent in physicians who are having these troubles, and they may consider suicide an option.

It is important to note that some personality traits—including perfectionism, compulsiveness, emotional control, conscientiousness, and deferred gratification—help young physicians accumulate facts and acquire skills. These traits are fostered and rewarded. However, these same qualities are predisposing factors for apathy, mediocrity, burnout, and depression.

One word that summarizes the feelings of apathy, burnout, mediocrity, and depression is OVERWHELMED.

But there may be some good news: These problems, along with stress, have some newly recognized, measurable abnormalities that can be classified in the psychoneuroendocrinology specialty (more information is available in *Psychoneuroendocrinology*, the official journal of the International Society of Psychoneuroendocrinology). This specialty broadly covers the immune system, inflammation, and the HPA (hypothalamic-pituitary-adrenal) axis. Psychoneuroendocrinology findings may lead to more exact diagnoses, coping measures, and specific treatments *(see the latter part of the chapter that focuses on stress)*.

APATHY

Apathy is often a precursor to burnout and more quickly reversible if the right action is taken. Some blame apathy on a person's leaders rather than considering it an isolated individual phenomenon like burnout or mediocrity. Apathy is an air of resignation that is infectious and contagious among a work group, while the other disorders tend to be more specific to an individual. Some describe apathy as a "release of freedom from passion, excitement, or emotion resulting in a feeling of 'who cares.'" It becomes a lack of concern and indifference. Pride is one of the first things to go when a person is apathetic, and teamwork soon follows.

Apathy relates more to a loss of control compared with the rest of the problems discussed in this chapter. The apathetic physician thinks, "Why should I work harder than the rest do?" This is a form of mental laziness. As a professional, you tend to have some control, or at least that was the expectation when you joined your division, group, or organization. But if you thought you had some control and then it was taken away, it is worse than never having it in the first place.

Apathy gets worse if there is a lack of communication (transparency) between the leadership and the workforce. Then it becomes "we" and "they." Not good! Collegiality diminishes, and apathy becomes infectious. Indifference permeates the group.

If you, the leader, stop rowing, don't be surprised if the rest slack off!

Apathetic professionals find excuses for not attending conferences and committee meetings. When they do travel to national meetings, they use their time to sightsee rather than attend educational conferences. Their colleagues begin to notice and say, "Why not?" and then do the same.

The apathetic physician seems to want to talk to his peers about what is bothering him/her more than a burned-out physician does. Burnout seems to be more personal. But if others listen to the apathetic physician, they may start to feel the same because of the problems confronting many of them, which embellishes what they already think and leads to more apathy within the division.

Since apathy doesn't become as ingrained, it is more easily reversible than burnout with the proper recognition by leadership. A fun group function can go a long way toward dealing with apathy (assuming everyone participates). The AHP will see apathy before the other physicians do.

Mediocrity and Burnout are Very Closely Aligned

MEDIOCRITY

The definition of *mediocrity* is just what the word implies. It describes an individual who is not performing up to expectations and showing a decline in his/her quality of work. Mediocrity is just as prevalent in physicians as it is in any occupation. It is estimated that at least 10 percent of all medical professionals are guilty of mediocrity. This is reflected most often in deteriorating patient care because the doctor has stopped learning and "doesn't care." Mediocrity is usually permanent if it is not recognized and treated—so the sooner, the better.

Mediocrity almost always begins insidiously and rarely manifests before the fifth decade, but with retrospective analysis, early signs may have been evident for years—maybe even during a physician's residency. Some might describe mediocrity as a loss of passion for the job but not necessarily for life itself. It isn't uncommon for those afflicted to continue with hobbies and other interests outside of work.

Mediocrity is one of the negative attributes that peers watch for during a physician's first three untenured years at Mayo Clinic. Mayo Clinic appoints new staff members as Senior Associate Consultants (SAC), and about 10 percent of them are not appointed to the active staff per a vote of their peers.

Loss of mindfulness (inattention; not thinking) is an attribute of mediocrity. Physicians who suffer from mediocrity just don't care, will come to work late and leave early, and won't attend conferences or division meetings. These individuals also won't return phone calls or emails. They don't contribute to the culture of the institution. They have crossed the line. Their supervisors should be documenting their absences, late arrivals, and early departure times.

The physician with mediocrity most likely won't have close friends in the division and maybe not even in the entire medical center. Word of this person's reputation has spread, and division members and others in the institution have lost respect for him/her. Their feelings also may reflect on the respect they have for your division, department, etc., especially if the chair doesn't do anything about this person.

According to a national newspaper report, dysfunctional workplaces that are the result of mediocrity and disinterest are estimated to cost the country $300 billion a year.

Mediocre people just want to be told what to do; they don't think "outside the box" (in fact, they also don't seem to think "inside" the box). They lack any personal incentive toward continuous improvement. If anything goes wrong, they find someone to blame. Sooner—rather than later—this person will make medical mistakes, and there will be complaints to the leadership. Incompetence has nothing to do with intelligence unless early dementia is setting in. We think mediocrity is more common in men than women.

Smaller departments within a large institution may provide the needed closer supervision that would help prevent mediocrity. But the large size of any institution, medical or nonmedical, can be a major factor in the tolerance of mediocrity because a mediocre person can stay "under the radar." When an institution is large, communication among the staff falters and relationships are superficial. We now rely too much on emails that are without a face. There is a loss of personal touch; the family concept is eroded. Mediocrity flourishes.

The early stages of mediocrity usually aren't evident to the surrounding personnel, and the mediocre person may not recognize it either. Unfortunately, it is tolerated in its early stages because others will think that the individual is just having some bad days. Maybe he/she is having problems at home. Eventually, the individual's colleagues will begin to note an attitude of laziness and almost boredom in their cohort, especially when they realize that they are carrying some of his/her load. When diagnosing the problem, the first possibilities to consider and exclude are depression, followed by alcoholism, and then substance abuse.

At this point, the support personnel also will recognize mediocrity in the person, but they may be afraid to discuss this with their leaders. They'll talk to other staff members about the little things the mediocre person is or isn't doing. It bothers them because they'll see deterioration in patient care. Patients may mention something to the allied health personnel; they may say that they felt the physician was disinterested in them because he/she did not engage with them. It may be nothing specific, but a patient may say that he/she didn't especially like the physician and didn't think the physician liked him/her. The patient asks to not see this physician again.

Now the chair needs to get involved. If a member of the allied health team has witnessed mediocrity, the chair should take and record a statement from this person and have him/her initial it. The chair also should reassure the AHP that there is no possible retaliation for this.

Some Things to Watch for That May Lead to Mediocrity

• **Tenure** is the guarantee that a job is secure except in the event of fraud, breach of confidentiality, sexual harassment, etc. Tenure begets a lack of incentive. Tenured physicians may coast along doing the minimum and kind of lose themselves in the system. They know all the tricks on how to do this.

• **Not being supervised.** Mediocre physicians slowly, over the years, slip into areas of work or locations where they can avoid supervision or look busy at the right times without drawing attention. They falsely elevate their relative value units (RVUs) to match busy physicians. If they work in a research lab, no other department or division members may be nearby so they can easily "hide out." They can go home early because only the lab techs would know, and they might not say anything because they don't want to lose grant support for their jobs. But, eventually, the grants will be lost. The chair needs to regularly make unannounced stops in the labs, which must be documented.

• Mediocre physicians don't read medical literature or attend CME conferences, except to attain the minimum hours needed to relicense. Then they usually won't stay for the entire conference. These physicians then feel insecure about and lack confidence in their own medical knowledge.

• **Coasting:** passing time by doing the least possible work until they can retire.

• Mediocre physicians avoid taking really good care of patients because they don't want patients to request them again or have to work them in as extras if they need to return on short notice.

• **Laziness.** These physicians respond to gentle or overt nudging by their peers or chairs but gradually slip back to their old ways. Laziness isn't new to them—they have just fooled everyone. They're not dumb. Their fifteen-minute coffee breaks usually last thirty minutes or longer.

• **Entitlement.** They believe that the institution/employer owes them something. There is a lot of anger behind this. Many don't see patients as important and only want to see the "diseases" they are interested in and researching. They are "organ"-oriented rather than "people"-oriented.

• They don't recognize the **value of role models**—"I'm better than any of them."

• They have poor people skills and don't care.

• **Negative attitudes.** Are they depressed?

• **Blames others.** Not a team player—lacks loyalty. This should be a clue; these people are very critical of everything.

External Factors for Mediocrity

• **Feeling unappreciated.** This person was a team player but not anymore. A little tiff between the chair and the person may preclude the chair from saying anything positive to the person. The chair may have selected his/her favorites and ignores the rest. The person may feel that he/she is too old to consider changing jobs so just coasts.

• **Depression, anger, ineptness, and stress at home (divorces are common). Alcoholism** is a significant risk before or after slipping into mediocrity.

• **Tolerance of mediocrity by leadership; never letting the person go (firing the person).** The pre-mediocre person sees this and figures that if others can get away with coasting, "Why should I work so hard?"

• **Lack of effective, respected leadership.**

• **Dysfunctional workplace** because of all the above reasons.

• Those who are around the physician may become aware that there is a problem before the physician admits it to himself/herself. Colleagues must keep this in mind. The physician's secretary may recognize all this but initially may be reluctant to say anything out of loyalty. The receptionist may know more than anyone because the patient goes right to him/her after a doctor visit to unload. The chair should discuss what others are seeing with the supervisors of the AHP.

• Prevention means not hiring mediocre people in the first place. There frequently are clues in physicians' residency records that point to mediocrity without the word "mediocre" or similar ones even appearing. Leaders should talk to interviewees' former program directors or chairs if they are coming from a different institution. If they trained at your institution, review the record from their training period.

• When interviewing anyone for a position, leaders should point out their expectations for loyalty, dedication, going the extra mile, attitude, carrying your load (and more), collegiality, and all the positive buzzwords. The leader should document in the interviewee's file that these were mentioned, and the interviewee should be given a copy of this document *(see Chapters 9 and 10)*. The leader now has a reference during a 360 review. The new person can't come back and say, "You never told me."

• Leaders should be cautious when granting tenure/partnership, etc., because they could be stuck with an undesirable employee who will take far more of their time than they ever imagined.

• **Laziness.** This condition permeates all the conditions discussed in this chapter. Everyone is lazy at some time during his/her work life, but it becomes a real problem when it is chronic. "Couch potato" is one description for laziness; "procrastinator" is another. It isn't a medical condition, but it sure contributes to nonproductivity. And it can become a habit. Laziness is always associated with having the flu, significant anemia, uremia, chronic pain, medications, sleep deprivation, and depression. Yet no one has ever measured anything in the blood or neuromuscular system that might explain the cause of the inability to act on something, or to exert, or of the feeling that "I just don't have the energy to do anything." As Hal Cranmer said, "For all these arguments against laziness, it is amazing we work so hard to achieve it. Even those hard-working Puritans were willing to break their backs every day in exchange for an eternity of lying around on a cloud and playing the harp."

• **Unhappiness** is another condition that could play a significant role in burnout, etc. Books are written and courses are given on achieving happiness, and there are even sections on happiness within psychiatry/psychology departments. What are the happiness and contentment levels of the spouses of physicians? Could their feelings play a significant role in the psyche of physicians?

BURNOUT

Burnout is mostly a result of loss of control, impaired coping skills, no one to talk to, no regular exercise to metabolize stress endorphins, excessive workload (partly self-induced), poor sleep habits, no vacations, alcoholism, and/or not being recognized or awarded for hard work.

Burnout is reversible. If depression is a factor with burnout, the patient likely will respond to treatment that may include medications and counseling. It is hard to know what roles *boredom* and *loneliness* play in all these negative attributes.

Burned-out Physicians Should Take the Following Measures:

1. Recognize and accept that they are burned out.
2. Reestablish a meaningful philosophy of life.
3. See their physician (they must get one now if they don't have one) for a general exam. The chair should inform the person's primary care physician of the division's concerns and possibly suggest that the primary care physician consider making a referral to a psychiatrist.
4. Correct the imbalance in their lives and reestablish some values (write them down). They should enjoy their hobbies and take up to a month's vacation soon or, better yet, a leave of absence so they will not use all their vacation time, which they may well need.
5. They need to share their feelings with others and may want to consider joining a study group, such as "Doctoring to Heal." If there isn't a local group, they should start one and stop operating in isolation. A discussion with the spouse by the chair could be very rewarding.
6. **Smile.**
7. Redevelop their **positive attitudes**. If they do, they can't feel sorry for themselves.
8. Try to do at least one small act of **kindness** every day.
9. Exercise (including yoga) at least five or six days a week.
10. **Laugh.** Join a laugh group; celebrate the little things.
11. **Friends.** Get together with different friends and do something every week. Go to lunch with three to five friends, for example. Have some *fun*—this is mandatory.
12. **Spirituality.** There are no atheists in a foxhole.
13. **Volunteer.** This is therapeutic.
14. **Count their blessings!**

External Factors for Burnout

• **"Burn-out" is listed in the 10th revision of ICD-10 under "Factors influencing health status and contact with health services."** There has been much written about physician burnout; an extensive survey of several thousand physicians confirmed that some division/department chairs were part of the problem. Since two of us (authors) were chairs, we appreciate the roles that chairs have in relating to staff. We have a few observations about chairs who may be part of these problems: (1) they accepted the invitation to be a chair to pad their CV; (2) they limit their time in administration and, instead, do research and see only patients related to it; (3) since they won't see any patients who aren't involved in their research, they won't see patients who don't have an appointment but have a semi-urgent problem—even though the division's receptionists are begging to have someone see them; (4) they seem to spend an inordinate amount of time in institutional and national committee meetings; and (5) they won't see the unhappy patient who wants to ventilate to only the chair; these patients can be time-consuming and demanding, but usually an empathetic physician is eventually able to appease them. *(Note: ICD-10 is the 10th revision of the International Statistical Classification of Diseases and Related Health Problems[ICD], a medical classification list by the World Health Organization [WHO]. The diagnosis code for "Burn-out" is Z73.0.)*

• Burnout can be differentiated from similar presenting disorders with morning plasma cortisol; it is low in burnout and chronic stress but elevated in significant depression.

• Burnout is a factor of stress in a workplace when combined with poor coping skills and a sense of loss of control. It has been reported in approximately 40 percent of physicians at some time in their careers. It is almost always preceded by apathy and stress—it is actually more of an advanced stage of apathy. One sign of a physician with burnout is that **he/she has stopped smiling**. Think about this. Some characteristics of burnout are a low sense of personal accomplishment, emotional exhaustion, and depersonalization.

• Although we see apathy as the immediate precursor to burnout, burnout seems to be more related to a loss of control—particularly the loss of control over the physician's calendar. As professionals, they had assumed that they would be "in charge" when they got out of training, but they aren't. They come to their jobs without having developed a "meaningful philosophy of life," which studies have shown to be very important to a physician. The burned-out physician suffers more from arrogance than apathetic doctors. Maybe they are angrier (generally suppressed anger).

• **Emotional detachment becomes a form of self-defense.** Symptoms of burnout can be fatigue, exhaustion, insomnia, and difficulty concentrating. Burnout always is associated with stress, which usually precedes it. Burned-out physicians don't take care of their health (one-third of all physicians don't have their own physician). Many physicians don't have or take the time for hobbies and nonprofessional *fun*. "All work and no play ..."

• Burnout also is associated with symptoms of anxiety, boredom, indifference, and depression. Alcoholism may not be far behind, and suicide may even be on this person's mind. At this point, physicians with burnout should make an urgent appointment with their primary care physician, which means they need to get one if they don't have one.

• What these physicians need is a feeling of connectedness with their patients. They need to believe that **they do exist for a purpose and they do make a difference in people's lives.** They need to feel that they are important to the work "family" and not "a waste of space" as some have described.

• Repeating this: Studies show that the physician-patient relationship is the most important stimulus to physician satisfaction. The burned-out physician needs to reflect on this, perhaps by writing about different patients they have bonded with. They should put these notes on their smartphones or computers so they always can look at them.

• The burned-out physician may need some time off, his/her workload cut back, and help with stress management (seeing a life coach or psychiatrist would be appropriate).

• Because of their occupation, physicians are at great risk for burnout. When they are working toward their career, they live on the kudos of good grades while they devote themselves to getting into medical school, working in their residencies that can take up to seven years, and finally getting into their subspecialty training that takes three to five more years. Physicians-in-training never really are able to learn how to bring balance into their lives because they spend their "free time" writing papers and preparing for board exams. They are constantly asking themselves if it is worth it.

The qualities that lead to success are the same qualities that lead to burnout.

• Burnout in medical students has been reported to lead to cheating/dishonest behaviors, along with misunderstanding appropriate relationships with industry, attitudes about physicians' responsibilities to society, and other criteria for the practice of professionalism. This all reflects on the integrity of the profession and, eventually, the person's employer/institution.

Dealing with Mediocrity and Burnout

Mediocrity and burnout, just like most other problems, are usually easier to prevent rather than deal with afterward. But someone must recognize the problem first. The individual will almost never ask for help, except maybe for depression. The chair must meet with the individual and discuss the situation. Can the chair get permission to talk to the physician's primary care physician and/or psychiatrist? Has leadership ever complimented the person? Are there any positive letters or comments in the person's file? It may be too late, but are there other members of the work group who deserve kudos that they haven't received?

If you are the chair, you must get involved once you and others recognize mediocrity or burnout in a staff member. Deal with it quickly with a one-on-one meeting. Explain what you know and **document**! If you don't document, it didn't happen. **Document** the meeting in the person's record, and give him/her a list (keep a copy) of your expectations. After this meeting, a thorough physical examination and possible psychometrics may be indicated.

Start a file of the documents. Consider sending copies—marked "confidential"—to the human resources liaison or the chair of the institutional personnel committee, if there is one. Better yet, hand-carry the file yourself. This is one of the most important things you will have if you get to due process because you'll need all the necessary documentation. It must be factual as this is discoverable. Discuss this physician's qualities with other physicians in your division in private. We don't think it is necessary to document these conversations.

Holding a pay increment is a possible first step to get a person's attention. If the problem persists, it may be time to begin due process toward dismissing the person. It likely isn't going to get any better and probably will get worse. Ignoring the problem is what a lot of "leaders" do. The personnel committee has to continue to be involved.

This may seem a little harsh, but remind the mediocre or burned-out physician that he/she has a job but is on the verge of losing it. Does he/she have the resources to find another job with this record? You can't write a decent referral letter because it would be unfair to the next employer.

These physicians won't have enough "fire" to start a practice alone. Some go into concierge medicine where they can be their own bosses. Can they now develop a "meaningful philosophy of life"?

Mediocrity is not the same as depression, but that doesn't preclude the presence of both. Burnout also can overlap with mediocrity and depression. Burnout and mediocrity are more difficult to treat and motivate than depression. Depression and burnout have similar symptoms, but treating burnout with certain antidepressants may aggravate the burnout. Burnout and mediocrity almost can be considered **"deprofessionalized."**

Buzzwords That Describe Apathy, Burnout, and Mediocrity*

Coasting	Negative attitude	Entitled
Arrogant	Poor people skills	Defensive/blames others
Lack of leadership	Dysfunctional workplace	Doesn't learn from role models
Unappreciated	Feels sorry for himself/herself	Alcoholism
Depressed	Increased medical mistakes	In denial
Underachiever	Lacks incentive	Lazy
Only a few friends	Not a team player	Doesn't complete projects
Incompetent	Work ethic challenged	Suicide/Suicidal thoughts

Recognizing these characteristics of apathy, burnout, mediocrity, etc., may lead to earlier action. If you are the chair, share this chapter with prospective staff members to enlighten them to the fact that you are sensitive to the traits of these disorders and will deal with them if necessary.

SUPPRESSED ANGER

Suppressed anger is present in most of the disorders discussed here, and especially in burnout and mediocrity. Like all the other disorders, there is no blood test or imaging study that can diagnose it—but the anger is there. Depression is part of this anger, but not all depressed people are angry. Anger is probably present in most (all?) people contemplating suicide—it's just a matter of degree. Most people who are angry—suppressed or not—feel their anger is justified toward who they blame for how they feel. Maybe they are actually angry with themselves.

The presence of anger is what keeps some people going. Anger energizes them, but it doesn't motivate them enough to be part of the team, to go the extra mile, or to seek help. Motivation is missing in the apathetic, burned-out physician.

THE IMPAIRED PHYSICIAN

This is a separate category as it is a reportable condition to state licensing boards. It is most often associated with alcohol and drug addiction; they are the most common conditions that lead to physician impairment. The allied health staff may be the first to suspect an addiction; patients will tell them that "Dr. X" is acting strangely and they think they detected alcohol on his/her breath.

According to the American Medical Association, *Physicians have an ethical obligation to report impaired, incompetent, and unethical colleagues.* You may be liable if you don't report them. Get help from your personnel committee and/or human resources committee. There is much more specific and effective help for impaired physicians from various sources than there is for the other disorders discussed earlier in the chapter.

Physician impairment is "the inability to practice medicine with reasonable skill and safety to patients by reason of psychiatric or general medical conditions." Prescription opioids are among the most prevalent sources of abuse. Denial is a feature of abuse. Unlike burnout, mediocrity, and stress, alcohol and drugs affect the central nervous system in areas that rely on "reward." Suicide is a greater risk for impaired physicians compared with physicians who suffer from some of the other disorders. It is estimated that one-third of impaired physicians are suffering from depression—we are surprised it isn't higher!

Signs that a physician may be impaired are patient complaints, an unprofessional personal appearance, tardiness, mistakes, impaired judgment, blaming others for his/her problems, and outbursts of anger. These are insidious and, in retrospect, may be present for years before they are recognized. The spouse will note these early on but be reluctant to tell anyone.

A physician with one or more personality disorders often has one divorce to his/her name. Can suicide be far behind? (**National Suicide Prevention Lifeline: 800-273-8255**) "Whom do I turn to for help?" Alcohol and/or drug addiction might be a (bad) solution!

Internal and external pressures on physicians are greater causes of stress than the stress associated with patient care. Arrogance becomes a defense mechanism for depersonalization and emotional exhaustion, especially if the physician is challenged in any way.

TURNING STRESS INTO A CHALLENGE:
Stress Management with Powerful Healing Measures

Stress is ubiquitous and present in every one of us. The World Health Organization (WHO) has called stress "The health epidemic of the 21st century." The American Medical Association has reported that stress is a major factor in 90 percent of medical illnesses! Billions of dollars are spent on treating stress; fortunately, it can be treated without medication.

We need more study on biochemical markers that might lead to the development of safe drugs to treat stress; this is especially true regarding post-traumatic stress disorder. Some stress begets more stress. Millions of people worldwide, probably hundreds of millions, turn to alcohol and/or psychotropic/illicit drugs for temporary relief, only to discover that they feel even more stressed when their "high" is over. But some stress is necessary for success, and we can't forget this. Many of us prefer the term "pressure" as the main form of stress when it is subacute, such as during a sports competition or giving a talk, i.e., "stage fright." This is usually self-limiting. For years, performers of any kind have taken a beta blocker before going on stage.

This section that focuses on stress supports the earlier part of the chapter regarding apathy, mediocrity, burnout, suppressed anger, and the impaired physician. There is considerable overlap. Every leader must be able to recognize increased stress in his/her employees and do whatever possible to relieve it. The more we read about stress, the more impressed we are to learn that the sensation of stress is a significant part—if not the cause—of a multitude of disorders.

This section also focuses on the power of healing measures that help with stress management. Some of the measures seem to be off-the-wall, but they all have strong supporters attesting to their benefits and appear to be harmless. They attest to the resilience of the human mind!

The list of possible sources of an individual's stress could include job issues, financial problems, interpersonal conflicts (especially with family members), health concerns, guilt, bullying, and more. Interestingly, more and more people consider the stress at home to be worse than the stress at work. It may be that many are taking their stress home with them where it is further accentuated.

Since almost every person has varying levels of stress a great deal of the time, the description of stress takes on many different forms, similar to the variances of pain. It seems that stress defies a clear definition. In fact, *we think stress should be classified in the same manner as pain: on a score of 0 to 10 as determined by the patient.* The average American reported a 4.9 level of stress in a recent study by the American Psychological Association. The association determined that stress above a 3.7 average was not healthy.

The following are situations, symptoms, lifestyles, health conditions, mental disorders, personality disorders, and diseases that relate to stress. It is very common for people to have two or more of these stressors.

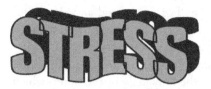

Feeling unloved	Bullying	Worry	Stage fright	Anticipatory concerns
Anxiety	Jealousy	Loneliness	Unhappiness	
Multitasking	NO FUN	Guilt	Excessive eating	
Social media	Debt	Lawsuits	Fear of any cause	
Family reunions	Giving a presentation		Absence of peace	
Procrastination	No mentors or role models		No exercise	
Not networking	DEADLINES		Hassles of any kind	
Unfulfilled life	Obsessive-compulsive disorder (OCD)			Burnout

Chronic physical and/or emotional abuse   Chronic anger disorder   Depression

Chronic frustration   Chronic pain   Chronic illness   Sleep disorders

Generalized anxiety disorder   Cyclothymic personality   PTSD

No obvious cause (we'll call this "idiopathic")   Hyperventilation syndrome

Tension headaches   Chronic tension state   Migraines

Withdrawing from tobacco and/or alcohol abuse   Hypertension   Asthma

Peptic ulcers   Colitis   Dementia   Cancer!

Predisposing Factors to Stress

Genetic response	Lack of coping skills/defense mechanisms
Lack of self-esteem	Trying to conform
Loss of control	No sense of humor
Loneliness	Expectations of family
Few friends; friends let you down	Unmet expectations
Holidays	Procrastination
Chronic stress begets more stress	Alcohol/drug abuse
Not recognizing normal circadian rhythm	Hormone surges
Coronary artery disease	Poor wound healing
Asthma	Increased frequency of colds

Pre-traumatic stress disorder (anticipatory anxiety/worry)

Most of you can add a few more that we haven't thought of. *It's everywhere!* Some of your friends will tell you they have most of the above!

Stress is different things to different people. We're believers that **most stress begins in utero**, and it worsens much earlier in children who don't grow up in a "normal" healthy atmosphere. Babies of stressed mothers have elevated levels of cord cortisol, which then become depleted with chronic stress. The baby of a mother who was subjected to physical and/or emotional abuse early in her pregnancy will show signs of stress earlier than other children. Some people "communicate" by yelling at times to levels above 100 decibels. Babies in utero can "hear" this loud and clear. This hardwires the neurons in their brains, which can take up to two years to reverse. But they can be reversed if the person wants to do so, perhaps with oxytocin, the "happy hormone."

A recent study describes "toxic distress" (also called "toxic stress"). This occurs in children after repeated emotional (and presumed physical) abuse that affects the amygdala in the brain, which controls emotions. These children develop emotional disorder syndromes with symptoms that may include hyperactivity, getting into fights, and the inability to be calm. This stress also disturbs the hippocampus, which affects memory and so impairs reading ability and test performance! Psycho-neuroendocrine seems to be a pathway for burnout, stress, and depression, which all affect the hypocampus pituitary adrenal (HPA) axis.

We believe that stress is much more prevalent in loners. What comes first, the stress or the loneliness? We think that loners suppress their stress more than others. We know about a study of Eastern European babies who were never held, almost never touched, and were fed by an aide who stood between two cribs and held a bottle for a baby on either side. Right from the beginning, these babies are loners. Their amygdala shrinks and never returns to normal size. They become social outcasts for the rest of their lives. It is hard to assess how stressed they are because they communicate poorly. They almost certainly are victims of bullying.

How affected are you by peer pressure? The attempt to conform is a tremendous source of stress. *Just be you*. This takes away some of the sting of a bully.

We think that a baby could have innate stress before he/she is born. The pregnant mother should laugh and smile a lot. We think mothers ought to begin reading out loud in a quiet room for thirty minutes a day from the beginning of their pregnancies; their babies can certainly "hear." An interesting study would be of mothers who read stories in a second language before their babies are born (could the babies become bilingual sooner in life?). Parents should continue to read to their children well into grade school. Studies show that if a mother causes stress in her child by yelling, scolding, and/or hitting, the child will no longer feel bonded with her.

This brings up the question of nature versus nurture. What about genetics? We don't know. There are endorphins and peptides, such as oxytocin, which can be measured in both a mother and child. A newborn "happy" child has high oxytocin levels, as does his/her mother, and an fMRI of the baby will highlight the left prefrontal cortex of the brain. The right prefrontal cortex will be highlighted in an unhappy baby. A mother's happiness sets the stage for a happy baby that, hopefully, will continue into adulthood.

We call oxytocin the "happy hormone" for good reason. Studies using intranasal oxytocin in autistic babies have shown some encouraging results. Drug companies certainly see this as a game winner and are actively studying its use—maybe for everyone!

Think about how children react differently when confronted with uncertain situations. When some children see Santa Claus, for example, they reach for "mommy's" hand—other kids don't hesitate to jump on Santa's lap. Is this stress related? Adults have told us that they still have their "blankies" and resort to holding them during times of stress.

"Stress" was termed **"shell shock"** in World War I. The same term was used in World War II and the Korean and Vietnam Wars, along with Chronic Nervous Exhaustion (CNE) or combat fatigue. Then the term "post-traumatic stress disorder (PTSD)" took hold following the Middle

Eastern wars and became a recognizable and treatable disorder. It is interesting that we haven't recognized—at least we're not aware of—PTSD in World War II veterans. Are we wrong?

Some anger is brought on purely by stress. These people have reached a "boiling over" point, and it is often quite uncharacteristic of them.

Problem stress is more prevalent than diabetes, hypertension, obesity, heart disease, and chronic obstructive pulmonary disease. Television is a big factor in this—commercials bombard you with instructions on what you need to buy to be happy, and you need to do it today! During an average day, people watch four hours of TV that includes more than fifty minutes (almost an hour) of pure commercials. In a year, you will have seen about 300 hours of commercials. Some are subliminal; you don't even have time to think!

Social media controls our lives because we allow it. We are afraid to *not* respond to a text or tweet immediately, or we'll become stressed thinking we may have missed something "important." Chronic stress is frequently associated with extra heartbeats, which is the same result as smoking tobacco. After fifty years of stress (or smoking), a person could have accrued more than 14 million extra heartbeats. What kind of reserve does your heart have? The chronically anxious person recognizes these extra heartbeats; these are a significant form of cardiac awareness.

> *Regarding non-aerobic tachycardia: the IndyCar driver typically has a per-minute heart rate of approximately 120 just sitting in the car waiting for the imminent start; however, pilots average 150-plus on an aircraft carrier landing!*

Experts differentiate between "uncontrollable stress" and "controllable stress," which is frequently self-induced.

We must accept that some stress is normal; we wouldn't get anywhere without it. It serves as a motivator and as a "challenge." The question is not *if* we have any stress (0 on the 0-to-10 stress-level scale), but how we handle it. *Wind bending the tree strengthens the trunk.*

Our distant ancestors had tremendous stress that has evolved into how we handle it today. It is easy to understand the "flight or fight" phenomenon when you think about it. Our very distant ancestors only knew "flight" because clubs, fire, and spears weren't developed until hundreds of thousands of years later. They were constantly on the alert for flight. They slept in trees or caves that could be closed off with rocks or downed trees.

One expert, after giving a talk on stress, was asked to define it. He said, "Funny, no one has ever asked me that question!" We can narrow the definition to the biochemistry of the release of epinephrine (adrenaline), norepinephrine, cortisols (cortisone derivatives), many endorphins (most of which we don't know much about), and other substances from the HPA. Their acute release, plus the rapid firing of millions of neurons in the brain, sets the stage for fight or flight. But acute reactions are uncommon now compared with generations ago. The chronic stage of stress is so common that it has become a permanent part of many people's lives. The *hurry factor* plays a large role in this. Why do people drive sixty miles per hour in a forty-five-mile-per-hour zone? And are on the cell phone at the same time? Why?

Terms related to stress are anxiety, nervous breakdown, chronic fatigue, pressure, extreme exhaustion, wired, and on and on. Stressed people always are worried and on edge. They can't think clearly or concentrate, which is mindful thinking. Stress seems to be worse around 8:30 a.m. and 3:30 p.m., however, some new studies are finding that stress levels for nearly half of the population peak after 4:00 p.m. on Sundays. We're not sure what shift work does to this, but it doesn't help.

Stress is different for the underprivileged. They may not know where their next meal is coming from or where they will sleep. Plus, crime and a dysfunctional family may surround them.

Some people seek immortality but don't know what to do on a rainy Sunday afternoon!

They're bored! Stress adversely affects most inflammatory diseases, such as asthma, coronary artery disease, inflammatory bowel diseases, rheumatoid arthritis, and others that are mediated through the immune system. About 80 percent of the U.S. population report to having at least one major new stress each year. Some claim they suffer up to fifty minor stresses a day! If so, this would amount to a low-grade constant stimulation of inflammation through interleukin 6 (IL-6) and other mediators. Is the new stress added to the old stresses or parallel to the old stresses for these people? Until we can better quantify stress, we will have to wait for this answer.

There is an entity worth mentioning here: hyperventilation syndrome. This is more common in young women who reach a breaking point in their stress and begin very rapid shallow breathing. They breathe off a lot of carbon dioxide, which quickly results in paresthesias (tingling) in the hands (less so in the feet) as well as around the mouth. They become very lightheaded and may have some chest discomfort, which could lead them to believe they are having a heart attack. All this is very scary, so many go to the emergency room. The standard treatment is breathing into a paper bag (re-breathing the person's own carbon dioxide), along with a lot of reassurance and explanation. Although we've seen many patients experience the syndrome, we haven't seen as many lately because the public has learned how to deal with it.

Stress leads to worry, and your mind becomes full of negative thoughts. You dread the recurring anxiety when the events provoking the previous threats appear on the horizon. The unpredictability of situations and the potential lack of control and coping mechanisms play significant roles here. *Centenarians will tell you they don't worry about anything!*

The only trouble with success is that the formula for achieving it is the same as the formula for a nervous breakdown.

A nervous breakdown occurs when you've depleted your calming endorphins and your mechanisms of coping aren't working. You probably never have been advised on how to cope!

"How stressed are you?"

"I didn't know I was stressed."

"What do you mean you're not stressed? You should be stressed—everyone else is!"

"Well then, when did you stop beating your spouse?"

The truth is that if you keep talking about the thing that is stressing you and, worse yet, thinking about it, you are only further hardwiring your brain to the negative pole. We know now that the brain is, indeed, hardwired. This can be seen on an fMRI, which also shows that dysfunctional areas of the brain can be re-hardwired over time. However, it can take at least six months and up to two years to completely get negativity out of the brain. And you have to want to do it! This will involve an **attitude change** *(see below)*.

Stress consumes a large amount of energy, which leads to physical problems including exhaustion, disordered sleep, the inability to concentrate, and emotional lability. Is it worth it? It is very reasonable to believe that many of our young people could live past the age of 100—but they won't if their bodies are full of stress.

Unappreciated chronic stress is almost always the precursor to burnout, which is described earlier in this chapter as a low sense of personal accomplishment, emotional exhaustion, and depersonalization. Mediocrity is not necessarily related to stress. Mediocre physicians just don't care *(this also is discussed earlier in the chapter)*.

With this in mind, we're changing the word **"Stress"** to **"Challenge."** Dealing with a challenge gives you energy as opposed to sapping it. A challenge motivates rather than depresses and gives you a great feeling of confidence to face and overcome it. This doesn't mean that you can't fail—successful people will tell you about their failures and setbacks and how they learned from them and went on to be successful. As this chapter continues, the word "stress" will slowly switch to "challenge."

Stress Versus Challenge

STRESS	CHALLENGE
Energy (–)	Energy (+)
Exhaustion, fatigue	Fired up
Accomplishes little	Achieves goals
↓ Self-esteem	↑ Self-esteem
↓ Confidence	↑ Confidence
Attitude +/-	Attitude +++

Stress is associated with worry 100 percent of the time. This is a big negative and must be overcome.

More Problems with Stress That Require a "Challenge" Response

• **Sleep problems?** Obstructive sleep apnea (OSA)? Your brain works 24/7. Sleep is the only way to restore it, and some people require more sleep than others. While you sleep, your brain is processing what went on during your day; not enough sleep and low oxygen levels in the blood (hypoxemia) affect this necessary processing. There is no upside to a lack of sleep—absolutely no benefit. It will compound all the above-mentioned problems.

• Is your reason for stress worth the worry? How will it affect you in a week, a month, or a year from now? You need to put this in perspective. Most likely, you will look back and wonder why you put in so much time and worry about an issue.

• **Are you ever stress-free? Most likely.** Do you ever stop and reflect gratitude for this? You can't be happy if you don't express gratitude.

• More than 90 percent of medical students say that they were abused in medical school; we submit that much of this is stress and reactions to critical but constructive comments misinterpreted as abuse. We educators must keep this in mind. Recall from Chapter 6 *(The Art of Educating)* that the secret to successful teaching is respect for your students. Think back to medical school and how you hung on to any comment from your professor that could be interpreted as praise. Students: Your faculty really does want you to succeed. The future of medicine in this country depends on the success of medical students. Remind yourself how good you are.

• Are you a Type A or Type B personality?

• Stress can be the result of **deadlines** and **multitasking**. You cannot multitask—it doesn't work and you just don't know it. Multitasking may be the biggest part of the stress of meeting deadlines. You don't know how to manage your time to "beat" a deadline. It is estimated that we all have more than 10,000 thoughts (most are fleeting) a day. And your brain has to process all these thoughts while you sleep.

• More about deadlines. How much is your procrastination at fault? Procrastination is a huge problem but preventable most of the time. So first do the thing you dislike the most.

• Time constraints/pressure for any reason. Again, how much is your fault?

• Outside noise, including loud music. When you listen to music that you like, does it calm or hype you? Bach and Mozart are said to be the most calming—some experts think their music is synchronized with brain waves to a positive effect. This is the so-called "Mozart Effect." If you are listening to a song's lyrics and studying at the same time—multitasking—change or stop the music. *Again, you cannot multitask.* Your mind can't do it. Turn off the TV if you are studying or preparing a report. However, if you are feeling low with your stress, maybe you need to hype it up a bit with some hard rock music for a short time.

• When you are studying for an exam, take a break every sixty to ninety minutes and do some exercise. Put your mind on something else.

• **Can't say NO?** You must learn how to do this. If you don't, too often you will be caught off guard and, before you know it, say "yes" to something you don't have any time for—or interest in—doing. For the next few weeks, you will be even more stressed thinking about what you agreed to. "How can I get out of it?" Always be prepared to say "I'm involved in too many projects now, but thank you for thinking of me," or "I promised my family I wouldn't take on any more projects," etc. You must do this with some empathy. An alternative is to say that you would like to think about it overnight. If your "friend" really pressures you at this point, you pretty well know that he/she is trying to dump this on you. When you finally work up the nerve to tell the person—with empathy—that you can't or don't want to do the task, you may lose this friend if you don't handle it right. But you are more important. Be cautious about accepting too many committee appointments—these never involve short-term projects.

• How much negative thinking do you do? Positive thinking? If you are sitting in a room and a certain person walks in, what is your reaction? Is it immediately negative because of something you know about the person? Then your brain is hardwired into the negative mode! Your brain can only be negative or positive at one time—it cannot be both. *You must begin—today—working on rewiring your brain to the positive mode.*

• **Sugar.** A lot of people resort to carbohydrates, including sugar, when they are more stressed. This has been shown to dull the brain! Sugar may relieve some stress for a short time, but then it comes back even more pronounced when the person's glucose level drops fairly rapidly to mild hypoglycemia. How fast this occurs varies by individual. But the faster it does, the more symptomatic the person will be. Then he/she would have to consume more sugar to get some relief. This is a yo-yo effect that alters insulin levels (endogenous insulin affects every system in the body) and plays some poorly understood mechanisms in stress. People on sugar-free diets say they feel great! High-fructose corn syrup, which is in many sugar products, is metabolized in the liver to form fat (triglycerides). *Students, minimize your sugar intake before a test or an interview. It is said that sugar dulls the intellect.*

• Worrying about anything before a big test also is likely to affect your thinking (and IQ). *We wonder if watching sitcoms does the same thing.*

• Are you not eating breakfast? This has been shown to have many negative consequences, including shortening a person's life span. We suspect this is related to insulin levels, which incite inflammation.

• Stress shortens the telomeres on the ends of your chromosomes, which also affects life span. Again, we suspect this is related to inflammation.

• **Social media!** Don't you already have more stress than you want? Medical-center studies report that regular social media use will cause stress and depression if you don't like what you see and read about yourself! Do you really need social media?

• Are you in debt? Keep a close eye on your credit rating; it may minimize future stress if you notice early that it has been lowered and then you deal with it.

• Did you loan money to a family member or friend? This often causes you to lose money (and sleep) as well as a friend. It has been shown that worry and stress over monetary affairs may decrease a person's IQ by 8 to 15 points, at least temporarily. This usually is reversible. Or it may drop some of us into the idiot level! If you loan more than $100, get an IOU in writing—although this doesn't mean you will be repaid. Above all, when someone owes you money, don't loan him/her any more until you are paid back. Since you already loaned money to this person, he/she sees you as an easy mark.

> ### *Always borrow money from a pessimist. He won't expect it back.*
> —Oscar Wilde

- Guilt, worry, depression, financial problems, family dysfunction, children in trouble, bullying, etc., are all major sources of stress. A psychiatrist once said, "It isn't love that makes the world go around, it is guilt." *"What lies we weave ..."* Soap operas are based on guilt.
- PTSD (chronic). This occurs not only in combat, but it also is very common in the workplace and schools. PTSD often is the result of bullying. Stress is a part of PTSD (acute and chronic). "Bad bosses" in the workplace, even in medical centers, are notorious for affecting work performance, even to the point of causing PTSD. This leads to a host of descriptions about the boss, such as hypercritical, inept, a blamer, a micromanager, and a sexual harasser, which can end up costing a workplace billions of dollars.
- **Apathetic boredom** (couch potato), which may be in response to chronic stress, is—surprisingly—associated with increased cardiac events, depression/stress, obesity, and shortened life spans. There is more to this than just not enough exercise; other likely causes are inflammation, insulin abnormalities, and poor sleep.
- Published studies confirm that stress in a marriage, especially when one person is not really committed, results in a very significant increased risk—nearly 50 percent—of coronary artery disease and congestive heart failure.
- **Tinnitus** (ringing in the ears) is said to be closely tied to emotional stress; emotional upheaval can be a trigger.
- **Oxytocin levels.** The "happy hormone" is elevated in happy mothers and their newborn babies. Low levels of oxytocin are found in stressed individuals. It is elevated in your pet dog!
- **Chronic pain** is a major problem for the people who live with it and also for society as it supports some of them with disability benefits. Valid or not, pain is hard to prove—and it is subjective. Pain that has been present for more than six months to a year resides more in the central nervous system, which is where pain specialists aim their treatments. Getting people off oxycodone medications and/or alcohol can be a huge challenge. Stress is a major component of chronic pain, and the stress on an afflicted person also can become a big problem for family members. Acupuncture treatment for chronic pain has shown very impressive results; we know of several friends who got great or complete relief after these procedures. Meditation also has been shown to relieve chronic pain by up to 60 percent and perhaps more.
- **Unable to empathize?** This is probably the result of not receiving sufficient love as a child, as well as not being touched enough as an infant. The power of caring brings the power of healing to others and yourself. Moms and Dads, touch your baby and young children a lot! Touch with your eyes. Continue with hugs. Hugging is good!
- **No close friends?** Lonely people without friends have a low pain threshold, studies show.
- No coping skills? A person may not like to socialize because of poor coping skills. Subjected to bullying? This is the description of a *loner*, but being alone is not always a cause of stress because some people prefer it and have adjusted well to it. They don't lack good self-esteem, which is the case for true loners.

- Watch too much TV.
- **Silence, serenity, and solitude: PEACE.** People need periods of calm and to just relax. Many people think that there is "not enough time to do this; too busy." People need to have fun (we're repeating this)! It is therapeutic to have silence and serenity, but many people are not accustomed to this. They can't exist without earbuds for music, being on their cell phones, or turning on the TV immediately after arriving home. Noise! There are many books on how to find some serenity. Learn to practice *serious silence*.
- **Simplify your life.** There are many books and magazines that will help you with this goal. Balance your life!
- **Practice patience.** Patience and empathy are the glues that hold society together. Patience is a habit. Being patient can help you become more effective, kinder, calmer, and tolerant. *Minnesota Nice!* You will be more empathetic and, in turn, be treated more empathetically by others. You also will be less overwhelmed, stressed, worried, and angry. The opposite is impatience, e.g., the guy behind you immediately honking his horn when the light turns green.
- Is **self-image** a problem? Get a makeover. If you are overweight, try to find a weight-loss program that works for you. Consider joining a gym.
- **Exercise** regularly. Be sure to take in enough fluids.
- Emotional swings (ups and downs) are normal and can last two to three days. Everyone has them as part of our **cyclothymic personality**. They don't appear to be related to a woman's menses. Accept this. Stress is worse during downtimes. Some people recognize their swings and avoid making major decisions during these times.
- **Frailty.** Many of you may have older family members, usually women, with frailty. Symptoms of frailty include an unexplained weight loss of ten pounds in a year, exhaustion, stress, depression, decreased handgrip strength, a slower walking speed, limited physical activity, and osteoporosis. If no organic cause is found, experts prescribe exercise as standard therapy. Could frailty be an atypical manifestation of chronic stress? Is there a place for a trial of a beta blocker here? One-third of women over the age of seventy-five die within a year of a hip fracture. In retrospect, many (most?) were frail before the fracture and their conditions declined afterward.
- **Diagnosis of cancer.** Depression and stress are very common after a person receives this diagnosis (this is a no-brainer). Patients tend to bypass, or not even consider, previous effective coping mechanisms and, instead, tend to concentrate on their cancer. They need help. Recent reports show that beta blockers may minimize the spread of some cancers by inhibiting epinephrines and norepinephrines, which affect a tumor's blood supply. Beta blockers normally lessen hypertension and some tachycardia syndromes by working on these two hormones.
- The national media recently showed a man running naked down the street; he said he did it because he was very stressed. Don't try this at home or at work!

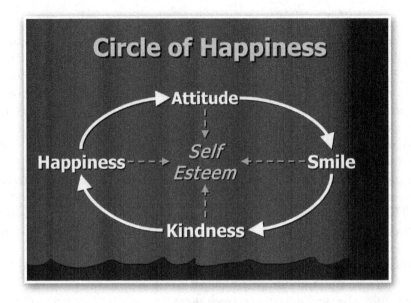

STRESS MANAGEMENT/CHALLENGE

This is our *ASKH—Attitude, Smile, Kindness, Happiness*

ASKH is our Circle of Happiness and attempt to prevent or manage **stress** as well as get more out of life. It doesn't allow for negative thoughts. *A positive attitude is mandatory—you can't complete the ASKH circle without it.* Every employer looks to hire people with positive attitudes. Don't allow a negative thought to reside in your mind!

> ### *The greatest discovery of my generation is that a human being can alter his life by altering his attitudes of mind.*
> **—William James**

• You can detect someone's attitude in his/her body language without a word being said. Patients frequently decide whether they like a physician within five seconds of meeting—even if the doctor hasn't started talking. Eighty percent of person-to-person communication is nonverbal!

• A **smile** is powerful. It releases endorphins, which may last for a few hours, in the person who is smiling and in the recipient. Smiles improve your mood and relieve stress. Smiles are contagious, express empathy, and help you stay positive. A smile is the same in all languages and the shortest distance between two people who are looking in each other's eyes. A smile is said to make you look younger!

• **Laugh every day.** This is different from just smiling and stronger in some ways. Laughing creates bonding and is thought to have healing powers. Join a laugh club.

• You can't think negatively while doing an act of **kindness**! Every person you encounter is an opportunity for an act of kindness.

Following the ASKH is a stress reliever.

Heroism isn't just about monumental feats of courage but about everyday selfless acts—both epic and small.

—John Gunyon

Happiness completes the ASKH circle. You can't be happy without a positive attitude, smiling, and kindness.

Every small act of caring in a medical center positively affects the health outcome of a patient. These acts of caring could come from physicians, nurses, allied health personnel (even if they are not in contact with patients), medical students, and residents. Many of our patients have said, *"Everyone was so nice at Mayo Clinic!"* Caring is another reason for Mayo Clinic's success—a true union of forces of all Mayo employees.

The needs of the patient come first.

—Mayo Clinic's Primary Value

If you want others to be happy, practice compassion. If you want to be happy, practice compassion.

—Dalai Lama

(We would add the importance of expressing gratitude. You can't have happiness without this.)

• **Stress.** Deal with it; don't succumb to it. Recognize that stress may be the cause of your physical symptoms—this is the first step toward dealing with it. *The JC mandates that hospitals promote the well-being of physicians.* This organization's officials can shut down a hospital if they don't like what they see in many areas; they are serious about their mandates.

• Follow the Serenity Prayer: *"God, grant me the serenity to accept the things I cannot change, the courage to change the things I can, and the wisdom to know the difference."*

• **Switch stress to challenge.** Consider every stressful event as a challenge that must be met—a challenge that will make you an even stronger, more confident, and better person. Write down the challenges that you are facing. There isn't anything you can do about some stresses, but you can calm yourself with some of the measures discussed later in the chapter.

• Rewire your brain. *The power of positive thinking!* Keep a list of the positive things you think or do, including nice things that have happened to you and/or your family, and look at these several times a day. Without a list to look at, these positive moments only last about two weeks in your memory.

• **Life isn't always fair. Believe this.**

• **Friendships** may be among your most important coping mechanisms. *You can't have friends without being one!* We're talking about good friends, not just casual ones. (It may be too late if you are suddenly in need of a good friend but don't have one. Good friends take nurturing and time.)

Don't unload on them. Nurture them, and some will last a lifetime. Have fun with these people. Socialize at least once a week; this is critical. Planning ahead is a distraction from stress. Celebrate anything you can: a promotion, birthday, holiday, etc. Make up an excuse to celebrate if need be.

• Your pets are among your best friends. Talk to them out loud! This is very therapeutic.

• **Volunteering** is one of the best stress relievers. But it needs to be more than just a one-time thing. Get involved in a project that has real meaning for you. Studies show that volunteering may significantly increase—by up to 90 percent in some cases—a person's mood and self-esteem. Volunteers also feel healthier overall, and their stress levels are lower.

• All of us will make mistakes. There are ways of dealing with this. What can you learn from your mistakes that will, hopefully, prevent you from making the same ones again? Learn to forgive and forget. You can't have happiness without being able to do this.

• You are as good as anyone. Believe this! Don't allow your mind to think otherwise. Write this down. You also have the potential to be great because you've already proven this by your accomplishments. Talk to yourself! Strive for excellence. Don't strive for perfection because you'll never get there, and it will just cause you more stress!

• Find a mentor *(see Chapter 4)*. If you are still in school, you must seek out someone for this role because a mentor shouldn't be assigned to you. You need to select your mentor. Learn **networking** from your mentor.

• Ask your school administration to offer a course in **time management**.

Active Means of Managing Stress

• Learn **mindfulness**—being present in the moment. Being focused. It is the opposite of multitasking. While focusing, you must not be judgmental or make assumptions. The ideal way to start learning about mindfulness is from an instructor—we think this should begin in third grade and be emphasized throughout schooling. Or attend lectures. Mindfulness more than triples a person's takeaway from a lecture compared with a person whose mind wanders (daydreams) or who is multitasking. You also can learn about mindfulness from books, articles, and the Internet. (There is plenty of information available about mindfulness, as well as about almost everything mentioned in this chapter.) *Practicing mindfulness is one of the most effective ways to deal with stress, depression, and almost everything that bothers you!*

• **Meditation** and **yoga** fall right alongside mindfulness. All three are powerful healers and help keep stress under control. The very quiet and stillness of meditation and yoga bring calmness and peace. We can't emphasize the importance of these three enough.

• Acute PTSD may respond to hydrocortisone and/or propranolol (a beta blocker).

• **Vibroacoustic disorder** is stress brought on or aggravated by loud music, e.g., a rock concert. The decibel level of hard-rock music through earphones can reach above 100. Perhaps you are subject to someone else's loud music, and it is significantly aggravating your stress because of the excessive decibels and your lack of control over the music. Deal with it. It has been shown that the higher the decibels, the more alcohol consumed!

• **Tai chi** has been practiced for millennia in the Eastern world. Tai chi enhances mindfulness, meditation, and yoga. Plus, it is good for strengthening muscles.

• Learn from the role models all around you. At Mayo Clinic, we think the quality and quantity of role models are the best in the world (we base this on our combined 100-plus years of experience). But you have to actively watch people around you. Write down what you see. *It's more what they do than what they say.* Good role models lead to a **culture of continuous improvement** for individuals and for groups of people who band together for the betterment of mankind. Role models also are major contributors to the culture of an institution.

• Be the kind of role model you look up to. Remember that role models may be younger than you and represent different aspects of your institution—they could be students, nurses, patients, custodians, etc. Write down a composite of what you see as the ideal role model. Note that most of them smile a lot and always are kind. This is a good place to start. Don't forget that you are also a role model to your children.

• Join or organize a group of people who agree to limit social texting. This should be part of a time-management course if you are still in school. You could organize a similar group of people who limit email and television use.

Sample Pact to Limit Texting/Emailing, etc.

• The group would include 10 to 100 people who commonly communicate with you.
• The group members would mutually agree to
  ■ not gossip.
  ■ limit "reply to all."
  ■ call the other person if the matter is important.
  ■ not ask open-ended questions.
  ■ limit social chat.
  ■ establish text holidays, e.g., Sundays.
  ■ limit most correspondence to between five o'clock and seven o'clock at night—and never in the middle of the night!
  ■ not consider it a sign of rejection if the recipient does not respond immediately.
  ■ prioritize correspondence from school, work office, family, and close friends.

Specific Aids to Help Deal with Stress Until You Rewire Your Brain

• Alcohol? No! Valium or a different antianxiety medication also is a "no," unless it is prescribed for a limited period. Marijuana? We're sure that everyone who uses marijuana will say it greatly relieves stress, but they don't say anything about how their addiction affects their IQ. Studies show that regular marijuana use by teenagers lowers IQ by 8 to 10 points, which may not be reversible. Remember that the brains of teenagers, especially boys, are still growing and maturing.

• **Smell/odor/fragrance/aroma.** We have lost our conscious brain-sensing "smell" mechanism through evolution because we don't need it anymore. One expert thinks that our individual fragrances are as unique as our fingerprints. People used to call this an "aura," however, we call it our "chemistry." Some people will pick up on your stress or other nonverbal messages and make decisions related to personal interactions—good and bad. They don't know why, but they might call it "intuition." Some bad judgments are made based on this "chemistry."

• **Don't sweat the small things!** And most things are small. Read Richard Carlson's books.

• **Deep breathing.** Every book and article about stress that we've read mentions the value of slow deep breathing. They don't explain why it helps—and it does—but just state that ten repetitions will take your mind off what's bothering you (a form of mindfulness) and relax your muscles. We have a theory relating to the Hering-Breuer reflex: as the nerves in the lung tissue stretch, they automatically stop deep inhalation when reaching a certain volume. We think the breathing receptors in the brain stem are very near some neurons that deal with anxiety and depression and go on up to the cortex and other areas. Impulses from the Hering-Breuer reflex carry over to the anxiety/depression receptors. When you are waiting to give a speech or go into a meeting that you are very anxious about, try taking ten (or as many as you want) slow deep breaths while concentrating on your breathing. While you are deep breathing, let your shoulder muscles relax and think good thoughts. Exercises that stretch your large muscle groups may offer similar benefits.

• **Resilience, i.e., "this too shall pass."** Resilience is really the result of a prolonged positive attitude and good self-esteem. Resilient people see problems as real challenges instead of succumbing to them.

• **Talk to yourself—but only in positive terms**. Actually, talking—quietly or otherwise—is more reinforcing than just thinking.

• Time heals a lot. Ask yourself if what you are stressed about will be of any consequence in five years? Or even one year?

• **Employee assistance program (EAP).** Most moderate-sized and all large employers have these programs available to their employees and their families. Mayo Clinic has had one for many years. EAPs are staffed by psychologists, social workers, and other experts who help those who are distressed due to relationship issues, dysfunctional family dynamics, financial problems, emotional health, grief, job stress, etc. They reference many websites and offer classes. EAP counselors frequently will guide employees to specific resources (both within and outside the institution) for help. They are not psychiatrists.

• **Life coaches.** These individuals have advanced degrees in sociology or psychology. They also are not psychiatrists, so they can't prescribe medications. They work with you at regular intervals.

It's not a sign of weakness to ask for help.

National Suicide Prevention Lifeline: 800-273-8255

• **Visit with a psychologist.** Psychologists teach behavior modification and may direct you to tapes for use at home.

• **Adequate sleep** is imperative—mandatory. We've mentioned this before! There is no substitute for sleep. Your subcortical area is working overtime to process what you put in it during your waking hours. Don't shortchange this. Impaired sleep can alter nearly 700 genes that affect inflammation, immunity, and metabolism.

• Sitting quietly for fifteen minutes while thinking good thoughts may be therapeutic. People who can't sit still this long should start with five minutes (this is a great time to meditate).

• **Exercise** is important, however, be aware that too much exercise depletes you of needed endorphins and catecholamines.

• Schedule fifteen minutes of "worry time" each day and then move on.

• **Write therapy.** It works and it is painless! Sit quietly and write for twenty minutes about everything that bothers you. Write rapidly; don't fuss with grammar or punctuation. Do this for three straight days—and then throw away or shred the papers. One study showed that those who kept a journal reported marked improvement in their rheumatoid arthritis or asthma compared with those who wrote about incidental things.

• **PETS**, especially dogs. A dog's sense of smell can be thousands of times and upward stronger than ours. We have no doubt that a dog can sense an owner's stress. We think some dogs can "respond" by sending a message back that says they are there to support you. Listen to them! There are numerous examples of these communications, and they have tremendous bonding powers. It is well known that pets can sense when a terminally ill patient is near death. Emotional Support Animals, which aid people with disabilities, are usually dogs and cats, but they also can be other animals.

• **More on pets.** Talking to someone, including your pet, has great healing power. We're thinking that talking to your pet out loud, when it is just the two of you, actually may be more therapeutic than talking to a human. You have no worries that your pet(s) will tell anyone. They love you unabashedly, unconditionally, and no matter what you say. They love that you are paying attention to them. They know you are unloading your stresses on them. Talk as long as you wish. We think this may be more effective than write therapy (journaling) since writing is just one pathway to ameliorate symptoms while talking out loud is both vocalized and heard through your auditory system. Who knows where these thoughts go when they are spoken out loud, but it's possibly different than just thinking or writing about them!

• **Touch.** Hand massage. Holding someone's hand. Putting your arm around another person. We know very little about touch, but there is no question that it is a form of bonding (see "Rubbing Velvet" and "Reiki" later in the chapter). Some people don't like to be touched or to touch, which may tell you something about them. But genuine touch is powerful. A physician should recognize that touch during a physical exam creates a sense of bonding and is an important part of healing. High-fives, pats on the back, and handshakes—all touch—during sporting events increase team effort and lead to more success.

• Some people are natural huggers, even with people they just met. This is very positive. Don't fight it!

Make Lists of ...

• All the things you are grateful for. Write these "gratitudes" on the backs of photos of your family, a pet, a beautiful place you love, a nature scene, etc., and carry the photos with you. Look at them regularly and especially when you are stressed and tired. Look at them while you are deep breathing or alone for a few minutes (like waiting for an elevator) and aren't on your smartphone! (But you could make a "gratitudes" list on your smartphone, and then you *should* look at the phone!)

• Your stresses. How important are they? Small? Prioritize them.

• The challenges you are working on (even better than listing the stresses).

• Things you need to do, such as shopping for specific items, etc. Life is complicated enough and gets more stressful if you forget to do something.

• People whose name you want to remember.

• Your good qualities and nice things that have happened to you. These "heartwarmers" will only last approximately two weeks in your memory bank, which is why writing them down is important.

One of the most important philosophies every physician should follow is the Platinum Rule of Medicine:
Treat every patient like you would want a member of your family treated.
(The Platinum Rule of Medicine is more important for physicians than the Golden Rule.)

Remember: Every stress should be looked at as a challenge!
And don't forget: *This too shall pass!*

Powerful Healing Actions by the Physician
(i.e., healing your patient's stress)

• Providing peace of mind.

• Saying "I'm sorry," "I don't know," and "I care about you."

• Anesthesiologists who whisper reassuring words in patients' ears as they induce anesthesia. These patients have fewer complications, and their hospital stays decrease by a day. Patients don't remember hearing the words.

• More words: "I understand your anger at your disease," and "I cannot begin to feel what you are feeling, but you must know (or it is important for you to know) that I care."

• "What other questions can I try to answer for you?"

• A phone call to a patient's home—**powerful!**

• Doesn't interrupt inappropriately.

• Essentially, every patient who comes to a physician, including the worried well, is worried and a little more stressed than he/she will let on.

• Smile, touch, listen to understand, and maintain eye contact.

• **The Platinum Rule of Medicine.**

• No other profession has the healing power of the physician just by being in a room.

• Empathy, caring—a must.

• Able to laugh (patients like to see their doctors laugh) and to make patients laugh.

• Handwritten notes.

• Not being arrogant.

• Pet therapy. The National Institutes of Health (NIH) has a program on the caring offered by animals. We put them in the class of the "powerful." "If my pets don't go to heaven, then when I die, I want to go where they are."

• When the situation is appropriate, tell your patient that you don't know yet what is causing his/her symptoms, but you know what isn't. Then tell him/her that there is no evidence of cancer, early dementia, or whatever might be bothering him/her (when that is all true).

• Consult with a colleague by phone in the presence of the patient.

> *Never take away hope; the clergy, nurses, and physicians can offer hope, but only the physician can take it away. The hope of many patients is that their physician(s) will not abandon them.*

Some Unusual Treatments for Stress

• *Rubbing Velvet (author ECR's favorite).* This is based on a ten-week Italian study of forty-five women who were eighty years old and above. They first answered questions about depression, stress, quality of life, and outlook on life. The women in one of the study groups rubbed canvas twenty minutes a day, another group rubbed Velcro, and the third rubbed velvet. After the ten weeks, the participants again answered the questionnaires, and only the velvet group's members improved in all aspects. Our theory is that rubbing the soft material stimulated peripheral c-nerve fibers, which go to the brain's frontal lobe where emotions (such as happiness) reside. We contacted the author, and she told us she had no money for further studies. If this holds, we see many possibilities, such as for soothing crying babies, calming demented people, reassuring pre-op patients, and on and on.

• *Tapping.* The Tapping Solution: A Revolutionary System for Stress-Free Living is a 256-page book that describes Emotional Freedom Techniques, which use acupressure, the noninvasive counterpart to acupuncture. "Tapping" yourself with your fingers in various places is said to be able to relieve just about everything! (*The Tapping Solution: A Revolutionary System for Stress-Free Living*, by Nick Ortner, 2013, Hay House, Inc.)

• *Eye movement desensitization and reprocessing (EMDR).* This sounds like snake oil but is reported to work in PTSD! There is an EMDR journal. A therapist directs the patient to rapidly move his/her eyes laterally while initially thinking about a problem and then switching to positive thoughts.

• *Reiki.* This is a Chinese therapy that relies on control of chi, i.e., "spiritual energy" or the "life force energy," which we all have but have lost in this world. It must be "real" because an acquaintance swears by it. Reiki practitioners are at different levels of expertise and may become master teachers. A practitioner's energy transfer is facilitated through the systematized or intuitive sense of hand placement. This is "palm healing" or "hands-on healing." The hands either touch the skin or are held just above it in many positions. A session takes fifteen to forty-five minutes and is repeated as often as necessary.

Treatments Not Covered in This Chapter

Hypnosis	Humming
Acupuncture	Subliminal behavior modification
Aromatherapy	Laughing/laugh therapy groups
Rocking chair	Music therapy by a certified therapist

Medical Students and Young Physicians Need to Know:

• Your deans, faculty, professors, etc., very much want you to succeed. They want you to make them (and the school) look good. Learn to accept appropriate constructive comments.

• We know that the first year in medical or osteopathic school is very stressful! *Look to your classmates to be your "family."* Family is one of the secrets of Mayo Clinic's Culture of Caring! These bonds of friendship will help you considerably with any stress (*see Chapter 13 on* The Art of Medicine).

• Try to exercise at least thirty minutes a day three or four times a week. This is imperative.

• You will be at the bottom of the pecking order for maybe the first time in your life, and you may be worried about being bullied by residents and nurses. Learn to not be overly sensitive when people are rude to you or if you think they are rude.

You can't manage stress and meet your challenges without good physical and mental health.

Self-love, my liege, is not so vile a sin as self-neglecting.
—**William Shakespeare**

• You must have a sense of humor. Find a way to have a good laugh every day.

• You must have your own physician and see him/her at appropriate intervals.

• You are the most important person in your life. If you don't believe this, how can your family and friends believe in you? It is the same with your patients. This isn't arrogance.

We're here to put a dent in the universe. Otherwise why else even be here?
—**Steve Jobs**

Chapter Thirteen

The Art of Medicine

The Culture of Caring in a Medical Center

In these times of rapidly advancing technologies and pressure for increased throughput, we have to remind ourselves that it is an honor and privilege to care for the patient. Yet patients see, hear, and read about technologic advances, which could raise their expectations beyond reason. They also know how third-party payers have come between patients and their physicians, and this change has greatly eroded the trust that has developed over the last 100 years. Patients also tell us that changes in the delivery of health care have added to their lack of trust in the system. This challenges our inherent capabilities to practice the Art of Medicine—the very core of our covenant with the patient.

This chapter, which focuses on how to better serve our patients, is a result of our combined involvement of more than 100 years in medicine. We learned a great deal from our experiences with role models and mentors as well as from our patients. This chapter also includes a short history of Mayo Clinic because the original personnel practiced a Culture of Caring, even though they may not have realized this almost precedent act's value in healing.

> ### *You will never go wrong by practicing*
> ### *the Platinum Rule of Medicine:*
> ### *Treat every patient like you would want*
> ### *a member of your family treated!*

We think that one of Mayo Clinic's secrets for success is the **Mayo Culture of Caring**, which permeates the institution and is reflected in its primary value: *The needs of the patient come first.* This culture is part of Mayo's history and helps explain its 150-plus years of success.

Mayo Clinic's Culture of Caring

Dr. W. W. Mayo (father of Dr. William J. "Dr. Will" and Dr. Charles H. "Dr. Charlie" Mayo) came to Minnesota in the 1850s and moved around within the state until he and his family settled in Rochester during the Civil War. In 1883, a tornado struck Rochester, and more than a dozen people were killed and many more were injured. Dr. W. W. sought nursing assistance from the Sisters of Saint Francis, who had an order in Rochester. Later on, Mother Mary Alfred Moes, the mother superior, asked Dr. W. W., who was an Episcopalian, if he and his sons would staff a hospital if the sisters were able to have it built. Indeed, they did. The sisters opened Saint Marys Hospital in 1889 with twenty-seven beds. Dr. Will had graduated from the University of Michigan Medical School in 1883, and Dr. Charlie graduated from the Chicago Medical College of Northwestern University in 1888.

The year 1901 was momentous in Mayo Clinic's history with the arrival of Dr. Henry S. Plummer, a true genius. Many of Plummer's ideas are still being used at Mayo Clinic including the patient records with individualized numbers that began in 1907 and later evolved into electronic medical records. The year 1907 could be considered another "beginning" of Mayo Clinic. Maud Mellish was hired that year to develop a medical library (another first?), and a library was built two years later. In 1914, the first building in the world to house the first integrated group practice (at least we think Mayo Clinic is the first) was completed.

The format of integrated health-care delivery had begun in 1892 when the three Mayos hired Dr. Augustus Stinchfield, a family physician referred to as a "diagnostician," to take care of nonsurgical patients. Over the years, Mayo Clinic continued to hire many more physicians of every subspecialty interest. The definition of integrated health-care delivery is self-explanatory. We don't know what the three Mayos were thinking, but integrated medicine was one of the greatest advances in health-care delivery. Mayo Clinic physicians do not sign contracts, and they all are salaried.

Any one of these events—Dr. W. W.'s new practice in Rochester during the 1860s, the Mayos' and the sisters' response after the Rochester tornado, the opening of Saint Marys Hospital, or the hiring of a diagnostician to begin integrated health care—might be considered the beginning of Mayo Clinic. Mayo Clinic certainly wouldn't have made it if it weren't for the sisters who worked eighteen-hour days. They did all the laundry and cleaning, learned nursing on the job, grew food for the hospital on a nearby farm, cooked that food, and on and on. If we were to begin a project like this today, we would have to outsource it and start with many dozen committees!

The concept of family is one of the strongest of Mayo Clinic's strengths. In the early 1900s, the Mayo Clinic and Rochester were growing fast. Because of the industrialization of farming, women had less work on the farms, so Mayo began drawing these women to Rochester to work at the outpatient practice and the hospital. They came to work at Mayo Clinic from numerous farms and from small railroad and grain-elevator towns that were up to 100 miles away. These young women came from non-dysfunctional families that had ten to fifteen children. In these churchgoing families, the older children helped care for their younger siblings and had additional chores. The families socialized with their multiple cousins, aunts, and uncles who lived close by. These family-centered employees brought a spiritual dimension to Mayo that was the rock foundation of their existence— their very souls. They never preached their religions—they didn't have to—but they did express them in their caring attitudes toward patients and each other—their new *family*. They knew only love toward other people. With the exception of those in nursing, Mayo Clinic didn't have to train these employees—they came trained! It might seem impossible today to get a large group of people with such a strong work ethic and caring attitude!

In 1910, Dr. Will spoke at a commencement exercise at Rush Medical College in Chicago with the pronouncement: *"The best interest of the patient is the only interest to be considered, and in order that the sick may have the benefit of advancing knowledge, union of forces is necessary."* This leads to the **Mayo Culture of Caring** or, should we say, the continuation of the Culture of Caring. Maybe the Drs. Mayo realized the importance of a Culture of Caring when a member of their family became a patient.

There are thought to be six classes of genius: music, math, spatial, athleticism, languages, and interpersonal relations. The Mayo brothers likely had great interpersonal skills that incorporated emotional intelligence and equanimity. (Sir William Osler said that equanimity could be one of a physician's greatest virtues.)

Mayo Clinic's Strengths
- The geniuses of Dr. Will and Dr. Charlie, along with Dr. Plummer who joined the practice in 1901.
- The Sisters of Saint Francis who opened Saint Marys Hospital in 1889, which was staffed by Dr. W. W., Dr. Will, and Dr. Charlie Mayo.
- Integrated health-care delivery (1892).
- The needs of the patient come first (1910).
- Physician leadership per the Mayo Clinic bylaws.
- Salaried positions.

Family
- Allied health personnel
- Nurses
- Role models

The combination of all the above has led to the

Mayo Culture of Caring.

The power of caring! It may be curative! Voltaire said, "The art of medicine consists in amusing the patient while nature cures the disease." We think that someday there will be a recognized science of caring.

The future of the Mayo Clinic depends on the quality of care given.
—Leonard L. Berry, PhD

It is the patient who carries the burden of illness,
but the compassionate physician shares that burden,
lifting it when possible and lightening it when that is
all that can be done. This sharing of the burden has
always been the hallmark of the medical profession.

—Richard S. Hollis, MD

We have discussed various *powers of healing*, and what follows are a few others.

Empathy and **patience** are the glues that hold society together. They are forms of bonding and of trust. In medicine, trust is essential in order to create and maintain a covenant with the patient. Empathy is thought to be evolutional and begin at birth. But we also suspect that a fetus picks up on it from the mother talking softly and reassuringly, laughing, smiling, and thinking good thoughts. We know that a baby and mother may have elevated oxytocin, the "cuddle hormone," at birth. It enhances bonding and is associated with happiness (the science of caring again). An absence of empathy may be found in people with autism and sociopathia. Something as simple as a genuine smile is an act of empathy and raises endorphins in the recipient as well as in the person who is smiling. We know that some babies born in Eastern European countries are never held and then grow up without any social skills. Their amygdala is atrophied, and this is permanent.

There is no such thing as an arrogant compassionate physician. The feeling of emotion can't be taught, but it can be learned—hopefully from being with parents, family, and good role models. Empathy in any form is powerful.

Oftentimes, peace and empathy offer more to a patient than hours of traditional "doctoring."

Empathy is expressed in your body language by a warm smile (we don't know what *warm* means exactly, but you know it when you see or feel it), eye contact while touching and leaning toward the patient, complete engagement by you, the tone of your voice, and—so importantly—listening intently.

Butterfly effect. In the 1960s, a meteorologist was asked if a butterfly's flap of its wings could affect the weather 1,000 miles away. After thinking about this for a few moments, he said he couldn't state that it wouldn't. If a patient encounters ten to more than 100 AHP in the course of a medical visit, would each of these AHP "flapping their butterfly wings of caring" enhance the healing effect of the patient's medical care? Absolutely, as we'll find out in the brief discussion of body language that follows. Just one negative "butterfly-wing flap" (negative encounter) may take a number of successive positive "flaps" of caring to overcome.

Peace of mind. What is peace of mind? We know it when we don't have it. Any worry, including a worry about your or a loved one's health, is very stressful. The very presence of worry is an absence of peace of mind. Although reassurance offers peace of mind, telling someone that everything is going to be OK without all the facts can be misleading. So reassurance must be given very cautiously.

148

But reassuring the patient and the family that you'll be there to help them is "priceless." *Hope* can provide peace of mind.

The mind. We don't even know what the mind is. Is it synonymous with conscience? Is it the source of all psychiatric illness? With wellness? Happiness? Healing? We know that the brain is rewiring (plasticizing) 24/7, which means that it is working while you sleep and dealing with what you put in it during your waking hours. How does it influence your physiologic health? The mind will certainly play a role in a science of caring. It has to play a role in stress *(see Chapter 12)*.

Names of people. Greeting people by name, both those you have known for some time and new acquaintances, is a form of bonding and social intelligence. It means that you cared enough to remember and say their names. If you add a smile to a greeting, you could make a person's day. It may be very important to some people. When you encounter patients, always say their names and use Mr., Mrs., etc., unless they are under twenty-five or so. However, if patients insist that you use their first names, we usually then insist that they call us by our first names. This gives them the sense of engagement that they are looking for.

Placebos. When it was learned that patients' symptoms might respond to a placebo even when they know they are getting one, then you have to believe that the *mind* has taken over some of the control of healing powers. Some of these studies have shown that measurable parameters, such as pulmonary function in the asthmatic, didn't change much in spite of the fact that the patient felt much better with a placebo. We're not sure how to explain this. Patients with rheumatoid arthritis have symptoms that are more subjective (pain and stiffness), but they do improve with placebos, namely write therapy.

Words. Powerful! Therapeutic. This means not only using specific words but also talking in a soft, soothing, never-irritating tone of voice. A speaker's inflection and body language may make a huge difference in the outcome of an encounter. The physician begins by saying the patient's name (as discussed two paragraphs above). It has been shown that patients have shorter hospital stays and less post-op complications when their anesthesiologists whisper soft, reassuring words into their ears while sedation is induced. Patients don't remember this. Where are the words going from the ear to the brain?! And why does this affect the physiology of healing?

When you are in the office or at the bedside, always choose your words. In the stress of the moment, the patient (and the family) may misconstrue what was said. This is very common. Sitting on the edge of the bed is OK most of the time. Look the patient in the eye, softly smile, and touch him/her as appropriate. If you have bad news, empathy is critical. Silence is OK. Let the patient think about what you said, and let it soak in. Ask the patient if he/she understands and has any questions. Be sure that you, the residents, nurses, and other direct caregivers are on the same page. Put the information given into the record.

Words: It's not what's said; it's what's heard.

Some Helpful Phrases

- *"What is your main concern that brings you here?" "How may I help you?" "What bothers you the most?"*
- *"How have your symptoms affected your life and your family members' lives?"*
- *"Tell me more." "Is there anything else?"*
- *"What do you think is causing your symptoms?"*
- When talking to a patient who understands a limited amount of English, speak slowly and maintain eye contact.
- *"Try not to worry. Let me do that."*
- *"I imagine this must be very uncomfortable for you."*
- It is OK to carry on the conversation and answer more questions while examining the patient.
- *"Let me make sure I have it right, you ..."*
- A sense of humor is OK when used appropriately.
- *"I'm sorry."*
- *"I was wrong."*
- *"I made a mistake, and we need to talk about it."*
- Say something complimentary.
- *"I share your burden."*
- Nod in understanding (you're engaged). Frown accordingly.
- *"I know how worried you are about this, so I'm going to expedite the testing and call you as soon as I get the results."* And keep your word; this engenders trust and bonding. It shows that you care.
- Don't explain away bothersome symptoms as "normal" or, worse, *"It's all in your head."* **Never.**
- *"I'm here for you."*
- *"Go on."*
- *"I think I know how difficult this must be for you."*
- Be cautious about reassuring patients if you don't yet have an answer to the cause of their symptoms. If you turn out to be wrong, it will make you look bad.
- *"I'm sorry I don't have better news for you."* Or *"I wish medical science had come further along to allow us to find a cure for your husband's serious illness." "Even if a miracle drug had just been discovered, it would be at least five or more years before we could try it."*

You, the physician, should do more listening than talking.

Cringe words. As a patient starts to tell you about his/her conversation with another physician, you start to cringe because you know what is coming next. We've collected many dozens of these cringe words. It is hard to imagine that physicians even say these things because they don't just reflect poorly on them but on the whole profession. The patients will never forget them. They will tell a lot of people what was said and who said it. Most of these examples are self-explanatory.

- *"If you weren't so fat, you wouldn't need to be here."*
- *"Shut up; I'll do all the talking."*
- *"When you get an MD after your name, then I'll let you talk."*
- *"I can't do any more for you. You might as well go home and prepare to die."*

- *"Well, you have one foot in the grave."*
- Nurse to a patient and family: *"The surgeons don't have time to talk to you."* (To this, we would answer: *"Maybe they'll have time to talk to my lawyer."*)
- From a cardiologist to an obese fellow physician: *"You look disgusting. Have you no shame?"*
- Patient says, *"I'm about to be told by a physician I've never met that I'm going to die." "I was kept waiting more than an hour, and after I was brought into his office, he took two personal phone calls that ate up another twenty minutes of my time."*
- *"My doctor was not as sympathetic as I **needed** him to be."*
- *"I didn't really understand what the doctor was saying, and I was too embarrassed to ask."*
- *"I left my doctor's office feeling worse than when I went in."*
- Surgeon to a nurse: *"You killed my patient!"* The nurse quit her job and dropped out of nursing entirely.

And on and on! These are totally inexcusable and an embarrassment to the profession. They are all examples of masterful arrogance! These words are from angry, arrogant physicians who never would say, *"I'm sorry."* Other terms that would describe these physicians are **insensitive**, **disrespectful**, **callous**, **disinterested**, **impatient**, **worst physician I've encountered**, and more. They all are very unprofessional.

What if a physician said cringe words to a member of an arrogant physician's family or close friend? Remember the **Platinum Rule of Medicine**!

Body Language. Your body language! The more we learn about this, the more powerful it appears to be. Some of this is covered in previous chapters but is worth repeating. Some patients will judge you within five seconds of your entering the room for the first time, even though you haven't said a word. They can sense if you are angry or arrogant. This may set the tone for the physician-patient encounter and affect whether the patient will comply with your recommendations. Experts estimate that 80 percent to 90 percent of person-to-person communication is by body language! Yet we'll wager that less than 5 percent of physicians and other health-care providers have any idea what their body language projects. Textbooks about body language define more than 1,000 positions that a student needs to look for! And more than 1,000 different facial expressions!

The Mayo brothers must have instinctively understood body language in regard to paying close attention to their patients—the desk chairs they purchased for physicians didn't recline!

The desk in a physician's office shouldn't be between the patient and the physician—the patient should sit beside the desk, not on the other side of it. When you are at the desk, do not stare at the computer, which is one of the most common patient complaints. But you can turn the computer screen toward the patient and family so they can see what you are looking at, and you can explain the results of blood tests and imaging. Until computers became standard in all offices, the Mayo brothers showed their wisdom by putting double-view boxes for imaging in every office/exam room. The patient could see any abnormalities reported by the radiologist. Today, all images are on the computer screen, and a patient can clearly see them. Patients are now part of decision-making.

A friend told us that he wanted to come to Mayo Clinic because his physician didn't seem "engaged" in his care. Another word for engaged is **mindfulness**. Another patient told us about a surgeon who was visibly upset after getting this patient's pathology report from a biopsy. This surgeon was upset because the patient *didn't* have cancer—apparently that meant he lost a chance to perform surgery and enhance his income! We asked these people how they knew their physician wasn't engaged or seemed upset. They said that they could just see it in the physicians' body language! This was from two people with no training in body-language interpretation.

It has been shown that patient satisfaction tends to correlate with a physician's nonverbal communication skills.

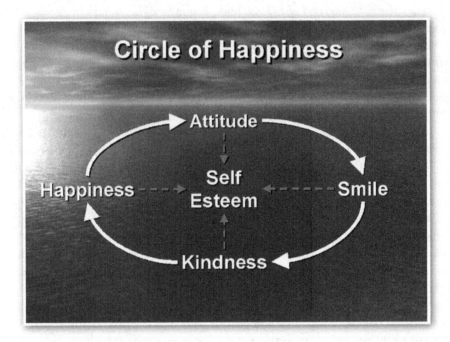

As we again look at the Circle of Happiness, remember that attitude is everything. You can't hide your attitude—faking it is a dead giveaway—so don't try. The fMRI has opened our world to just a fraction of what goes on in our brains, but we do know that you can change just about everything—including your attitude—through re-hardwiring your brain. This is *plasticizing* your brain through positive thinking. It may take six to twelve months or more but is very doable. This leads to ...

Smiling. Here are more thoughts on smiling because it is so useful and powerful.

- It expresses empathy, is a form of bonding, and, in turn, creates *trust*.
- It changes our mood, boosts the immune system, and relieves stress. And you don't have to be with someone to smile.
- It is contagious; it disarms the angry patient.
- It can be perceived even if it lasts less than a second.
- It may make you look younger and more attractive.
- Studies have shown that people who smile (10 percent of us have beautiful, natural smiles) are happier and more successful. They are healthier and live longer, and they have fewer divorces and more friends. There is no downside. A fake smile doesn't involve the muscles around the eyes.
- A frown is a negative that reflects disappointment, surprise, anger, sadness, and/or disgust.

On the **Circle of Happiness**, the next quality is **kindness (empathy)**. You can't smile without increasing your tendencies toward acts of kindness, and you can't have **happiness** without a positive attitude, smiling, and kindness. They all enhance your self-esteem, which is a great reducer of stress and will brighten your own day. All happiness experts state that *gratitude* is essential for happiness, and you can't just think about it. Write down a few things you have to be grateful for every day. Have you personally thanked the person(s) responsible for your gratitude?

Facial expressions. In addition to smiling, your face is capable of making more than 1,000 subtle changes in expression that may last only 0.1 second. These changes are easily detected by slow-motion computer cameras and by people skilled in body-language interpretation. One or both eyebrows moving almost imperceptibly may be a clue to a quick attempt to frown that is retracted. But the patient might pick up on this.

Voice. Some people think that an electronic recording of a person's voice is almost as sensitive as a lie-detector test. Certain emotions, such as sadness, guilt, anger, and stress, are perceptible to some people; you have almost no control over this. If you add lack of eye contact, not smiling, and looking bored, it may all add up to a significant message to the patient. How does your voice sound over the phone? Condescending? Angry?

Body position. As stated previously, there are more than 1,000 ways of "speaking" body language. These include crossing your legs or ankles, fidgeting, looking at your watch, folding your hands, nervous twitching or tics, where your eyes are focused, and on and on. A composite of these and other body-language positions projects your self-confidence and attitude, which leads to a patient's perception of you and whether he/she feels there is any possibility of bonding and trust.

Eye contact. This may be one of the most underappreciated—but most important—communication skills. You can't listen with the intent to learn without eye contact. Look your patient in the eye while you nod in agreement and empathize with him/her.

Touch. Touch is another sensation that is probably more powerful than we have ever imagined. We were impressed with a fellow physician's story about being admitted into his own intensive care unit. He was in shock from multiple bee stings. He partly attributed his survival to the people in the unit who continuously held his hand until he was out of the woods. He said this comforted him and greatly reduced his stress. But what did the skin-to-skin contact accomplish? Was a message mediated through the peripheral nervous system? What words of reassurance were said to him?

More touch: hugging and kissing. Hugging is OK—it is good! However, some people don't like to be hugged, so don't push it. Kissing family members and close friends is the oldest form of therapeutic touch. What about kissing our pets—what do we receive from this very common form of touch? We think that many forms of kissing produce a momentary act of smiling, which is enough to evoke the release of endorphins and oxytocin. Puckering the lips also might mimic the sucking reflex we see in babies.

Massage is another form of healing **touch**. Not too many years ago, nurses gave fifteen-minute back massages to patients every evening. When, why, and where was this art initiated? We know why it was stopped—it was "not cost effective"! Studies now confirm that massage is a great stress reducer even if just the hands are massaged.

Mindfulness. This is the engagement mentioned previously. It is giving your full attention to the patient. Patients can easily sense if you are engaged—or if you are not. Mindfulness is the opposite of multitasking, and a patient can see and/or sense the difference. "He spent most of the time on the phone or looking at the computer screen, and neither was about me." Mindfulness is taught in some medical schools—instruction should start in grade school!

Aura, chemistry, and olfactory. Of the senses mentioned, most have not been researched in terms of our understanding, but researchers in a science of caring will look into these someday. Chemistry is intriguing and may be very significant because of what we are learning from animals! We can train dogs to "sense" when their owners are going to have a grand mal seizure. When these trained dogs warn their owners, the owners have enough time to call someone and then lay on the floor with a protective mouthpiece in place. The aura of an epileptic patient is probably an odor the dog can detect. Maybe a researcher in the science of caring will come up with a device that can detect all kinds of "messages."

In 2011, ten highly trained German shepherd police dogs were part of a fascinating study. Two sets each of identical twins and fraternal twins under age thirteen were part of the test, so each set was then living in the same environment, eating the same food, etc. The eight children had their scents collected on cotton squares stored in glass jars. The dogs were introduced to just one of the scents (by sniffing) and then told to find the jar with that person's matching scent. Twelve trials were done by the ten dogs. The final score was 120 to 0! Not one mistake. (This study was done in case there was a murder by an identical twin with DNA left at the scene!) Some dogs have a sense of smell that is thousands of times greater than that of humans.

It has been shown that a dog can sense your oxytocin, and in turn, you probably can sense your dog's.

What we (and our dogs) may be sensing is in the breath. When highly sensitive odor analyzers are developed in the future, we may be able to diagnose many diseases beginning with the help of dogs. We know that dogs can be trained to detect melanomas directly and detect thyroid cancer in a patient's urine. In the meantime, the patient may be trying to figure out why he/she likes or dislikes the physician!

All animals have their own sense of smell, and we don't know exactly how they use it in their brains. Sharks can smell blood from a quarter of a mile away.

We talk of the chemistry between two people: "What does she see in that jerk? There must be chemistry between them." We postulate that we don't know what our brains smell; we have lost our protective sense of smell through evolution. We don't need it anymore. But the olfactory portion of the brain can perceive some odors that we can't detect consciously. Women may have an evolutionary attraction to a man's perspiration, e.g., "a hard worker is someone who will provide for me and our kids."

Listening. We saved this for last because it is one of the most important skills in effective communication—whether it is listening to a patient, family, friend, or customer. *It's as important to know how to listen as when to listen.* If a physician allows a patient to talk uninterrupted for up to three minutes, the patient estimates that he/she talked for at least ten. "My doctor actually listened to me. No doctor has ever done that before!"

The physician must listen with the full intent to understand. He/she must be *engaged* 100 percent to what the patient is saying. You have to give people time to ventilate. Many people listen with the intent to reply and give their opinion. They don't listen to understand. Listening is a learned skill and may be extremely therapeutic to the patient because it shows that you care. In a study, surgeons who spent an average of three more minutes with patients and their families were compared with a control group. The surgeons who spent more time with the patients were sued much less often than those in the control group. During this extra time, the physician was listening, providing a more thorough explanation of the intent of surgery, and answering the patient's and family's questions.

Listen with your eyes; listen for feelings! You must want to listen!

The patient will know if you are listening or not. Did you make eye contact? This is a *soul-to-soul* engagement. The patient is looking for empathy. Respond with facial expressions, nodding in understanding, saying "Go on," and so on. A frown is appropriate at this time to reflect your understanding of the patient's distress.

Listen to learn how the symptom or disease is affecting the whole of the patient.

Don't listen to what I say; listen to what I mean!

Before you go into a room to visit with a patient (and his/her family), remind yourself of the power of healing in your body language.

More on the Art of Medicine
(repeating some from previous chapters)

I don't care how much he knows until I know how much he cares!

• Always try to be on time; if you aren't, apologize.

• Remember that even the worried-well patient usually is apprehensive and anxious until you can tell him/her that his/her exam and tests are normal and there is no evidence of cancer, diabetes, hypertension, or any precursor of a chronic disease. This is the time to *educate* and *motivate* to maintain *wellness*. Adding that the tests "don't show any evidence" of a chronic disease is much better than saying that the person "doesn't have" a chronic disease. This is preferable because you can't know whether or not something will pop up showing a cancer, etc., in six months.

• Thoroughly examine the patient as appropriate; this may be therapeutic as it involves touch.

• **Never** put down another physician or the allied health personnel to the patient.

• Have you offered hope (hopefully, you haven't taken it away)? Would you want a member of your family to receive care from a physician who shows the same qualities as you do? Ask yourself that.

• Are you caring with dignity? With a sense of warmth and kindness? With compassion? Are you sure? Remember the Platinum Rule of Medicine.

• Don't hesitate to unmask a depression. It may be the cause of a patient's symptoms. Are you depressed?

It's not a sign of weakness to ask for help!

• Ask, "Have I answered your questions?" "What do you think your problem is due to?"

• Explain things in nonmedical jargon.

• Ask patients if they want copies of their tests and your summaries of their workups. Remember, people travel more than ever, and it could save them a lot of lost time and money if they take these documents (or know how to access them online).

• Talk about Living Wills with your patients. Encourage them to complete one and send you a copy. If you don't receive it, remind them the next time they come in. Give them a blank copy. Do you have a Living Will? Travel with it.

• After a woman has a mammogram, try to give her the results the same day—just like you would want for a member of your family. This applies to any test result that your patient is especially anxious about. (We've known of patients who had to wait two weeks for the results of a biopsy!) If the result is negative, your nurse may call the patient, but if it is positive, you need to make the call. Do not send an email.

• An unsolicited phone call from you is a tremendous demonstration of caring.

• Return phone calls and emails promptly—*today*. This is integrity. This is the Platinum Rule.

• Treat the allied health personnel the way you want them to treat your patients—with respect!

• **Think!** Always be self-critical. "Am I missing something?" "Have I made the right diagnoses?" "Is the patient trying to tell me something?" "Is this the right medication?" "Could the medication be the problem?" Self-questioning tends to protect physicians from arrogance.

• Realize that the day is coming when patients will grade you and the results will be public. Ask yourself, "How will this patient grade me?"

YOU!

• You and your family are the most important substances in your life. Your health is your most important asset—never take it for granted. You must have your own physician; get an exam every few years depending on your age and risk factors. Do not self-diagnose and self-treat. Deal with a depression that will affect 15 percent to 25 percent of us.

• Are you a good role model to the people around you? To your kids?

• Your life and your work are not two separate things—your work is part of your life.

• Balance your life!

• Don't postpone joy! Savor the little things. Have fun. Laugh every day! You alone are responsible for your happiness. **Be happy!**

• Maybe you are enjoying life and don't know it! You're too preoccupied with the past and the future. Try to live and think only in the moment—in today.

• You will make mistakes—it's 100 percent guaranteed. Learn from them, and then forget them! Be gentle on yourself!

• **Learn to say "no."** You owe this to yourself. Learn to say it gracefully.

• Learn to accept normalcy in mood swings. Don't make major decisions when you are in a low mood as *this too shall pass.*
• Practice time efficiency.
• Don't sweat the small things—and they are all small.
• Slow down to enjoy the speed of life.
• **Have fun!**

The following is a synopsis of a few articles that is told by a patient after meeting with a male physician who practices the **Art of Medicine**.

The receptionist and clinical assistant seemed unusually friendly and happy. The physician came in the room, called me by name, and introduced himself. He smiled. At no time did he seem to be in a hurry. Right away, I knew he was engaged with me. We made small talk as he asked about my family and occupation. He carefully reviewed the questionnaires I had completed. He was interested! "How can I help you?" As I talked, he rarely interrupted except to fill in some of my gaps. He was relaxed, and I felt like I was his only patient that day. He didn't wear a watch. He nodded frequently. I felt comfortable with him and opened up easily, something many are afraid to do. I already noted that I felt better even before we were done. He looked like he had been practicing his body language. He examined me thoroughly and then answered all of my questions. I listened. I had more questions; he listened. He outlined the program for further tests. I left his office feeling good. I knew that I was in the hands of a doctor who really cared and who would care for me just like he would want a member of his family cared for.

Remember: *Always practice the Platinum Rule of Medicine.*

Chapter Fourteen

Palliative Care, End-of-Life Issues, and Medical Ethics

Palliative care is the care of patients with advanced chronic illnesses who usually have heavy symptom burdens. Palliative care clinicians align patient management with a patient's values, preferences, and goals of care using advance care planning, conversations, and a shared decision-making model. The goal of palliative care is for patients to live as long and well as they can and to remain at home if that is their desire. It is unlike hospice care since these patients could live several more years—frequently with a "new lease on life."

Objectives of Palliative Care
- Provide relief from pain, dyspnea (shortness of breath), and other symptoms
- Affirm life and regard dying as a normal process
- Intend to neither hasten nor postpone death
- Integrate the psychological and spiritual aspects of patient care
- Offer a support system to help patients live as actively as possible until there is a resolution of symptom(s) or death
- Offer a support system to help families cope during their loved one's illness and in their own bereavement
- Use a team approach—a **strength** of the palliative care approach—and require that everyone be on the same page so there are no mixed messages given to the patient and/or the family members
- Enhance the quality of life, which at times may positively influence the course of a disease
- Palliative care is applicable early in the course of an illness and in conjunction with other therapies intended to prolong life. Patients who may be candidates for palliative care could have advanced heart failure, chronic obstructive pulmonary disease (COPD), amyotrophic lateral sclerosis (ALS), stage III or IV cancer, and other conditions.

Hospice is one facet of palliative care. *Hospice, which is a Medicare benefit, is offered to patients wherever they live and whose life expectancy is judged to be less than six months.* One of the huge benefits of hospice is its 24/7 nursing availability. This keeps patients from having to go to the emergency room and be admitted to the hospital where they will have to start afresh with a new team that may not understand their narrative or their goals.

A Brief History of Palliative Care

A holistic approach to patients with advanced illnesses is as old as the medical profession itself. A resurgence of interest in this approach evolved in the United Kingdom in the 1960s, while Dame Cicely Saunders simultaneously began the modern hospice movement at St. Christopher's Hospice in London. In the early 1970s, Dr. Balfour Mount coined the term "palliative care" from the Latin "palliare," which is a term that describes a priest's cloak. Thus, to "palliate" is to "cloak" or "surround" an illness rather than cure it.

Palliative medicine's official recognition as a specialty by the American Board of Medical Specialties, with its own written board exams, came about in the 2000s. The specialty was first recognized in the United States in the 1980s. For many palliative care physicians, the specialty represents the reason they chose medicine—to comfort and alleviate suffering.

Ethical Issues in Palliative Care

Ethical issues and challenges are not uncommon at the end of life. Physicians should be guided by ethical and moral tenets, some of which include the following:
- Respect for human life and dignity
- The acceptance of a dignified and comfortable death
- Truthfulness in communication
- Fidelity to trust
- Humility
- Intellectual honesty
- Non abandonment

Four basic ethical principles that apply to the practice of Western medicine have been formulated and affirmed. These are the following:
- **Autonomy.** Patients have the right to truthful information and self-determination while working with their physicians using a shared decision-making model.
- **Beneficence.** Doing good.
- **Nonmaleficence.** Do no harm.
- **Justice.** Consider the needs of society as well as the patient's. Be fair.

The physician also may have the ethical dilemma of judging a patient's capacity for understanding the extent of the illness and for decision-making, as delirium and somnolence frequently occur. After receiving accurate information, a patient must be able to perform the following to demonstrate adequate capacity to give consent:

• Capacity is task specific. For example, a patient may exhibit the capacity to make decisions regarding his/her living situation but not have the capacity to make decisions regarding the risks and benefits of chemotherapy.
  • The patient must understand the risks, benefits, and alternatives to what is being proposed.
  • The patient must make a decision logically.
  • The patient's decisions must be consistent.

Euthanasia is derived from the Greek "eu," which means good, and "thanatos," which means death. Euthanasia, in the modern context, refers to the intentional and deliberate ending of life. In most contexts, a physician performs euthanasia at a patient's request and with his/her permission to relieve pain and suffering. **Euthanasia** has its proponents, but it is illegal in the United States. Some believe that physician aid in dying or assisted suicide, which is legal in a few states (and being deliberated in a number of others), is equivalent to a physician performing euthanasia.
  Importantly, euthanasia is not:
  • Withholding or withdrawing life support.
  • Using excessive opioids to treat pain at the risk of inducing respiratory failure.
  • Palliative sedation, which is discussed at the end of this chapter.
  • "Do not resuscitate" or "Do not intubate" orders.

Suffering

Pain is inevitable—suffering is optional.
—Anonymous

In medicine, we often equate suffering with physical pain, but suffering also includes emotional, psychological, social, and spiritual components as well. It is important to recognize suffering because the manifestations can be subtle and hidden. *Suffering comes from the soul—it is not a disease.*
  • Patients with unremitting and untreated suffering may lose hope and feel isolated and abandoned. Always remember that the effects of illness and suffering may extend to the patients' families, loved ones, friends, and coworkers.
  • It is said that *the most difficult part of communication is hearing what isn't said*, and to detect and alleviate suffering, one must be an *intentional and reflective listener.*

Hope, Resiliency, and Dignity
  • Hope is a feeling of longing and desire for something that usually lies in the future. Thus, hope can be precarious in patients with an advanced or life-limiting illness. Hope is often tied to faith as written by Paul in Hebrews: *"Now faith is being sure of what we hope for and certain of what we do not see."*
  • A loss of hope is associated with a fear of *abandonment*, thus, it is inexorably linked to *trust*. A patient's ability to maintain hope is linked to the trust that he/she has in the physician. The patient trusts that the physician will treat his/her pain and suffering and act in his/her best interest.

• *In people with advanced illnesses, hope almost always changes over time*, and as a physician, it is imperative that you help your patients redirect hope when need be. When a patient is faced with a life-limiting illness, the initial reaction often is hope for recovery. As death approaches, hope may take another direction. At this stage, patients almost always want to spend time with their families and die with dignity and resilience, free of spiritual and existential worries.

Common themes are a connectedness to God, a search for spiritual meaning and significance in life, and resolving any conflicts that may exist with family and loved ones. Most patients desire the ability to thrive in the face of adversity and suffering and do not want to burden others. Patients must have trust in you, their physician, in order for you to help them through these different stages and processes. *This trust usually takes time to develop* and is incremental in nature. You must learn your patient's personal narrative—everyone has one. And once again, this requires the skill and experience of *listening* to your patient.

Listening is the ultimate form of communication.

Never take away your patient's hope by saying, "There is nothing more we can do," or "We are withdrawing care." We always, always care for people. **There is always more you can do. You can continue to care. And listen.**

The Palliative Care Team's Benefits and Services

• Because suffering is multidimensional and composed of more than just physical pain, palliative care is based on an interdisciplinary team. In addition to physicians, the team usually is comprised of advanced practice clinicians, such as nurse practitioners and physician assistants, along with nurses, social workers, and chaplains.

• Other health-care providers, such as massage therapists, counselors, and patient care assistants, are sometimes involved. A coordinated system of care increasingly makes sense with patients growing older and having more complex issues—all within the setting of technological advances and a fragmented health-care system. *Communication among members of the team is not just beneficial but critical to success.*

• The palliative care team strives to provide the right care, at the right time, and at the right place by focusing on symptom management in the context of a patient's illness burden and goals of care. Studies are beginning to show the *value* of this type of care. For instance, patients with metastatic lung cancer have been shown to live longer while having a better quality of life when palliative care is involved **early** in the course of their disease. Likewise, patients with COPD and congestive heart failure (CHF) who received in-home palliative care reported greater satisfaction and were more likely to die at home with peace of mind compared with those who received usual care. Not only can palliative care involvement improve outcomes, but it also has been shown to lower costs.

• Various models exist for the implementation of palliative care. In the hospital, a traditional consultative model is often utilized. An integrative approach with the palliative care team embedded into the primary team, especially in the ICU, also may be very effective.

• Palliative care that is based in the home also has been shown to provide greater patient satisfaction with lower utilization of hospitalizations and procedures. Many patients express a strong desire to get home whether to heal or to die.

• Palliative care is not without its barriers and challenges. Both patients and physicians may wrongly assume that "palliative care" means "giving up," "withdrawing care," and "all hope is lost." Additionally, a team-based approach, for all its positive attributes, may be challenging to physicians. Medical doctors have traditionally viewed their role as "captain of the ship" and "the buck stops with me." While these maxims can still be true in palliative care, a flexible, inquisitive, and inviting disposition with colleagues is most helpful.

• If your institution has an instructional pamphlet on palliative care, it would be beneficial to give a copy to the patient and the family before their first meeting with the palliative care team.

• It is important that medical students, residents, fellows, and nurses be part of the team; this may be the only "formal" education they get in end-of-life issues.

While doing the right thing for the patient, palliative care also can help with resource utilization and cost avoidance. By 2030, the number of people in the United States over age eighty-five is expected to double to 8.5 million while, at the same time, the number of people with chronic medical conditions is estimated to be 170 million. Currently, fully 20 percent of Americans die in an intensive care unit, often with prolonged suffering.

The sickest 10 percent of the nation's population accounts for 64 percent of health-care expenditures. The palliative care team helps patients focus on what is important to them and make wise decisions while providing relief from their suffering; palliative care consultation in Medicaid patients in New York showed an average cost savings of $6,900. The Center for Palliative Care estimates that the typical palliative care consultation saves $2,800, representing a savings of $2.5 million for the average academic medical center.

Palliative Care: The Conversation

• Initiating a conversation about palliative care can be challenging because many people have never heard of the term, or it may generate negative emotions about dying and hopelessness. Most often, it is best to proactively address this problem by explaining what it is we do in palliative care. After receiving a consultation, talking with the person who placed the referral is always helpful, provides insight, and is a mark of professional courtesy.

• After speaking with the referring clinician and reviewing the record, the next step is to meet the patient. After brief introductions, consideration should be given to *explaining palliative care and why you are being consulted*. Some examples include the following.

■ **Symptom management.** *"Your doctor wants me to see if I can help reduce and treat your pain and shortness of breath."*

■ **The "Big Picture."** *"You have lots of wonderful doctors and nurses taking care of many problems, and I want to be sure that we take a step back and focus on what is important to you." "Your doctor is still going to be your doctor."*

■ **Transitioning to a supportive and comfort approach.** *"Your doctors want us to talk about where you are in the course of your illness and options moving forward for your care."*

■ **Advance care planning.** *"Sometimes we do what we call preparedness planning. It's kind of like a fire drill—we don't expect to have a fire, but if we do, we want to know what to do. The same with your health. If for some reason you could not make decisions for yourself, we want to know your wishes and who would help make decisions for you."* *"So far, what questions do you have for us?"*

■ **Shared decision-making**. *"Sometimes you get so much information that it's hard to keep it all straight and make any sense of it. Even as a doctor, I have trouble sometimes understanding all of it. At times, people want us to work with them to help them make decisions about their health that would be best for them."* While respecting *patient autonomy*, most patients will benefit from a shared decision-making model and are desirous of your recommendations.

Following your explanation of the consultative process, making a *nonmedical connection* and learning a bit about your patient and his/her family is almost always beneficial. You begin learning the patient's story and narrative, which imparts to the patient a sense that he/she is not just another "case." *"So before we talk about your medical issues, tell me a little about you."* By listening carefully, you will get a sense of the patient's fears and understanding of what is going on, along with his/her worries about how the family is coping.

After spending a few minutes getting to know your patient, you will begin to redirect the discussion. *"Thanks for sharing a bit of your personal story with me. Would it be OK if we now talked some about your health issues?"* At this point, utilizing the Ask-Tell-Ask method of communication can bear fruit, especially since palliative care often involves goals of care and focusing on the big picture. Ask-Tell-Ask is simply what it says: *"Just to be sure we are on the same page, can you tell me how you understand your medical condition?"* or *"What have your doctors told you is wrong with you?"* Then "Tell": *"OK, would it now be all right if I told you how I understand your health-care issues?"* Then, *"What questions do you have?"* *"If you had to call your spouse now and summarize what we have just been over, what would you say?"* This typically leads to a more detailed discussion of symptom management, goals of care, and the like.

Some Specific Palliative Care Conversations

Advance Care Planning (ACP)

ACP often carries the connotation of end-of-life planning, use of life support, artificial hydration and feeding, and resuscitation status. While all these are part of ACP, advance care planning is simply a *conversation* about what medical treatment is right for your patient.

• Ideally, the conversation takes place over time and is both *incremental* and *iterative*. It is a conversation that should not only reflect the medical issues at hand but also the *patient's goals, preferences, values, hopes,* and *fears*. ACP should be part of routine medical care and revisited whenever there is a change in a patient's medical condition. Medicare has begun to reimburse physicians for the time spent with these discussions.

• As medical care becomes more fragmented, seamless transitions in care can be difficult to manage. If a palliative care consultant has a long-standing relationship with the patient's primary care clinician, a call to this doctor often may be immensely helpful.

• Good advance care planning has been shown to help with patient compliance, reduce hospitalizations at the end of life, and lead to greater patient satisfaction. Remember that the conversation is longitudinal, iterative, incremental, and almost always changes over time. Since patients and family members can only remember a small percentage of what you tell them, go slow, give them small chunks of information in nonmedicalese, check in for their understanding, and summarize—*and do all this frequently!* Keep in mind that some of these patients may have an altered sensorium. And also keep in mind that family members will hear different things. Some revert to the old school of thought of "not telling Pop that he has cancer." This works for only so long as the public (including the patient) is now quite savvy about medicine.

• Depending on the patient's illness, you may ease into the fact that chemotherapy and/or radiation therapy may not be curative, and in some cases, the risks may outweigh the benefits.

Advance Directives

Advance Directives are legal documents that help direct a patient's care when he/she is unable to make his/her own decisions. *They apply only to patients who have lost their decision-making capacity.*

• In broad terms, Advance Directives have two components: (1) naming of a surrogate decision-maker, i.e., *Durable Healthcare Power of Attorney*, and (2) a patient's preferences for future care, i.e., *Living Will*. Following Advance Directive instructions can decrease the use of life-sustaining measures when they are not warranted, increase the use of palliative care, and lessen family conflict.

• Ideally, an Advance Directive document flows out of an iterative conversation about advance care planning, and not vice versa. This document should be completed long before the patient gets sick—maybe even when the individual is in his/her twenties or thirties—with the expectation that it should be revisited every five or ten years. Asking a person to fill out a Living Will without having had a conversation about his/her goals and values, along with considering his/her health status, is potentially fraught with problems.

• It is important to know the law in the state where you practice as well as the different directives available. Patients' primary care physicians and attorneys will generally keep copies of Advance Directives.

• Directives that incorporate *values* and *preferences* ("Five Wishes" and "Values History" are two examples that may be part of an Advance Directive) are preferable over documents that focus primarily on legalistic terms, such as "If I have a terminal illness" and "vegetative state."

• Since we can't predict every possible clinical scenario, understanding a patient's goals, values, and preferences is much more elucidating. Patients also typically associate "terminal illness" with cancer but not with conditions such as multiple organ failure in a frail, elderly patient with multiple comorbidities.

• Surrogate decision-makers often are family members or close friends, but sometimes a caregiver who knows the patient's health situation is designated for this role. Be aware that there may be times when surrogate decision-makers are not aware of or don't understand their role. They also may not relish the idea. Their role is to make decisions about what is best for the patient and what the patient would want, and not make decisions based on their own preferences.

• After the patient chooses a surrogate, it is best that the patient help define that role. Does the patient desire for the surrogate to precisely follow the outlined medical treatments or use his/her own judgment in these matters? Does the patient expect the surrogate to make decisions independently or in consultation with other family members and loved ones? All this reflects the importance of the conversation about advance care planning. Again, the family may have other ideas. You must listen to them.

A Case

This fifty-eight-year-old woman was recently diagnosed with stage IV lung cancer. She was undergoing chemotherapy and radiation, and her oncologist wanted her seen by a palliative care team member because of her difficulties with pain and nausea. After the team and I (author JKM) were introduced to her and spent some time getting to know her, we then spent the rest of the visit focusing on symptom relief and management. After a couple of visits and phone calls, her pain and nausea were much improved and her mood had lightened considerably. She was actually able to smile and even told me a funny story about her grandchild.

*After a few more visits and second-line chemotherapy, we began to talk about her **hopes, fears, expectations**, and **goals**. On the next visit, her husband accompanied her. Since I knew that she did not have an Advance Directive, I asked if it was acceptable to talk some more about her goals and preferences. She expressed that she wished to continue chemotherapy and to live as long as possible. I affirmed her values and conveyed that I, too, hoped these things for her, but I also felt that we should talk about how to proceed if things did not turn out as expected. She was a bit emotional, and she and her husband told me they thought it best that they go home and continue the conversation.*

At her return visit, she and her husband expressed her desire to continue chemotherapy, to be as comfortable as possible, and to see their daughter graduate in about six months. I asked if they had conversed about who might make decisions on her behalf if she lacked the ability to do so, and they both articulated that her husband would be her surrogate decision-maker for health matters. I gave them a copy of an Advance Directive and asked them to look it over. I felt we had discussed most of the items in the directive and told them to take their time filling it out.

To be continued ...

Discussing Prognosis

Having an understanding of your patient's prognosis is an essential part of palliative care. Aligning a patient's goals of care with potential therapeutic options is dependent not only on his/her values and preferences but also on an expectation of survival. Determining prognosis as best you can, and then conveying this to your patient in a compassionate manner, is paramount when using an informed, shared decision-making model.

• Prognosis is discussed less often than in times past, probably for a host of reasons. Patients are older, have more complicated issues, and often have multiple comorbid conditions. As physicians, we don't like to be wrong, and this is sometimes a reason for being tepid when it comes to these conversations.

• Likewise, there is a feeling among some in the medical community that these discussions may "take away hope." A recent study revealed that the majority of persons with widely metastatic lung and colon cancers thought they were taking chemotherapy with a curative intent. People sometimes get these ideas from television ads that imply curative treatments for cancer while downplaying side effects.

• Patients who have chronic advanced illnesses and limited life expectancies are more satisfied and have less symptoms and less grief when their doctors have honest discussions with them about their prognosis.

• Many different prognostic models exist for various diseases. Often though, these illnesses don't happen in isolation—a patient may have COPD, CHF, diabetes, and chronic kidney disease, and *his/her organ systems could fail in a cascade of events. As a group, physicians tend to be overly optimistic when predicting survival.*

• Generally, *it is easier to predict short-term as opposed to long-term survival,* and we are more accurate when predicting the survival of a patient with cancer than a patient with multiple organ problems. It is helpful to look at a patient's *functional status,* especially with cancer. People who spend most of their time in bed just don't do well.

• Like all conversations in medicine, *setting and timing are keys.* Hopefully, the discussion is longitudinal, repetitive, and changing. Having the first conversation during a hospitalization for an acute problem is less than ideal but certainly imperative at times.

• Opening the talk with an *invitation* may be beneficial. *"Would it be OK if we talked some about what to expect as your illness progresses?"* Depending on the patient and your relationship, a follow-up question to learn how he/she likes to receive information might be in order. *"Some folks like to know the details and specifics when we talk, while others like to talk about the big picture. Do you have a preference?"*

• From here, the conversation usually should follow the *Ask-Tell-Ask* method. Get a sense of the patient's understanding of the prognosis before articulating your understanding.

• When conveying the diagnosis, think about presenting the information in both a positive and a negative light. *"Out of 100 patients with your condition, twenty-five will die within six months and seventy-five will live longer than that. It is difficult for us to predict the outcome for an individual."* Sometimes, unexpected complications of treatment occur that shorten the time span.

• Very often, it is useful to talk in terms of hours to days, days to weeks, and weeks to months *"I am not as smart as I would like to be about this, but if things go as expected, I would judge your survival in terms of weeks to a few months."* More often than not, these discussions do not happen in isolation and are part of a broader conversation about goals of care that may include patient preferences, recommendations from you and his/her other physicians, and responding to emotion. If you are talking about drug therapy, you must tell the patient that the side effects could shorten his/her quality of life and life span, if that is the case.

• One question that sometimes arises at the end of life is *"Doctor, what would you do if you were me?"* It is important to listen and attempt to discern the real meaning of the question. Sometimes the family wants a simple answer, e.g., what they really want to know is whether to continue statin drugs in a dying family member. However, what they are often asking for is an affirmation of a decision, e.g., withdrawing life support in a dying parent. It is usually helpful to go back to the values, preferences, and goals of the patient.

Discussing the "Do Not Resuscitate" (DNR) Order

• Like most other physician-patient interactions, conversations about cardiopulmonary resuscitation (CPR) should be timed appropriately and occur in the right setting. Talks about DNR orders often flow naturally out of discussions about goals, values, preferences, prognosis, and limitations.

• CPR in hospitalized patients—and especially those who are toward the end of life—is associated with very poor outcomes. While respecting patient autonomy, the treating physician usually makes a recommendation about CPR: *"Would it be OK if I made a recommendation about what to do if your heart stops beating or you quit breathing? Based on what we have discussed about your goals and prognosis, I would not recommend CPR for you because I do not think it will either prolong your life or improve your quality of life."* Or *"Based on what we have talked about, CPR in your case is not a good idea because it would only induce and prolong suffering."* This is supported by extensive statistical studies in the medical literature.

• It is wise to stay away from phrases such as *"Do you want everything done?"* and *"Do you want us to restart your heart, or do you want to die?"* These tend to place a patient in an either-or situation with the sense that he/she is giving up hope, which only induces anxiety in your patient and family.

• **Almost all patients want an honest, forthright, and compassionate discussion with your recommendation**. They want to know what their doctor thinks.

• Don't forget the importance of *responding to the patient's and his/her loved ones' emotions*, as they are usually present. If the discussion about DNR does not go well or your patient does not wish to have the conversation, this does not mean that you should not continue to talk about goals, prognosis, and possible therapies.

• You may encounter differing opinions from the spouse and children—this is not a rare occurrence. You have to decide if you want to get involved, but you may have to if there is an inordinate delay in decision-making about further care while waiting for input from other family members. Guilt or suppressed anger often is a significant factor in the emotions of family members. You may not appreciate this and further confuse the situation. The patient's clergy may be the best person to intercede here.

Our Case (continued ...)

Several months later, I saw my patient in the hospital. She had completed her Advance Directive. Unfortunately, she had failed second-line chemotherapy and had entered a clinical trial. Despite this, her disease was progressing with new bony and hepatic metastases. She was spending the majority of her time recumbent and had lost about twenty pounds. She was hospitalized for pneumonia and seemed to be responding to antibiotics.

As I sat on the side of her bed, I asked her how she saw the big picture of her illness. She cried and said that although no one had told her, she suspected that she was nearing the end. I asked her if it was OK to talk some about her prognosis and goals, and she said, "Of course," and that she wanted to talk about these things. I briefly summarized her clinical status and explained that my best judgment was that her life expectancy could best be measured in weeks to months. Based on this information, I asked what she was hoping for—What were her goals? What were her fears? She talked about being free of suffering, dying at home with her family, and her desire to see her daughter graduate in a couple of weeks. I affirmed all of these, and we talked some about her fears as well as her faith and the love of her family. I asked if I could make some recommendations, and so we discussed transitioning to hospice, getting care at home, and the fact that CPR would do nothing to meet her expressed goals. She died at home one month later under hospice care after witnessing the graduation of her daughter ...

Family Meetings

Family meetings are an integral part of care at the end of life. A couple of things are *different* with family meetings. First, there are usually several different services involved with the patient, and it is almost always a good idea to have a *pre-meeting meeting with everyone who is working with the patient from all the clinical services.* This helps delineate the opinions of all who are caring for the patient, get their sense of prognosis and options, and formulate a general outline of the family meeting. This is often the only time that the various teams will meet face-to-face and talk outside of the medical record. This can be an immensely fruitful and insightful time and provides a great service for your patient and family.

Be aware when planning a team meeting with family members that everyone may not be available. During the actual meeting, emotions can run high, and patients and their families are generally desirous of information regarding symptom management, prognosis, and what to expect. The meeting begins with introductions and is followed by an assessment of the patient's and family's understanding of the patient's health status and an explanation by the medical teams of the patient's current clinical status. This may be followed by recommendations, a plan moving forward, responding to emotion, and a summary.

• It may be helpful to have the meeting in the room with the patient even if he/she is comatose or sedated. This emphasizes to all present that the meeting is about the patient. Though sedated patients may not have the ability to communicate, they may "hear" (hearing is the last sense to disappear) and recall some of the conversation. Sometimes, however, families prefer to meet in a separate room, and it is usually best to defer to their wishes. Be sure the room is large enough with seating for everyone. Although it is important to have all the pertinent teams present, too many people in the room can sometimes be overwhelming to the family. Use your judgment, and ask the family members what they prefer.

• A family meeting is different compared with other physician-patient communications because you are dealing with a host of people who have varied relationships with the patient. Disagreement among family members is not uncommon, and it takes experience and wisdom to be sure that everyone is heard yet no one dominates the conversation. *Self-awareness* and *mindfulness* are keys to running a good family meeting. We all have emotions, and you also must be in tune with your own feelings and emotions during this time.

At the Bedside

• Clinical assessment and management of patients with advanced chronic illnesses and those approaching the end of life are dependent upon the same clinical tools used in practice. A thorough history, physical examination, and discussion of therapeutic options are all part of the physician's skills and acumen.

• What tends to be different is that suffering and pain are part of *total pain*, as described by Dame Cicely Saunders. Total pain is not just physical suffering but also emotional, social, psychological, and spiritual suffering that are often intertwined and not easy to discern at times. Additionally, the patient's family and loved ones, along with friends and coworkers, often share the burden of suffering. Every individual has a different pain threshold.

• Patients in palliative care may question the meaning of their illness and become withdrawn and socially isolated. Their self-image may change. *Anticipatory grief* is common and expected as patients begin to visualize their death. Physician attributes that are keys to caring for these patients are clinical discernment and experience, good communication, reflective listening, the ability to ask the right questions, and understanding and responding to emotion with empathy and caring. Touch the patient, hold his/her hand, and pull the covers up. Fuss a little.

• It is important to distinguish between grief and *depression*. Palliative care patients with depression will often experience *anhedonia*, the inability to find pleasure in anything—and they certainly cannot from a hospital bed. Two helpful questions are the obvious: *"Have you felt depressed lately?"* or *"How depressed are you?"* Then *"Tell me about it."*

• Symptom burden usually is high and multifaceted at the end of life and may include pain, nausea, dyspnea, delirium, fatigue, anorexia, anxiety, depression, a total sense of loneliness, and insomnia, among others. Focusing on symptom control is essential. *If you neglect patients' pain or nausea, they won't think you care much about them.* Since symptoms are subjective, a detailed and discerning history is paramount when caring for patients in palliative care.

• Before evaluating specific symptoms, such as pain and nausea, it is usually helpful to obtain a global assessment of your patient. Some things to look for during the assessment include the following:

Mental state	Functional status
Mood	Stamina
Eye contact	Nutritional status
Socialization	Anger

• Some things to think about when evaluating symptoms:
  ■ Most patients have multiple symptoms. Try to determine which ones bother them the most.
  ■ Symptoms should be rated and recorded. A 1–10 scale is easy with "0" being symptom-free and "10" being the worst they can imagine.
  ■ Symptoms should be reassessed at each visit.
  ■ Try to find out how the symptom is affecting your patient and how he/she is coping with the symptom burden. How does the patient judge his/her overall quality of life? Does the person feel isolated from others because of the symptoms? Has the patient's self-image changed? We all have different families of origin, and sometimes our diverse cultural backgrounds may convey different meanings and etiology to suffering.
  ■ Remember that patients may downplay their symptoms because they are afraid that the symptoms could portend a worsening prognosis. Listen carefully and ask the right questions with honesty and compassion.

■ Because suffering and symptoms are so multidimensional, seek input from other members of the care team. Nurses, social workers, chaplains, and massage therapists may have insight that you aren't aware of.

■ The financial well-being of a patient's family after his/her death may be weighing heavily on your patient and exacerbating other symptoms. Do not neglect this topic as part of your inquiry into suffering.

■ When inquiring about symptoms, ask about location, description, aggravating and alleviating factors, associations (opioids for pain may induce nausea, for example), and diurnal variations (pain may be worse at night and dyspnea in the early morning).

The Actively Dying Patient

• **Being present at the bedside of a dying patient is one of the most meaningful acts a physician can perform.** Medical students, residents, and even fellows should be involved on the team; we are talking about the *Art of Medicine*. Remember the Platinum Rule of Medicine: Treat every patient like you would want a member of your family treated. Treating symptoms of the dying, alleviating suffering, and educating patients and families about the dying process are some of the most venerated traditions of the medical profession. Seeing the dying in their homes, touching those close to death, and even a quiet presence are all sources of healing. *Kindness, a smile, and a touch*—or tears for that matter—are acts that communicate nonverbally (and powerfully) your compassion and humanity.

• Patients desire, expect, and deserve to be as comfortable as possible as they die. Spend time at the bedside looking for clues of suffering. Grimacing, tachypnea, increased work of breathing, delirium, secretions, mottling, pulses, and body temperature should be noted and serve as guides to treatment. Some ophthalmic scopolamine drops in the mouth can reduce secretions. Sit on the bed, *touch* your patient during your evaluation, and explain to your patient (if he/she is alert) and others present what you are finding and what to expect.

• **Does the patient have a cat or dog that he/she would like to bring to the hospital or hospice?** If the pet is allowed, having the animal on the bed next to the owner is very therapeutic. Dying will be more peaceful. The family will never forget you.

• Families want your assessment and to know that their loved one's suffering is being treated. Ask about the concerns and needs of all present, including for spiritual support from the hospital chaplain or a member of their clergy.

• Some appropriate comments by the physician at this point include *"Let us know when you want us to quit,"* and *"It's OK to let go. You don't have to fight anymore. We will all see you soon."* One of patients' most common requests at this point is *"I want to go home."* When it is possible to get your patient back home, arrange for it.

• On occasion, families may have *seemingly small concerns* when dealing with a dying loved one: *"I don't like the energy in the room; that painting in the room makes me sad."* These concerns should not be overlooked, and attempts should be made to address them.

• After a patient's death, try to be present for some period. Even a small amount of time will seem like a lot to family members and loved ones. If you are asked to pray with the family and are comfortable with this, it is fitting and appropriate to do so. It also is acceptable to decline if you are not comfortable. It is OK for the physician to cry. If you should notice the tears of an AHP, put an arm around him/her. If appropriate, do the same for members of the family. Use your own judgment about funerals and visitations, but it is usually the right thing to do if it feels congruent with your sense of propriety. Call your patient's widow/widower a few months after his/her spouse's death. If your hospital has a grieving service, try to attend.

• A handwritten condolence note to the family after the death of their loved one will never be forgotten. Sending a card signed by the team members who cared for the patient is a kind gesture. *Likewise, don't forget the potential grief that may be experienced by the allied health staff and especially the nursing staff. A number of nurses, as well as your physician colleagues, may have spent many hours with the patient.* A soft word of caring to those colleagues who are grieving and *a phone call to the local physician* are acts of kindness and courtesy that are marks of your *professionalism* and *compassion*.

A Case

I (author JKM) was asked to see an eighty-year-old man with Parkinson's disease who was hospitalized with a complete bowel obstruction. His Parkinson's disease was complicated by dementia, and his quality of life was poor. A very bright and accomplished man, he had always been fearful of losing his cognitive abilities. After conversations with his wife and son, arrangements had been made to get him home with hospice when he had an episode of aspiration pneumonia. Now septic and tachypneic, it was obvious that he would die in the hospital.

I spent a considerable amount of time at the bedside treating his tachypnea and excessive secretions, along with his vomiting and other symptoms. All the while, I attempted to nurse the emotions of his family and provide a road map of what to expect. For some reason that was unclear to me, his wife was agitated about his hospital room, and I could not allay her emotions. I offered a transfer to another room, albeit smaller. It turned out that the new room happened to have a painting of a canoe on a lakeshore—and the couple had spent most of their vacations canoeing and camping with their children at Minnesota's Boundary Waters Canoe Area Wilderness. His wife felt he could now die in peace. If only I had known.

He died the next day, and I visited his family in their home afterward and exchanged letters with them. When I saw them at the annual Mayo Clinic bereavement service (Mayo Clinic now has a semi-annual service for the families of patients who have died within the past six months), his wife was most appreciative of his nursing care and the fact that they could spend their last hours together by the still waters ... Seemingly small things can make such a difference at the end of life ...

Psychological, Social, and Spiritual Issues

Your patient's psychological, social, and spiritual needs represent critical domains of palliative care, and as a physician, you must be proficient in screening for these issues and also in providing general care related to them. As with the other aspects of your care, addressing these concerns appropriately is dependent upon a trusting relationship, along with compassionate listening.

• Treating a dying person's symptoms is critical. Those with unremitting physical pain will have difficulty coping with their emotions and spiritual distress during an already vulnerable time.

Existential distress, matters of faith, family conflict, unresolved guilt, a loss of dignity, and concerns about one's legacy are all issues that may arise in persons with advanced illnesses. *Reflective listening* is needed—and is a required skill.

It's not what's said; it's what's heard.

- Caring for patients at the end of life requires **intellectual humility**. *"I wish I knew precisely how long your mother has left, but my best judgment is a few days, though I have been wrong many times before."*
- *Reflection, silence* when appropriate, an *inquiring countenance*, and a *healthy sense of your own emotions* are needed. *"I can't imagine all that you are going through." "How are you coping?" "Is there anything I need to know about you that we haven't talked about to help me care for you?"* **Remember, you will never go wrong with practiced silence while holding the patient's and spouse's hands.**
- The ability to properly screen for a patient's psychosocial and spiritual needs is a key role of the physician. Some issues to consider when taking a patient's history include the importance of faith or spirituality to help him/her find meaning and support, along with a sense of the family structure and their support. You also should find out if the patient's history includes emotional problems, neglect or abuse as a child, substance abuse, personality disorders, and unresolved conflicts.
- After you take a spiritual history, you should be able to identify who can help the patient with his/her spiritual concerns. You might encourage him/her to contact a clergy member from his/her place of worship and/or suggest a visit from the hospital chaplain. A visit from someone who can connect to the patient in a spiritual way may be an integral part of care.
- Since anticipatory grief at the end of life is common for both the patient and caregivers, don't forget to ask about this. *"Grieving about your loved one's dying is normal and expected. How are you doing?"* It is vital that you have effective communication with and referrals to social workers and chaplains who are colleagues on the interdisciplinary team. Lean on them when need be. *More often than not, they will have insights that you don't possess.* Dying patients also may benefit from other components of palliative care. Massage therapy, music therapy, etc., may all provide solace and comfort.
- Caregivers are sometimes the forgotten ones when dealing with patients at the end of life. They, too, are your patients, so don't forget them. They also may have an illness and could become physically and emotionally exhausted. They may need a respite from caregiving.
- After the death of a loved one, grief and bereavement are normal processes of loss. One of the beauties of hospice is that the hospice staff provides bereavement services for many months after the death of a patient, and it is usually helpful to acknowledge this with your patients. *Hospice can be a gift of love that a patient can give to his/her family because its staff will be with them and care for them after the patient is gone.* Some of the expected emotions of grief are denial, disbelief, anger, yearning, and, eventually, *acceptance. Complicated grief* is grief that lasts longer than expected and may entail frank depression—be on the lookout for it.

Ethical Concerns at the End of Life and Palliative Sedation

• Palliative sedation is sometimes necessary in terminally ill patients who are experiencing unmitigated suffering despite all conventional attempts to alleviate the symptoms at hand. Examples include pain, delirium, or existential suffering.

• Palliative sedation is only undertaken when all other avenues of therapy have been exhausted and all domains of palliative care, such as spiritual distress, depression, and emotional issues, have been addressed. Before embarking on palliative sedation, there should be a consultation and review with another palliative care physician. The other physician also should note this in the patient's records.

• There are two important ethical principles to consider about palliative sedation. The first is **proportionality**. The degree of sedation should be enough—but only enough—to abate your patient's suffering. At times, it will be appropriate to decrease the sedation to allow the patient a period of awareness to communicate with family and friends, as long as the symptoms don't recur. The second principle is that of **double effect**. The goals of palliative sedation are to alleviate suffering and to neither prolong life unnecessarily nor hasten death. Knowing that, it is possible that the use of drugs to induce sedation may have side effects that hasten death. This is double effect. The difference between sedation and euthanasia/physician-aided death is intent. Our intent with palliative sedation is to treat symptoms and not to hasten or cause death.

• Keep in mind the patient's cultural and spiritual beliefs; seek advice from his/her minister/spiritual leader.

Withholding/Withdrawal of Care, Artificial Hydration, and Feeding and Futility

• Though not initiating some type of care and withdrawal of that care are ethically and legally without difference, it is sometimes emotionally more trying for families to stop care, such as dialysis, mechanical ventilation, or artificial feeding. Hopefully, this is covered in the Advance Directive. Trust, listening, knowing your patient's narrative and understanding of his/her illness, and the use of a shared decision-making model should be your building blocks to help guide your patient and family.

• Honed communication skills, recognizing and responding to emotion, and self-awareness are essential tools for the physician in this setting. While you should acknowledge patient autonomy—"Do you want me to do everything for your husband or let him die?"—your patient might be better served by a recommendation, such as "Based on what you have told me about your husband, I don't think continuing life support at this juncture will reverse the course of his illness nor achieve his goal of always living independently at home."

• Likewise, if you suggest that IV fluids and tube feedings be stopped, the family may be concerned that this could lead to hunger and thirst in a dying patient. This may be best addressed during a compassionate conversation during which you articulate the fact that thirst and hunger abate as death nears and continuing these measures may lead to more symptoms, such as secretions, edema, and dyspnea.

A Case

A sixty-four-year-old man with widely metastatic pancreatic cancer was hospitalized for unremitting pain and delirium. Despite doing all that we (author JKM and the palliative care team) knew to do and consulting with our physician and pharmacy colleagues, his symptoms continued unabated. Both he and his family were suffering—physically and emotionally.

I discussed his status with another palliative care physician. I told her that I was considering palliative sedation and asked if she would review the record of my patient. After her review, we both agreed that he was dying and suffering, and palliative sedation was in order.

I sat down with his family and conveyed compassionately and honestly my concerns for his suffering, our failed efforts thus far, and the idea of palliative sedation. Though he was dying, I did not want to do anything to hasten his death but was aware that intravenous sedation could potentially lead to a more rapid demise. They understood, and we all spent some time with the chaplain discussing the plan. They voiced their concerns about his physical and spiritual suffering and the need to do whatever we had to do to alleviate his symptoms.

We proceeded with sedation, and actually, the dose required to keep him comfortable was quite small. His breathing was regular, and he showed no untoward complications of palliative sedation. During the next two days, his family spent time remembering him, telling stories, and actually laughing and celebrating his life. He died sixty hours after undergoing palliative sedation.

Never forget the
Platinum Rule of Medicine:
*Treat every patient like you would want
a member of your family treated.*

Chapter Fifteen

Life After Medicine

Medicine will always be in your heart and mind, but at the rate new knowledge and increasing government oversight about everything are occurring, you most likely will have to *quit* sometime. Can you just quit and not turn back? Do you want to? Can you afford to? Can you keep up continuing medical education (CME) for your state medical licensure? What feedback do you get from your professional colleagues and especially from your family? Is there a possibility that you can work part-time and ease out of medicine? Is there an element of burnout that might play a role here? Does the extreme loyalty you have for your patients affect your thinking about retirement? Have you started making plans for retirement, no matter what your age? The following are some thoughts about retiring related to the above questions.

• **Plan ahead.** When we are in our forties, very few of us begin serious thinking about retirement. But by the time you turn sixty, you need to give the idea some serious consideration. Maybe you are still in the thinking stages, but discussing your options with your financial advisor could be very worthwhile. If you have a spouse, what does he/she think? This may clarify what your future holds. Will you be supporting a family member in college after retirement?

• Many medical centers offer yearly or every-other-year preretirement programs that feature experts in retirement, finances, etc. Spouses are welcome. Take advantage of these.

• **To many of us, our work is our image—our self-identity**. It may seem that is gone in retirement. But it doesn't have to be (see what follows for ideas about teaching, mentoring, and volunteering).

• **What do you want to do in retirement?** You can only watch so much television or spend so many hours reading. Now that you will have the time, consider taking up or resuming a sport (tennis, golf, etc.). Do you have any current hobbies or possible hobbies that you seriously want to spend time on? If you haven't tried any of your possibilities, you had better look into them before retiring in case they don't turn out as you wish. Then you won't have to wonder what to do with a basement full of woodworking tools.

• One way of dealing with the dilemma of what to do in retirement is to make a list of the pros and cons regarding your possibilities and give each of them a relative value.

• You might be thinking about moving out of state to be near your children. This would be a big move. And what if they move?

• Maybe you want to spend six months every year in a warmer or cooler climate; what preparations do you need to arrange for this? Is your spouse ready for this? If you are working part-time, you may find that you feel "out of date" when you come back after six months.

• There are tremendous and rewarding opportunities in **volunteering**, both medical and nonmedical. Regarding medical volunteering, it can be very gratifying to volunteer at a health clinic, e.g., the Salvation Army. If you are considering this, be careful that you don't let your state medical license expire. It can be a lot of work to get it back. You likely would need to continue your CME. Check with your state licensing board to see if there is a reduced fee if you don't plan to see any paying patients. Also, check on malpractice insurance needs and who might pay for this.

• **Teaching!** Just think about your lifetime of experience. Find ways of passing this information on to young physicians. You will get more out of it than they will!

• **Mentoring!** Talk to local high-school counselors about the possibility of meeting with students who are interested in the medical/nursing field. Who can tell it better than someone who has been there? When you visit the school, you will likely get to know some students who you can personally mentor either individually or as a small group. This is tremendously rewarding!

• We have been surprised to discover how few senior people have started writing their life history. It is so easy when you use the computer since you can stop in the middle of a paragraph and start up later. When you think of something, you can just add to your story. Your life history will be of its greatest value in 100 and 200 years. No one will believe that all cars were black for decades! Searching your genealogy also can be rewarding, as well as a lot of fun.

• Studies now show that nurturing good friendships is more predictive of a long and healthy life span compared to almost anything else. Spend time in your retirement with old and new friends. *Don't wait until you need a friend to be a friend!*

• One way to stay in medicine at least partway is to get involved with fellow medical retirees in an emeritus quarters (this isn't the same as an alumni quarters). If your medical center doesn't have such an area, ask your administrators to find a place where retirees can meet and have their own space with file drawers and computers. If this isn't possible, ask for a room with several computers available to all emeriti. Inquire about secretarial support.

• You can maintain your CME and stay in touch with medicine by attending educational conferences or your division's education meetings.

• Finally, another way to maintain collegiality is to have lunch once a week (or at least once a month) with fellow retirees from the same division or department and/or any other medical friends. Limit the lunch group to eight or nine so everyone can fit around the table. If possible, find a restaurant with a small meeting room since some retirees may be hard of hearing—meeting in a noisy place will defeat the purpose of being able to hear everyone at the table and not just the people sitting nearby. These meetings can be very therapeutic. Another option is for group members to invite their spouses to join them at a monthly dinner at a restaurant that has a quiet meeting room.

The choice of food and method of payment could be worked out ahead of each meal. One addition to these monthly meetings could be a twenty- to thirty-minute slide show on a hobby, travel, etc. But don't include anything medical-related routinely unless those in attendance request it.

Chapter Sixteen

Women in Medicine

Adamarie Multari, MD

In 1849, Elizabeth Blackwell became the first woman to receive a medical degree in the United States. In her book *Pioneer Work in Opening the Medical Profession to Women,* published in 1895, she reported that what helped motivate her to become the first woman in America to earn a medical degree was a dying friend who said, "You are fond of study, have health and leisure; why not study medicine? If I could have been treated by a lady doctor, my worst sufferings would have been spared me."

Blackwell was a visionary. She and others established one of the first infirmaries for women and children in New York City. The facility was operated by women and also provided clinical training for women.

Throughout history, women have been portrayed as healers. They bring forth life. They care for their children, families, and communities. Many healing traditions have been passed down from mother to daughter.

In early Egyptian wall paintings, the goddess Isis is painted "as [a] magical healer, she cured the sick and brought the deceased to life."[1] According to Dr. Marjorie A. Bowman in *Women in Medicine*, discrimination against women in medicine began as early as 1421 "when a petition was presented to King Henry V to prevent women from practicing medicine."[2]

In the 1840s, men continued to dominate the medical profession. Women were restricted from entering some medical schools in the United States. It would take 130 years before laws would be written to lift these restrictions. In 1970, the Assembly of the Association of American Medical

---

[1] Tyldesley, Joyce. "Isis: Egyptian goddess." Britannica.com.
[2] Bowman, Marjorie A., MD, MPA; Erica Frank, MD, MPH; Deborah I. Allen, MD. 2002. *Women in Medicine: Career and Life Management,* 3rd ed. New York: Springer Science+Business Media.

Colleges expressed support for equal rights in the medical field. Soon thereafter, the two laws that specifically ban discrimination on the basis of gender were approved: Title IX of the Education Amendments of 1972 and the Public Health Service Act of 1975.

During the 1970s, American culture was changing, and single-income families were unable to sustain a middle-class living. This economic change mobilized women from the home to the workforce, and their employment numbers in the United States increased dramatically. Women accounted for approximately 30 million employees in 1970, and this increased to 73 million during the years 2006 to 2010.

In the 1970s, the nation saw an increase in women entering and graduating from medical school as their access to medical training increased. In the United States, women represented 9 percent of total medical-school enrollment in 1969, and this increased to 20 percent by 1976. In 2014, the total female medical-school enrollment was up to nearly 50 percent.

Fellow women, we have come a long way!

From 1970 to 1980, more than 20,000 women graduated from medical school in the United States. This was a dramatic increase from the previous forty years (1930 to 1970) when the total number of female medical-school graduates was only 14,000.

In the United States today, female physicians outnumber male physicians in certain specialties: family medicine, pediatrics, psychiatry, and obstetrics and gynecology. However, this mix is changing. I have observed recent increases in women staff and fellows in general, vascular, orthopedic, and cardiothoracic surgery.

During my medical career, I have witnessed many changes in medicine with the most in the last ten years. I began medical school in 1979 and completed my residency in internal medicine in 1986. I spent the majority of my career in academic medicine, and I was privileged to work at the Mayo Clinic in Rochester, Minnesota. I retired from the Division of Executive, Preventive and Aerospace Medicine in 2013. Just like many other physicians in academic medicine, I was involved in teaching and research in addition to working a full clinic schedule. Mayo Clinic physicians are provided many opportunities to pursue personal areas of academic interest. I became involved in the Mayo Breast Diagnostic Clinic at its inception in 1995. I served as an associate editor for the Mayo Clinic Women's Health Letter. I trained many residents and lectured on Communication in Health Care to staff, fellows, residents, and medical students. And in retirement, I continue to teach as a member of the Program in Professionalism and Values faculty.

The Mayo Clinic supports women (and families) in medicine. It has childcare facilities for sick children of employees and backup child daycare. Many of my Mayo colleagues, including both male and female physicians as well as the allied health staff, take advantage of part-time clinical practices to provide a work-life balance that is sustainable.

At the Mayo Clinic, we women have the opportunity to hold high leadership positions, including as chairs of divisions and departments and as members of the Board of Governors. Many women have achieved the academic status of Professor. For the Clinical track, one can be awarded the Distinguished Clinician Award.

I have enjoyed my career in medicine, which I considered very rewarding. I practiced during what I feel was one of the greatest times in the history of medicine. We had time to talk to our patients, time to develop lasting relationships, time to discuss cases with our colleagues, and time to engage in academic discussions.

The physicians of today face many challenges. Today's medicine is fast-paced—there is an explosion of knowledge. I see new staff members choose professions with a single focus, such as adrenal carcinoma, mesothelioma, or melanoma. As I see it, the biggest challenge facing those who come after us is time. Time is needed to build relationships and establish trust in those under our care.

In conclusion, women have a presence in medicine and have made many changes to advance it. Together with our male colleagues, we will face the challenges that are before us. I am hopeful that we remain committed to the values passed down to us by our founding fathers: "The best interest of the patient is the only interest to be considered, and in order that the sick may have the benefit of advancing knowledge, union of forces is necessary," which Dr. William J. Mayo stated in 1910. The foundation of the Mayo Clinic is teamwork, which is defined by the talents of the individual members and not by gender.

For further reading about the history of women in medicine at Mayo Clinic, an outstanding source is the recently published Women of Mayo Clinic: The Founding Generation, *by Virginia M. Wright-Peterson, 2016, Saint Paul, Minnesota: Minnesota Historical Society Press.*

Chapter Seventeen

The Patient-Physician Relationship

Edward C. Rosenow III, MD
J. Keith Mansel, MD
Walter R. Wilson, MD

*For, ultimately, it is our respect for the human soul
that determines the worth of our science.*

—Norman Cousins

How to Be a Patient—the Patient's Half
of the Patient-Physician Partnership

You also might call this **"The Art of Being a Patient."** As physicians, we think we have an obligation to teach our patients how to visit the doctor. Ideally, this would be taught in school health classes, but don't count on that, so it's not really the patients' fault. When patients give an orderly, succinct, well-thought-out presentation that outlines the reasons they have come to the doctor, it can smooth the patient-physician encounter and, ultimately, lead to better patient compliance. It certainly will reduce some physician frustration—it has been shown that not getting the information needed from the patient can sometimes be a source of friction. The history provided by the patient—the "interview"—is perhaps the most important aspect of this encounter.

You, the Patient

Physicians want you, the patient, to understand what information they need and how to present your history without adding extraneous side comments like "I think my problem began the day we went to visit Aunt Minnie, or was it the day before that?" or "Let me think now." In fact, rehearsing your "presentation" either to yourself or with a family member will greatly benefit you and your doctor. It also will help clarify in your own mind what is going on. Then after meeting with the doctor, you will come away with a feeling of some control over your health care and a better feeling overall about the quality of the visit. The physician will see that you are truly interested in your health—sometimes we physicians get the feeling that a patient isn't interested or, at least, not until he/she doesn't seem to be getting better.

Patients should be encouraged in responsible participation!

The day is past when a visit to the doctor could be part social/part "business." The name of the game now is **time**. One of the most common patient complaints is "The doctor never seemed to have enough time to spend with me," followed by "The doctor didn't communicate with me." These two complaints are usually interrelated because there isn't enough time in the ten or fifteen minutes allotted by third-party payers. It greatly improves the efficiency of a visit if you learn how to present a series of related symptoms in the order they occurred.

When you go to the doctor with a complaint that doesn't have clear meaning to you and you want some relief and reassurance, you need to plan ahead (we're not talking about routine visits for test results or a blood pressure or blood sugar check). Before the visit, think about why you are going and your expectations for the appointment. Write down a list of your concerns. Some patients tend to put their most important concern part way down the list or save it until last! **It should be first**. Your information should include a time sequence of events—sort of a diary in a nonsentence format.

Once you are in the doctor's office, it is almost too late to try to sort out a complicated problem. Too often, the spouse (usually the wife) will pop up and say, "You've got it all wrong. Your abdominal pain began three weeks ago and your fever one week ago, and you did have chills!" You should never have to turn to your spouse (in our experiences, again, it was almost always the husband turning to the wife) and ask, "Where was my chest pain?" Or "How long did it last?" Or "Was it sharp or dull?" We are firm believers that it is the patient's—and only the patient's—responsibility to know his/her medical history unless he/she is incompetent. *You* should know where you felt the chest pain, how long it lasted, the nature of it, and if there were any precipitating factors, such as exercise, etc.! You must take control of your health, which includes being involved in major decisions. This is *patient autonomy*—ownership of your health.

One aspect of this ownership is knowing when to apply an appropriate amount of assertiveness. But you must approach the patient-doctor interaction with an open mind and not come to an appointment having already decided what is wrong with you and what is to be done about it.

You should have straightforward answers to all of your doctor's questions. It will be more difficult for him/her to help if you say, "Well, let me see now, I'm not sure what came first," or "I don't remember if I was short of breath with the chest pain or not." "I'm trying to think; did the symptoms occur before or after eating?" or "I don't know what medicines I'm on. I've been to so many different doctors!" The physician isn't a magician, and if it takes many minutes to sort this out in an allotted ten-minute office visit, extremely valuable time has been lost. Meanwhile, the patients in the waiting room are wondering, again, why they have to wait for the doctor—just as you have many times in the past!

Most of this chapter will help you prepare for a doctor visit when you have a problem you wish to address with a physician, as opposed to a "routine" office visit, such as for a blood pressure check, blood test, or prescription refill. If in doubt, come prepared!

Another problem that physicians encounter is some patients' perception of time. We might ask you when your pain began and how long it lasted—we want to know in terms of seconds, minutes, hours, days, weeks, months, and years! If you answer, "A while back," "Some time ago," "A while ago," or "Not very long ago," this doesn't mean anything to us. If you don't have the specifics available in your mind and on paper, it only slows down the interview. You need to think this out ahead of time and write it down. If you aren't organized with your thoughts and it takes too much time to sort through the information, you may need another appointment to continue the conversation.

While your doctor is examining you, it is important to be silent except to answer questions, but do wait until after he/she is done taking your blood pressure or listening to your heart or lungs with a stethoscope.

If you have medical records from other physicians, bring them in, preferably in chronological order. *Bring in all your medications in their original bottles, including over-the-counter (OTC) medications, herbal medicines, and eye drops.* (You don't need to bring these if you were in the doctor's office recently for similar problems, and no new medications have been added or deleted in the interval.) Do bring along any drugs you received from other physicians. You also should keep a list of your medications in your purse or wallet (or on your smartphone), and update the list as needed. Medical complications caused by prescription and OTC drugs, including medication interactions, are some of the most serious problems we (the patient and the physician) face. Just because a drug is heavily advertised doesn't necessarily mean it is any better than a less expensive, safer drug. Also, do not think that OTC drugs and herbal medicines are always safe just because you don't need a doctor's prescription to get them.

Use caution when asking for (demanding?) certain tests or drugs that your doctor feels are unnecessary. Physicians usually can tell which drugs have been blitz advertised on TV. Members of the medical community currently are greatly concerned about the overuse of antibiotics because we believe this overuse is causing a dramatic rise in antibiotic-resistant bacteria—and we have no alternative antibiotics. The usual antibiotics do not work on viruses, such as the common cold. But many busy physicians find it easier to prescribe an antibiotic rather than argue with a patient who demands one.

Please keep your doctor's phone number handy in case you need to reschedule or cancel your appointment. You wouldn't think of being a "no-show" at any other appointment. Being a "no-show" is not only disrespectful to the physician's practice but also to the sick patient who can't get in because you haven't canceled. So if you need to reschedule, make the call. This is common courtesy.

After your appointment, take your medicine as prescribed and for the full course. If you can't afford a medication, tell your pharmacist and your doctor because there may be a less expensive alternative or a way of getting it from the manufacturer.

The patient (you) should not offer a diagnosis with the symptoms as this confuses things. However, your doctor should ask you what you think if he/she isn't sure what is going on after the initial visit.

Eventually, at least 25 percent of the population will be significantly depressed; it can manifest different ways over and above feeling sad. Depression might be the cause of insomnia, back or abdominal pain, headaches, loss of interest in socializing, and many more symptoms. The patient is looking for a socially "acceptable" disease (cause of symptoms) and then a pill for an immediate cure. If there is the slightest chance you could be depressed, mention this to your physician. Many physicians are reluctant to "unmask" a depression because it can be very time-consuming if you are trying to avoid admitting to it. However, if you are depressed and it is diagnosed and treated sooner rather than later, you will ultimately save hours of time in office visits and probably many tests.

In the "old days," the diagnosis of a mental illness carried tremendous stigma—especially for men whose macho image couldn't handle it. In those "old days," most patients who received this diagnosis were referred to a psychiatrist, and patients had the mental image of being in a locked ward or of spending time on a couch talking about their childhoods. Nowadays, medications for most depressions are very effective and usually only needed for six to twelve months—not a lifetime. Ask yourself, "Are my symptoms possibly due to depression?" You don't need a reason to be depressed. Depression results from a chemical change in the brain. Don't fight it! Also, on a ranking of 1 to 10, estimate your stress level, keeping in mind that just about everyone has some stress.

We know that your time can be as valuable as the doctor's. Most physicians try to stay on time for your sake, but you also know that acute illnesses don't follow a clock (and babies come when they want to). You also know that your doctor may not be able to squeeze you in on a particular day unless openings are built into the schedule. (But appointment coordinators who work for busy and popular physicians may not build in those openings.) And if they do work in more patients, the physician may be delayed in getting to you.

Remember that you aren't the physician's only patient, and on some days, he/she sees numerous patients with very challenging medical—as well as social and mental—problems. These visits are difficult, if not impossible, to handle in the ten, fifteen, or twenty minutes allotted. You may need to return for a follow-up visit if your problem is challenging.

Third-party payers reimburse only a finite amount per standard office visit, which results in the time constraints. Physicians have tremendous office and professional overhead. Time constraints and other challenges are very stressful to physicians, especially compassionate physicians who carry many of these burdens on their shoulders and take them home. Too much stress on a physician leads to burnout—a big problem.

These reasons and more demonstrate the importance of making the visit with your physician as smooth and "businesslike" as possible—but not so businesslike that it discourages bonding.

You need to be aware that the physician's time is increasingly consumed by paperwork, meetings devoted to learning how to conform to federal regulations, getting permissions from insurance companies (sometimes this means that permissions are granted by employees who have little or no training in health-care delivery) for more tests or referrals for a patient, and answering frustrated patients who want to bypass an office visit and do medicine only by phone or email. This results in physicians having less time for their families, exercise, hobbies, and other diversions, and also for keeping up with the Science of Medicine at conferences and/or by reading medical literature. These pressures are causing physicians to retire "prematurely" or go into administration, which leaves less experienced physicians in the practice of medicine.

Physicians can get frustrated by patients who have unrealistic expectations about what the physician or the Science of Medicine can do because of what they have seen or heard in the media. When a report comes out stating that there may be a cure for cancer, the news reporter may not mention that it might be another ten years before it is available. Or too often, patients expect that their doctors will straighten everything out after they have abused themselves by not exercising, not controlling their weight, smoking, and/or not taking their medications.

We mention this because as a partner in your care, you need to know some of what is happening on the other side. We always have felt that our best allies are our patients—well-informed patients. The third-party payers and government health administrators rarely do anything to make the patient-physician encounter more precious. They are only interested in the bottom line.

When your doctor returns your phone call, know exactly what you want answered. This is not the time to ask about your sister-in-law's or your neighbor's symptoms. The doctor may have ten or more calls to make, and it is 6:00 p.m.

You, the patient, may not realize that it is almost as important for the physician to establish some trust with you, just as you do with the physician. If the physician can't trust that you are interested in getting better, are honest with the facts, and are complying with recommendations, he/she loses some—and maybe total—interest. The mutual trust will be gone. In fact, a physician's overall feeling of satisfaction correlates with patients' adherence to his/her recommendations, as well as with patients' satisfaction with their care.

Studies show that the patient-physician relationship is most consistently reported as the main determinant of physician satisfaction!

Listen to the physician. We've observed many patients not listening to a thing being said, and their minds were wandering. In fact, they may have interrupted with an irrelevant question or statement while we were trying to explain something, give instructions on how to take a medication, or take care of their problem. They weren't being rude, but they weren't concentrating on what could have been a very important part of their visit. No wonder these people don't get better. You, the patient, need to be a part of the decision-making and the treatment plan.

None of us will live forever, and although we may not like to think or talk about it, it is very appropriate to do so well before the end is near. You should talk about this with your doctor after you have completed an Advance Directive (Living Will or Durable Power of Attorney) or designated someone, preferably in writing, as your proxy to make end-of-life decisions should you become incapacitated *(see Chapter 14)*. You need to be aware of end-of-life options that range from doing everything heroic to maintain life to just comfort care. In the 1990s and 2000s, the Terri Schiavo case in Florida brought all this out in a terribly agonizing way.

Talk to your doctor about what you've put in your Advance Directive, and you should have some reassurance that he/she will try to carry out your and your family's wishes during a difficult time. Leave a copy with your doctor, and give copies to your children after you have discussed it with them and are sure they are in agreement. But, at any time, you may change your mind about what is in your Advance Directive. However, if you wait until you are near death, it may be difficult to arrive at meaningful decisions that will make it easier on you and your family, as well as on your doctor who, unless otherwise directed by you, will tend toward performing heroic measures. You also should discuss costs (when known) with your physician.

Have your Advance Directive available to take to the hospital should you become acutely ill or when you are having an elective surgical procedure. You also should travel with a copy. The right age to write your initial Advance Directive is eighteen. It should be updated every five to ten years depending on your overall health.

There is no such thing as a "death squad" and never will be.

Keep your health records, including a copy of your Advance Directive, in a folder, on your computer, or in a notebook. Get copies of your laboratory test results and x-ray and pathology reports from your doctor, and file them chronologically (or know how to access them online). These medical records belong to you to keep according to the law. If you see a consulting physician who sends a report to your primary care doctor, ask for a copy. If you fill out forms that detail your history, family history, current problems, etc., make copies and file them as well. If your blood relatives have had health problems, record and file that information. This may be very important someday when genetics become a part of everyday medical practice.

You are responsible for your health, in partnership with your doctor. It is the privilege of physicians to help you in every way we can, but we can't do it without you!

By government decree, you must be given the Patient Bill of Rights *(see the end of the chapter)* when you check into a hospital. If you don't receive a copy, ask for one. You also will be asked if you have a Living Will; you don't have to have one, but you must be asked if you do.

It was simpler in the "old days" when patients were discharged from a hospital to go home or to transfer to a hospital nearer to their home or to a nursing home. You, as a patient, would have received instructions verbally and/or in writing regarding diet, exercise, limitations, and when to see your doctor at home, and perhaps you would have received some prescriptions. However, if you, as a patient, are discharged from a hospital today, there likely would be discussions about your medical problems, what to expect regarding your health, who to call with questions or problems, who might call you to follow up, and when to return. You also should expect to receive copies of your medical records to take home, along with copies to give to your family, your home care coordinator (if you wish), and your referring physician. Your home physician will likely receive a copy (and always will if he/she made the referral). You can get a report of your current visit and test results, but if you want copies of previous results, there may be a charge for them.

The importance of doing everything that we, your medical team, and you can do to minimize the likelihood that you will need to return to the hospital cannot be overstated! Medicare officials can penalize a hospital millions of dollars when they deem an unacceptable rate of return of patients for the persistence of or worsening of their disease. Always take your medications as directed.

What questions do you have? Now is the time to ask them.

The Patient Bill of Rights*

The right to ...

◆ respectful and compassionate care regardless of race, color, religion, sex, age, physical or mental impairment, or national origin.

◆ pain and anguish management.

◆ know the names of the physicians responsible for your care. You can have this in writing. You also can have the name(s) of other health-care providers, including nurses and those in supervised training (medical students, residents, and fellows) assisting with your treatment.

◆ understand and agree to the treatment recommended by the physician most responsible for your care.

◆ know the specifics and risks about your treatment or planned procedure.

◆ complete information about your diagnosis, treatment, and prognosis.

◆ have family members and surrogates be kept informed of your status, including the working diagnosis.

◆ make decisions with your health-care team about your health care, which includes the right to accept or refuse medical or surgical treatment. Your physician will tell you your prognosis and consequences if you refuse treatment or a procedure, as permitted by law.

◆ be told immediately of any medical mistake, including what has or hasn't been done and what is needed to correct it (your family members also have this right to be told).

◆ prepare a Durable Power of Attorney or Living Will and to receive written information about these rights.

◆ have your legally authorized representative make health-care decisions for you if you become incompetent according to the law or if your physician decides that you can't understand treatment(s) or procedure(s).

◆ be provided with an interpreter—preferably not a family member or close friend—if you don't speak or understand English.

◆ participate in discussions about any ethical issues affecting your care.

◆ have all your medical records kept confidential and available only to those responsible for your medical care, as well as those authorized by law or those responsible for paying part of or all of your bill.

◆ be informed of clinical research, which may provide you with an investigational drug, device, or other treatment available only through participation in an Institutional Review Board (IRB)-approved clinical research protocol.

◆ express what you think your medical problem is.

◆ examine and receive an explanation of your bill.

◆ be free of restraints imposed for purposes of discipline or convenience and not required to treat medical symptoms.

◆ express concerns about any aspect of your care without fear of retaliation.

* This is an incomplete listing of government-mandated rules for the patient's protection. Patients have access to the complete list from their hospital or physician.

Printed in the United States
By Bookmasters

The
Philosophers

The
Philosophers

The 100 Greatest Thinkers
of All Time

Denise Despeyroux

KONECKY&KONECKY

Konecky & Konecky
72 Ayers Point Rd.
Old Saybrook, CT 06475

Text copyright © 2008, Denise Despeyroux
Copyright © 2008, Editorial Océano, S.L.
English translation copyright © 2014, Sean Konecky

ISBN: 9781568528106

Table of Contents

INTRODUCTION
The Examined Life

All that we are arises with our thoughts
BUDDHA DIAMOND SUTRA

*Beyond its wars and scientific achievement, the history of the West has been
recorded by many great minds who from Ancient Greek times until today have
reflected on the significance of human existence and asked the quetsion, "What is
Reality?"*

Proposed by Lou Marinoff as a therapy, the philosophy of the last
three thousand years gathers the themes that have preoccupied and
still concern human beings. This book pays homage to them; it is a
school of philosophy where the readers will encounter thinkers such as
Plato, Descartes, Schopenhauer, and Russell, to name just a few.

Each philosopher in this anthology puts forth his vision of the world in
two pages. In addition to a brief biography, you'll find a selection of
their most important thoughts in their own words in order to give you
a significant taste of their work, and a select bibliography for those
who wish to learn more and gain a deeper understanding. In total,
there are 100 great thinkers ordered from A to Z for easy reference.

In this one volume, we bring together the most brilliant moments in
the history of thought so that the reader might uncover at his own

pace that which can be personally useful. From the reflections on existence and death, to advice regarding the art of living, *The Philosophers* provides lessons great and small to help us think more deeply about our world and be inspired to improve it.

I hope this book stimulates the most powerful muscle we possess—a thousand times more sophisticated and beneficial than any machine that has ever been created—the human mind.

F.M.

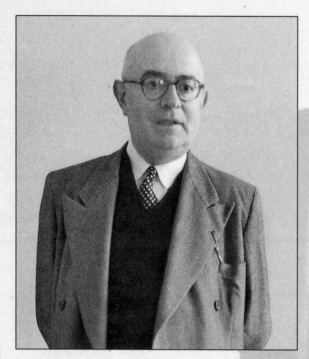

Theodor Adorno

(Frankfurt, Germany, 1903-1969)

Adorno, along with Horkeimer, is considered to be one of the principal representatives of the Frankfurt School. He was a friend and disciple of Walter Benjamin with whom he engaged in a long and fruitful dialogue. He dedicated himself to philosophy, sociology and music theory. One of his most original contributions was his defense of the negative dialectic, which emphasizes the incessant movement of thought in lieu of any definitive conceptualization.

Adorno had to flee the Nazis. In 1941 he moved to California where he joined his old friend and colleague Max Horkheimer. In his *Dialectic of Enlightenment* (written with Horkheimer), he warned that progress, instead of leading toward humanistic goals, threatens to plunge the world into a renewed state of barbarism.

Recommended reading:

📖 📖 📖 *Aesthetic Theory* (1970)

📖 📖 *Negative Dialectics* (1966)

📖 *Minima Moralia* (1951)

"We need to describe the mechanisms that make men capable of committing atrocities, demonstrate to them how they work and how to prevent them from taking hold, while displaying a general awareness of such mechanisms.

We are born with an innate responsibility. We are all heirs to past injustices: some inherit good fortune, others ill.

Fear and destructiveness are the major emotional sources of fascism, eros belongs mainly to democracy.

Writing poetry after Auschwitz is barbaric. And that requires that one know why it is impossible to write poetry today.

When I made my theoretical model, I could not have guessed that people would try to realize it with Molotov cocktails.

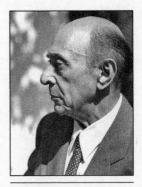

Influenced by Arnold Schönberg (shown above) and Anton Webern, in his philosophical essays on music, Adorno related musical forms to philosophical ideas.

Humanity had to inflict terrible injuries on itself before the self, the identical, purpose-directed, masculine character of human beings was created, and something of this process is repeated in every childhood.

The phrase, "the world wants to be deceived," has become truer than had ever been intended. People are not only, as the saying goes, falling for the swindle; if it guarantees them even the most fleeting gratification they desire a deception which is nonetheless transparent to them. They force their eyes shut and voice approval, in a kind of self-loathing, for what is meted out to them, knowing fully the purpose for which it is manufactured. Without admitting it they sense that their lives would be completely intolerable as soon as they no longer clung to satisfactions which are none at all.

Traditional philosophy's claim to totality, culminating in the thesis that the real is rational, is indistinguishable from apologetics.

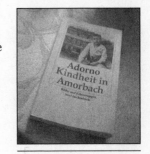

One of the books from the Frankfurt School.

Minima Moralia

Repudiation of the present cultural morass presupposes sufficient involvement in it to feel it itching in one's finger-tips, so to speak, but at the same time the strength, drawn from this involvement, to dismiss it. This strength, though manifesting itself as individual resistance, is by no means of a merely individual nature. In the intellectual conscience possessed of it, the social movement is no less present than the moral super-ego. Such conscience grows out of a conception of the good society and its citizens. If this conception dims—and who could still trust blindly in it—the downward urge of the intellect loses its inhibitions and all the detritus dumped in the individual by barbarous culture—half-learning, slackness, heavy familiarity, coarseness—comes to light.

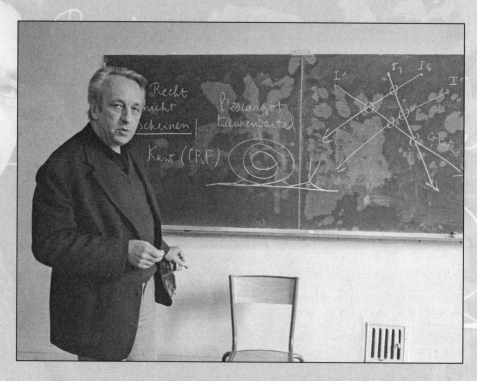

Louis Althusser

(Birmandreis, Algeria, 1918–Paris, France, 1990)

Althusser studied philosophy in Paris and became one of the leading academic thinkers of the French communist party. He fought in World War II, was captured by the German army and spent five years in a concentration camp.

Diagnosed with mental illness, he suffered many psychological problems through the course of his life and was hospitalized more than twenty times.

In 1980 he strangled his wife. He was put on trial but avoided prison for reason of diminished responsibility. The French Right accused the Left of conspiring to keep him out of prison.

Recommended reading:

📖 📖 📖 *Reading Capital* (1965)

📖 📖 *The Future Lasts Forever: A Memoir* (1994)

📖 *The Humanist Controversy and Other Texts* (1966–67)

An idealist is someone who knows from what station a train leaves and what its destination is. He knows this in advance, and when he gets on he knows where it will take him. The materialist, on the other hand, is someone who gets on the train while it is moving without knowing where it's going or where it comes from.

———

If someone were to ask me to state in a few words the essential thesis that Marx attempted to propound in his philosophical works, I would say: Marx founded a new science, the science of History. And I would add: this scientific discovery was an unprecedented theoretical and political event. To be precise: this event is irreversible.

———

Only one expression describes the practice of philosophy. It serves to draw a line of demarcation between true and false ideas.

———

Philosophy struggles with words: it fights against lying and ambiguous ones in favor of correct ones. It is a struggle for clarity.

———

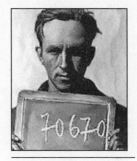

Althusser during his imprisonment in a German concentration camp.

Lenin shows that, 'spontaneously', the proletariat cannot but be influenced by bourgeois ideology, and that Marxism, far from being the subjective theory of the proletariat, is a science that must be taught to the proletariat. Lenin and his followers have often drawn attention to the fact that the proletariat had existed for a very long time, and endured a thousand different ordeals, before assimilating Marxism and accepting it as the science that could account for its condition within the overall framework of capitalist society, securing its future as well as all humanity's. Only later did the proletariat produce, in its class organizations, intellectuals of its own, who developed Marxist theory in their turn.

———

In the battle that is philosophy all the techniques of war, including looting and camouflage, are permissible.

———

One of the goals of philosophy is to wage theoretical battle. That is why we can say that every thesis is always, by its very nature, an antithesis. A thesis is only ever put forward in opposition to another thesis, or in defence of a new one.

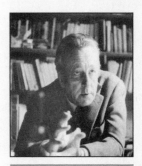

Althusser was a leading figure in post World War II French Communism.

Ideology and Ideological State Apparatuses

I ask the pardon of those teachers who, attempt to turn the few weapons they can find in the history and learning they 'teach' against the ideology, the system and the practices in which they are trapped. But they are rare and how many (the majority) do not even begin to suspect the 'work' the system (which is bigger than they are and crushes them) forces them to do, or worse, put all their heart and ingenuity into performing it with the most advanced awareness. So little do they suspect it that their own devotion contributes to the maintenance and nourishment of this ideological representation of the School, which makes the School today as 'natural', indispensably useful and even beneficial for our contemporaries as the Church was 'natural', indispensable and generous for our ancestors a few centuries ago.

Anaxagoras of Clazomenae

(Clazomenae, Ionia c. 500-Lampsacus, Anatolia c. 428 BCE.)

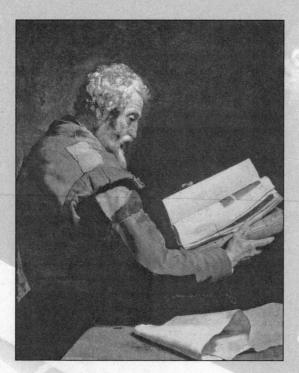

Anaxagoras is reputed to have been the first to bring philosophy to Athens. He was in all likelihood a disciple of Anaximenes, describing himself as such in a work entitled *Peri physeos* of which only fragments remain, quoted in the works of other philosophers.

Anaxagoras introduced the notion of *nous* (mind), as the active intellectual principle. Accused of blasphemy for asserting that the sun is a mass of incandescent metal, he was exiled to Lampsacus in modern-day Turkey, where he is said to have starved to death.

When he received news of the death of his son, he responded: "I know that I have bred mortality." His last words are reported to have been "Everywhere is equidistant from Hades."

Recommended reading:

Diogenes Laertius, *Lives of Eminent Philosophers* (1st century BCE)

Kirk, G.S. and J.E. Raven, *The Presocratic Philosophers* (1987)

Jonathan Barnes, *The Presocratic Philosophers* (1992)

The sun, the moon, and all the stars are merely incandescent rocks.

———

The sun is larger than the Peloponnesus.

———

The Greeks follow a wrong usage in speaking of coming into being and passing away; for nothing comes into being or passes away, but there is mingling and separation of things that are. So they would be right to call coming into being mixture, and passing away separation.

———

All things were together, infinite both in number and in smallness; for the small too was infinite.

———

And since these things are so, we must suppose that there are contained many things and of all sorts in the things that are uniting, seeds of all things, with all sorts of shapes and colors and savors.

———

As regards Anaxagoras, if one were to suppose that he said there were two elements, the supposition would accord thoroughly with a view which Anaxagoras himself did not state articulately, but which he must have accepted if any one had developed his view. (Aristotle, *Metaphysics*)

———

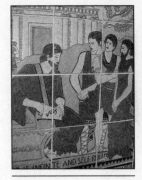

Anaxagoras and his disciples (of whom he had many, some celerbated) Anaxagoras followed Parmenides' teaching in many respects.

Anaxagoras of Clazomenae, who, though older than Empedocles, was later in his philosophical activity, says the principles are infinite in number; for he says almost all the things that are homogeneous are generated and destroyed (as water or fire is) only by aggregation and segregation, and are not in any other sense generated or destroyed, but remain eternally. (Aristotle, *Metaphysics*)

———

Everything has a natural explanation. The moon is not a god, but a great rock, and the sun a hot rock.

———

Appearances are a glimpse of the unseen.

———

Men would live exceedingly quiet if these two words, mine and thine, were taken away.

———

Then, I ween, there is Anaxagoras, a doughty champion, whom they call Mind, because forsooth his was the mind which suddenly woke up and fitted closely together all that had formerly been in a medley of confusion. (Diogenes Laertius, *Lives of Eminent Philosophers*)

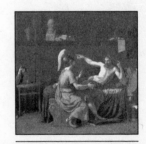

Augustin-Louis Belle, *Anaxagoras and Pericles*

Simplicio, *Physica Ausculatio*

All other things partake in a portion of everything, while *nous* (mind) is infinite and self-ruled, and is mixed with nothing, but is alone, itself by itself. For if it were not by itself, but were mixed with anything else, it would partake in all things if it were mixed with any; for in everything there is a portion of every-thing...and the things mixed with it would hinder it, so that it would have power of nothing in the same way that it has be alone by itself. For it is the thinnest of all things and the purest, and it has all knowledge about everything and the greatest strength; and *nous* has power over all things.

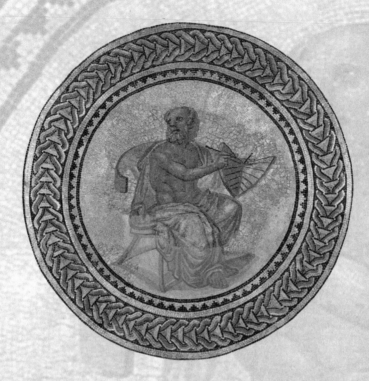

A naximander was a pupil of Thales. His thought comes down to us strictly through the commentaries of other authors. Attributed to him are a book on nature, a map of the world, and a meditation on the solstices and equinoxes.

To the first question that occupied philosophy, what is the principle behind all phenomena, Anaximander put forward the idea of *aperion*, a substance he considered indeterminate, indestructible, unborn, and imperishable.

According to Cicero, Anaximander warned the Spartans of an imminent earthquake and that they needed to leave their homes and get out in the open. "Then the city collapsed around them."

Recommended reading:

Martin Heidigger, " The Anaximander Fragment," from *Early Greek Thinking* (1975)

Kirk, G.S. and J.E. Raven, *The Presocratic Philosophers* (1987)

Jonathan Barnes, *The Presocratic Philosophers* (1992)

Whence things have their origin there they must also pass away according to necessity; for they must pay penalty and be judged for their injustice according to the ordinance of time. (Pseudo-Plutarch)

Anaximander said that the aperion is the cause of the birth and destruction of all things, the origin of the heavens and all the worlds, which are infinite. He affirmed that its destruction and long before that its birth produces the cyclical movement of eternity. (Pseudo-Plutarch)

He declares that what arose from the eternal and is productive of hot and cold was separated off at the coming to be of the cosmos, and a kind of sphere of flame from this grew around the dark mist about the earth like the bark of a tree. When it was broken off and enclosed in certain circles, the sun, moon, and stars came to be. (Pseudo-Plutarch)

The earth's shape is curved, round, like a stone column. (Hippolytus)

Anaximander says there is a circle 28 times the earth, like a chariot wheel, with its rim hollow and full of fire. It lets the fire appear through an orifice at one point, as through the nozzle of a bellows; and this is the sun. (Aetius)

Anaximander...believed that there arose from heated water and earth either fish or animals very like fish. In these humans grew and were kept inside as embryos until puberty. Then finally they burst, and men and women came forth already able to nourish themselves. (Censorinus)

The earth is in mid-air not controlled by anything, but staying put because of its distance from all things.

Anaximander related everything to wind; he said that thunder is noise produced by wind striking clouds. (Aecio)

Anaximander the Milesian, affirmed the infinite to be the first principle, and that all things are generated out of it, and corrupted again into it. His infinite is nothing else but matter. (Plutarch)

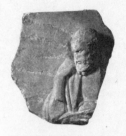

One of the few images of Anaximader of Miletus that still exists.

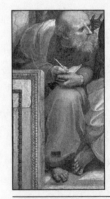

Depiction of Anaximader in Raphael's *The School of Athens,* 1509–1510 (Vatican Museum)

Wherefore they (the Syrians) reverence the fish as of the same origin and the same family as man, holding a more reasonable philosophy than that of Anaximander; for he declares, not that fishes and men were generated at the same time, but that at first men were generated in the form of fishes, and that growing up as sharks do till they were able to help themselves, they then came forth on the dry ground.

Anaximenes of Miletus

(Miletus, Asia Minor c. 585–524 BCE.)

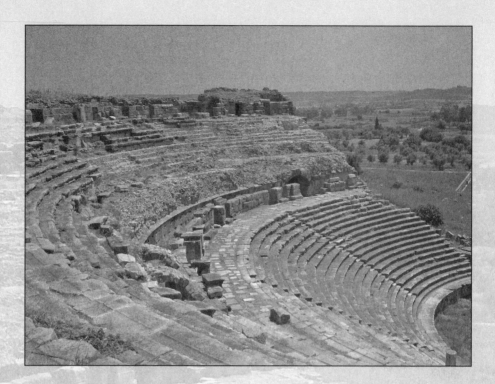

Anaximenes was a disciple of Anaximander and, according to some, of Parmenides as well. He agreed with his master that the first principle of all things is infinite, but he thought that it was a single element: air. He explained its transformation into other phenomena through the processes of rarefaction and condensation.

He composed one work entitled *Peri Physeos* (Discourse on Nature), which has not survived. Diogenes Laertius quotes from it in his *Lives of Eminent Philosophers*.

According to Pliny the Elder's *Natural History*, Anaximenes was the first to design a sundial using shadows to measure the passage of time.

Recommended reading:

Diogenes Laertius, *Lives of Eminent Philosophers* (1st century BCE)

Kirk, G.S. and J.E. Raven, *The Presocratic Philosophers* (1987)

Jonathan Barnes, *The Presocratic Philosophers* (1992)

Anaximenes...declared that air is the principle of existing things; for from it all things come-to-be and into it they are again dissolved. As our soul, he says, being air holds us together and controls us, so does wind [or breath] and air enclose the whole world. (Aetius)

Anaximenes of Miletos, son of Eurystratos, a companion of Anaximander, agrees with him that the essential nature of things is one and infinite, but he regards it as not indeterminate but rather determinate, and calls it air; the air differs in rarity and in density as the nature of things is different; when very attenuated it becomes fire, when more condensed wind, and then cloud, and when still more condensed water and earth and stone, and all other things are composed of these; and he regards motion as eternal, and by this changes are produced. (Theophrastus)

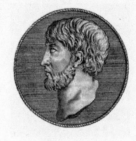

Some say that the universe always existed, not that it has always been the same, but rather that it successively changes its character in certain periods of time; as, for instance, Anaximenes and Heracleitus and Diogenes. (Simplicius)

Anaximenes of Miletus. The preceding page shows the ruins of the Greek theater in Miletus.

Anaximenes son of Eurystratus, of Miletus, was a pupil of Anaximander; some say he was also a pupil of Parmenides. He said that the material principle was air and the infinite; and that the stars move, not under the earth, but round it. He used simple and economical Ionic speech. He was active, according to what Apollodorus says, around the time of the capture of Sardis, and died in the 63rd Olympiad. (Diogenes Laertius)

Anaximenes determined that the air is a god and that it comes to be and is without measure, infinite and always in motion. (Cicero)

And the form of the air is as follows. Where it is most even, it is invisible to our sight; but cold and heat, moisture and motion, make it visible. It is always in motion; for if it were not it would not change so much as it does. (Hippolytus)

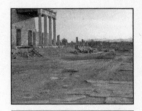

The agora in Miletus.

Winds are produced when condensed air rushes into rarefied; but when it is concentrated and thickened still more, clouds are generated; and lastly, it turns to water. (Hippolytus)

■ **Pseudo-Plutarch,** *The Doctrines of the Philosophers*

The sun, the moon, and other heavenly bodies are supported by the air...The heavenly bodies were produced from the earth from moisture rising from it. When this is rarefied fire comes into being and the stars are composed of fire raised aloft. There were also bodies of earthy substance in the region of the stars, revolving along with them. And he says that heavenly bodies do not move under the earth, as others suppose, but round it, as a cap turns around our head. The sun is hidden from sight, not because it goes under the earth, but because it is concealed by the higher parts of the earth.

Hannah Arendt

(Hanover, Germany, 1906–New York City, U.S.A., 1975)

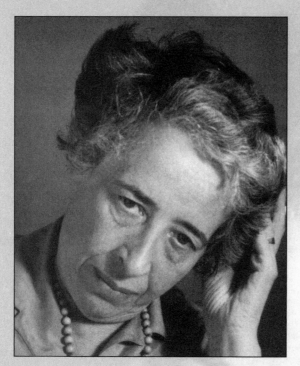

Born to a middle-class Jewish family, early on Arendt demonstrated intellectual brilliance and a love of philosophy. She attended the University of Marburg, where she studied under Martin Heidegger and soon became his secret lover.

The difficulties in continuing an adulterous affair (Heidegger was married with children) combined with the growing power of National Socialism, convinced her break off with her lover and mentor, and move, first to France and then to the United States.

In 1950 Arendt became a U.S. citizen. She considered herself a political theorist rather than a philosopher. Her works addressed themes such as political power, authority, and totalitarianism.

Recommended reading:

The Human Condition (1958)

Eichmann in Jerusalem: A Report on the Banality of Evil (1963)

The Origins of Totalitarianism (1951)

The sad truth is that most evil is done by people who never make up their minds to be good or evil.

When all are guilty, no one is; confessions of collective guilt are the best possible safeguard against the discovery of culprits, and the very magnitude of the crime the best excuse for doing nothing.

Man cannot be free if he does not know that he is subject to necessity, because his freedom is always won in his never wholly successful attempts to liberate himself from necessity.

Clichés, stock phrases, adherence to conventional, standardized codes of expression and conduct have the socially recognized function of protecting us against reality.

In solitude a dialogue always arises, because even in solitude there are always two.

Living beings, men and animals, are not just in the world, they are of the world, and this precisely because they are subjects and objects—perceiving and being perceived—at the same time.

No human life, not even the life of the hermit in nature's wilderness, is possible without a world which directly or indirectly testifies to the presence of other human beings.

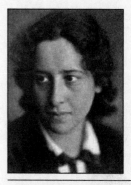

The totalitarian attempt at global conquest and total domination has been the destructive way out of all impasses. Its victory may coincide with the destruction of humanity; wherever it has ruled, it has begun to destroy the essence of man....And if it is true that in the final stages of totalitarianism an absolute evil appears (absolute because it can no longer be deduced from humanly comprehensible motives), it is also true that without it we might never have known the truly radical nature of Evil.

Hannah Arendt in 1928. In her work Arendt examined the nature of power and investigated themes such as politics, authority, and totalitarianism. A major preoccupation was the consideration of the Holocaust. Her subtle analysis of society as a humanly created environment earned her a place in the first rank of twentieth-century thinkers. Her coverage of the Eichmann trial stands as a powerful meditation on the nature of evil.

Eichmann in Jerusalem

The trouble with Eichmann was precisely that so many were like him, and that the many were neither perverted nor sadistic, that they were and still are, terribly and terrifyingly normal. From the viewpoint of our legal institutions and of our moral standards of judgment this normality was much more terrifying than all the atrocities put together for it implied—as had been said at Nuremberg over and over again by the defendants and their counsels—that this new type of criminal, who is in actual fact *hostis generis humani*, [an enemy to humanity] commits his crime—under circumstances that make it well-nigh impossible for him to know or to feel that he is doing wrong.

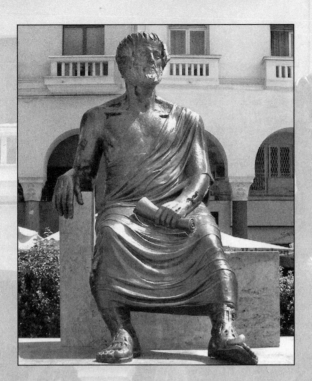

Aristotle

(Stagirus, Macedonia, 384–Chalcis, Eubea, 322 BCE)

Aristotle was a student at Plato's Academy. He spent the greater part of his life in Athens, where he founded the Lyceum, a school dedicated to philosophical pursuits.

Aristotle's oeuvre is vast and his surviving works, which are not dated, were destined for a very restricted audience. They include treatises on logic, physics, metaphysics, ethics, politics, rhetoric, and poetry. His division of all of knowledge into three categories—theoretical, practical and poetic—endured for centuries.

His philosophy superceded the monism of Parmenides and Platonic dualism. He bequeathed to succeeding generations the notion of man as a unitary being.

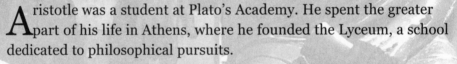

Recommended reading:

Metaphysics

Politics
The Nicomachean Ethics

Poetics

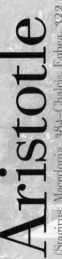

Knowing yourself is the beginning of all wisdom.

I count him braver who overcomes his desires than him who conquers his enemies, for the hardest victory is over self.

The whole is greater than the sum of its parts.

Man is by nature a social animal; an individual who is unsocial naturally and not accidentally is either beneath our notice or more than human. Society is something that precedes the individual. Anyone who either cannot lead the common life or is so self-sufficient as not to need to, and therefore does not partake of society, is either a beast or a god.

Learning is an ornament in prosperity, a refuge in adversity, and a provision in old age.

Fear is pain arising from the anticipation of evil.

The only stable state is the one in which all men are equal before the law.

Poetry is finer and more philosophical than history; for poetry expresses the universal, and history only the particular.

The gods too are fond of a joke.

Plot is character revealed by action.

Man is by nature a political animal.

If you would understand anything, observe its beginning and its development.

The aim of art is to represent not the outward appearance of things, but their inward significance.

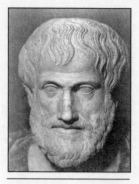

Aristotle's work was the precursor of the sciences of anatomy and biology. He was the first to create a taxonomy.

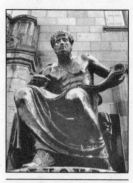

Aristotle was one of the greatest Western philosophers. He was the father of scientific study and academic rigor. Statue from Freiburg, Germany.

Preceding page: Statue of Aristotle from Thessalonica, Greece.

Nicomachean Ethics

By a passion or emotion we mean appetite, anger, fear, confidence, envy, love, joy, hate, longing, emulation, pity, or generally that which is accompanied by pleasure or pain; a power or faculty is that in respect of which we are said to be capable of being affected in any of these ways, as, for instance, that in respect of which we are able to be angered or pained or to pity; and a habit or trained faculty is that in respect of which we are well or ill regulated or disposed in the matter of our affections.

Augustine of Hippo
(Thagaste, Roman Africa, 354–Hippo, Roman Africa, 430)

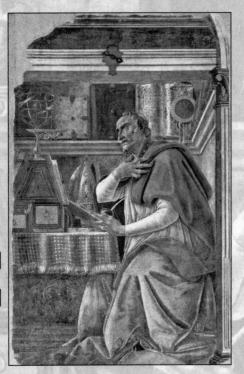

Philosopher and theologian, Aurelius Augustine is better known as Augustine of Hippo or Saint Augustine. His life was governed by his ardent search for the truth. Before his conversion to Christianity he was drawn to various philosophical schools of his time.

Augustine lived in a time of great instability that witnessed the dissolution of Roman hegemony. He made use of Platonism to support and articulate Christian dogma, transmitting Greek ideas to the culture of the Middle Ages.

His powerful body of work, written in Latin, was the vehicle through which early Christianity was able to maintain a vital connection to Greek thought. Augustine enunciated the idea of "original sin."

Recommended reading:

Confessions (397-400)

The City of God (413-426)

Letters (386-430)

Give me chastity and continence, just not yet.

Love, and do what you will. If you keep silence, do it out of love. If you cry out, do it out of love. If you refrain from punishing, do it out of love.

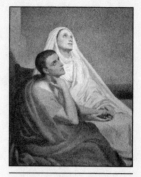

To love without measure is the measure of love.

There can only be two basic loves...the love of God unto the forgetfulness of self, or the love of self unto the forgetfulness and denial of God.

Where your pleasure is, there is your treasure; where your treasure, there your heart; where your heart, there your happiness.

Saint Monica with Saint Augustine, who is considered as one of the four doctors of the Catholic Church.

Have I spoken of God, or uttered His praise, in any worthy way? Nay, I feel that I have done nothing more than desire to speak; and if I have said anything, it is not what I desired to say. How do I know this, except from the fact that God is unspeakable?

Miracles are not contrary to nature, but only contrary to what we know about nature.

I have read in Plato and Cicero sayings that are wise and very beautiful; but I have never read in either of them: Come unto me all ye that labor and are heavy laden.

I was in misery, and misery is the state of every soul overcome by friendship with mortal things and lacerated when they are lost. Then the soul becomes aware of the misery which is its actual condition even before it loses them.

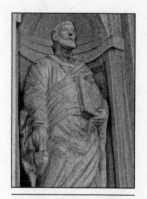

No one knows what he himself is made of, except his own spirit within him, yet there is still some part of him which remains hidden even from his own spirit; but you, Lord, know everything about a human being because you have made him...Let me, then, confess what I know about myself, and confess too what I do not know, because what I know of myself I know only because you shed light on me, and what I do not know I shall remain ignorant about until my darkness becomes like bright noon before your face.

Philosopher and Catholic thinker, Saint Augustine was one of the most important figures in Western Christianity. The statue shown here is from Manila in the Philippines.

Confessions

For what is more miserable than a miserable being who commiserates not himself; weeping the death of Dido for love to Aeneas, but weeping not his own death for want of love to Thee, O God. Thou light of my heart, Thou bread of my inmost soul, Thou Power who givest vigour to my mind, who quickenest my thoughts, I loved Thee not. I committed fornication against Thee, and all around me thus fornicating there echoed "Well done! well done!" for the friendship of this world is fornication against Thee; and "Well done! well done!" echoes on till one is ashamed to be thus a man.

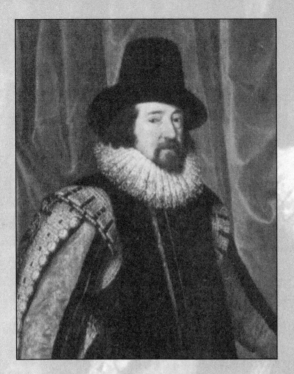

Francis Bacon

(London, England, 1561-1626)

Philosopher and politician, Bacon studied at Cambridge before traveling to Paris as attaché to the English ambassador. Returning to England at the age of eighteen he entered into a career in law and politics. He was elected to Parliament and became the confidant of Queen Elizabeth's favorite Robert Devereaux, Earl of Essex.

Elizabeth's successor, James I, appointed him Attorney General and then in 1618, Lord Chancellor. He published his masterwork, *Novum Organum,* in 1620. Two years later he was forced to stand trial on charges of corruption. He retired from public life and spent his remaining years devoted to study. A year before his death he completed the third edition of his *Essays.*

Recommended reading:

    Novum Organum (1620)

    Essays (1625)

    The New Atlantis (1627)

I confess that I have as vast contemplative ends, as I have moderate civil ends: for I have taken all knowledge to be my province....I hope I should bring in industrious observations, grounded conclusions, and profitable inventions and discoveries; the best state of that province.

Nothing is terrible except fear itself.

Hope is a good breakfast but a bad supper.

Knowledge is power.

Riches are a good handmaid, but the worst mistress.

God has placed no limits to the exercise of the intellect he has given us, on this side of the grave.

The greatest error of all the rest is the mistaking or misplacing of the last or farthest end of knowledge: for men have entered into a desire of learning and knowledge, sometimes upon a natural curiosity and inquisitive appetite; sometimes to entertain their minds with variety and delight; sometimes for ornament and reputation; and sometimes to enable them to victory of wit and contradiction; and most times for lucre and profession; and seldom sincerely to give a true account of their gift of reason, to the benefit and use of men.

Seek first for virtue; everything else will come or not be missed.

They that will not apply new remedies must expect new evils.

A little philosophy inclines man's mind to atheism, but depth in philosophy brings men's minds about to religion.

It is impossible to love and to be wise.

Imagination was given to man to compensate him for what he is not; a sense of humor to console him for what he is.

If we are to achieve things never before accomplished we must employ methods never before attempted.

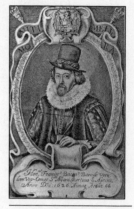

Bacon's pioneering philosophy included the idea that man is both subservient to and an interpreter of nature, that the truth does not derive from authority, and that knowledge is first of all the fruit of experience.

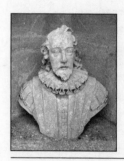

His *Novum Organum* was widely influential in its presentations of a scientific method of observation and experimentation.

Novum Organum

There are and can be only two ways of searching into and discovering truth. The one flies from the senses and particulars to the most general axioms, and from these principles, the truth of which it takes for settled and immovable, proceeds to judgment and to the discovery of middle axioms. And this way is now in fashion. The other derives axioms from the senses and particulars, rising by a gradual and unbroken ascent, so that it arrives at the most general axioms last of all. This is the true way, but as yet untried.

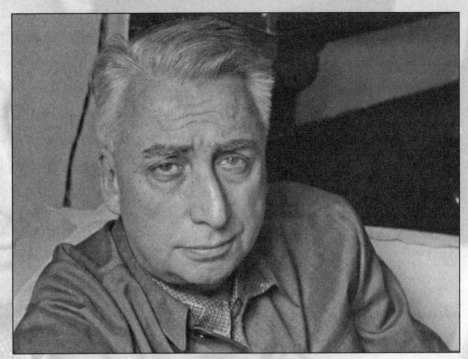

Roland Barthes

(Cherbourg, France, 1915–Paris, 1980)

Barthes studied at the Sorbonne where he received his degree in Classical languages. His work encompassed the fields of philosophy, literary criticism, communication and sociology. He is recognized as one of the most significant figures in French intellectual life in the twentieth century.

Barthes was one of the key representatives of poststructuralism and a critical voice in the development of semiotics. He was hit by a laundry van while returning from a dinner with French president, François Mitterand, and died a month later. In a sad irony this recalled the words of his friend Tzvetan Todorov: "I will die like a child, while crossing the street."

Recommended reading:

    Mythologies (1957)

    Writing Degree Zero (1967)
    S/Z (1970)

    The Camera Lucida (1980)

Am I in love?—yes, since I am waiting. The other one never waits. Sometimes I want to play the part of the one who doesn't wait; I try to busy myself elsewhere, to arrive late; but I always lose at this game. Whatever I do, I find myself there, with nothing to do, punctual, even ahead of time. The lover's fatal identity is precisely this: I am the one who waits.

———

Language is a skin: I rub my language against the other. It is as if I had words instead of fingers, or fingers at the tip of my words. My language trembles with desire.

———

What the Photograph reproduces to infinity has occurred only once: the Photograph mechanically repeats what could never be repeated existentially.

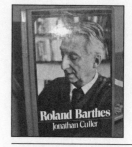

———

What I claim is to live to the full the contradiction of my time, which may well make sarcasm the condition of truth.

———

What the public wants is the image of passion, not passion itself.

Roland Barthes can be viewed as the originating spirit of semiotics. He was the author of a wholly original work of literary criticism, *S/Z*.

———

The politician being interviewed clearly takes a great deal of trouble to imagine an ending to his sentence: and if he stopped short? His entire policy would be jeopardized!

———

Language is legislation, speech is its code. We do not see the power which is in speech because we forget that all speech is classification, and that all classifications are oppressive.

———

I think that cars today are almost the exact equivalence of the great Gothic cathedrals: I mean the supreme creation of an era, conceived with passion by unknown artists, and consumed in image if not in usage by a whole population which appropriates them as a purely magical object.

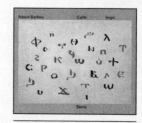

———

Ultimately—or at the limit—in order to see a photograph well, it is best to look away or close your eyes. "The necessary condition for an image is sight," Janouch told Kafka; and Kafka smiled and replied: "We photograph things in order to drive them out of our minds. My stories are a way of shutting my eyes."

This gouache created by Barthes exemplifies his semiotic discourse.

The Text is plural. Which is not simply to say that it has several meanings, but that it accomplishes the very plural of meaning: an irreducible (and not merely an acceptable) plural. The Text is not a co-existence of meanings but a passage, an overcrossing; thus it answers not to an interpretation, even a liberal one, but to an explosion, a dissemination.

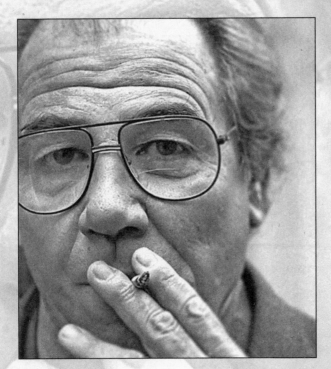

Jean Baudrillard
(Reims, France, 1929–París, 2007)

The work of this French philosopher is dedicated to the analysis of contemporary society. After his early texts, which were marked with the influence of structuralism, he denounced the process of dematerialization of reality, which, according to him, characterizes Western society.

Baudrillard notes that the gaze of modern man is fixed on television screens and communication has become an end in itself, an absolute value. Myth and its purposes have been discarded and the excess of information obstructs the search for meaning. Authenticity has been replaced by its simulacrum, nothing is real, and those involved in the illusion are unable to see it.

Recommended reading:

Fatal Strategies (1983)

The Transparency of Evil (1990)
Seduction (1979)

The Gulf War Did Not Take Place (1991)

The end of history is, alas, also the end of the dustbins of history. There are no longer any dustbins for disposing of old ideologies, old regimes, old values. Where are we going to throw Marxism, which actually invented the dustbins of history? (Yet there is some justice here since the very people who invented them have fallen in.) Conclusion: if there are no more dustbins of history, this is because History itself has become a dustbin. It has become its own dustbin, just as the planet itself is becoming its own dustbin.

It is always the same: once you are liberated, you are forced to ask who you are.

The sad thing about artificial intelligence is that it lacks artifice and therefore intelligence.

In addition, due to their omnipresence, due to the prevailing rule of the world of making everything visible, the images, our present-day images, have become substantially pornographic. Spontaneously, they embrace the pornographic face of the war.

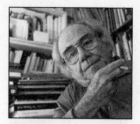

Even objective reality becomes a useless function, a kind of trash, the exchange and circulation of which has become more and more difficult. We have moved past objective reality into something new, a kind of ultra reality that puts an end both to reality and to illusion.

This retrospective compassion, this conversion of evil into misfortune, is the twentieth century's finest industry.

Television knows no night. It is perpetual day. TV embodies our fear of the dark, of night, of the other side of things.

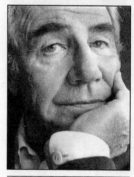

Governing today means giving acceptable signs of credibility. It is like advertising and it is the same effect that is achieved—commitment to a scenario.

Cowardice and courage are never without a measure of affectation. Nor is love. Feelings are never true. They play with their mirrors.

Philosopher and social critic, Baudrillard analyzed the "culture of the simulacrum," which he called "hyperreality." Baudrillard was a mong the most signicant of the postmodernist thinkers.

The Spirit of Terrorism

This is not a clash of civilizations or religions, and it reaches far beyond Islam and America, on which efforts are being made to focus the conflict in order to create the delusion of a visible confrontation and a solution based upon force. There is indeed a fundamental antagonism here, but one that points past the specter of America (which is perhaps the epicenter, but in no sense the sole embodiment, of globalization) and the specter of Islam (which is not the embodiment of terrorism either) to triumphant globalization battling against itself.

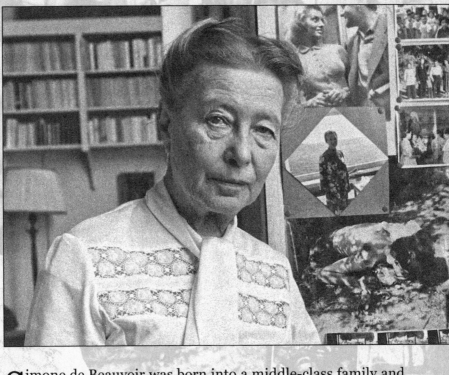

Simone de Beauvoir

(París, France, 1908-1986)

Simone de Beauvoir was born into a middle-class family and schooled according to strict Christian morality. However, early on she turned her back on the values she was brought up on.

She studied philosophy at the Sorbonne where she met Sartre and became his lover. She spent most of her life deeply involved with philosophy and the French intelligentsia. During the Second World War, however, she abandoned intellectual pursuits to become active in the French resistance against German occupation.

Her novels and essays are powerful meditations on existentialist ideas about liberty, action, and responsibility.

Recommended reading:

The Second Sex (1949)

The Mandarins (1954)

Adieux: A Farewell to Sartre (1981)

Representation of the world, like the world itself, is the work of men; they describe it from their own point of view, which they confuse with the absolute truth.

One is not born a woman but becomes one.

A woman's situation, i.e., those meanings derived from the total context in which she comes to maturity, disposes her to apprehend her body not as instrument of her transcendence, but an object destined for another.

Man is defined as a human being and a woman as a female— whenever she behaves as a human being she is said to imitate the male.

On the day when it will be possible for woman to love not in her weakness but in her strength, not to escape herself but to find herself, not to abase herself but to assert herself—on that day love will become for her, as for man, a source of life and not of mortal danger.

To abstain from politics is in itself a political attitude.

Change your life today. Don't gamble on the future, act now, without delay.

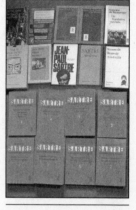

Books of Simone de Beauvoir and her companion, Jean-Paul Sartre.

Freedom is the source from which all significations and all values spring. It is the original condition of all justification of existence.

If you live long enough, you'll see that every victory turns into a defeat.

Legislators, priests, philosophers, writers, and scientists have striven to show that the subordinate position of woman is willed in heaven and advantageous on earth.

One can never know oneself; only tell one's own story.

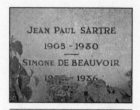

Few tasks are more like the torture of Sisyphus than housework, with its endless repetition: the clean becomes soiled, the soiled is made clean, over and over, day after day.

Tombstone of de Beauvoir and Sartre in Paris.

■ *The Second Sex*

The category of Other is as original as consciousness itself. The duality between Self and Other can be found in the most primitive societies, in the most ancient mythologies; the division did not always fall into the category of the division of the sexes....No group ever defines itself as One without immediately setting up the Other opposite itself. It only takes three travelers brought together by chance in the same train compartment for the rest of the travelers to become vaguely hostile "others."

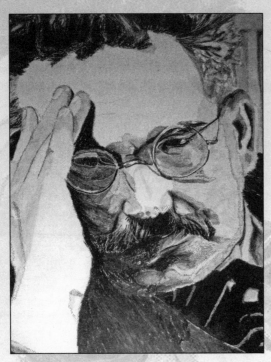

Walter Benjamin

(Berlin, Germany, 1892–Port Bou, Spain, 1940)

The fragmentary and poetic character of Benjamin's writings has come to be looked upon as singular expression of one of the most extraordinary minds of the twentieth century. His philosophy entails more of an atmosphere than of a system of ideas. He expressed himself through the medium of reflections and "illuminations" rather than with sustained argument.

Fleeing from the Nazi occupied France in 1940, Benjamin committed suicide in the town of Port Bou on the French-Spanish border, after being informed by the Spanish police that he was going to be deported back to France.

The bulk of his work was published after his death.

Recommended reading:

📖 📖 📖 *The Arcades Project* (1927–1940)

📖 📖 *The Work of Art in the Age of Mechanical Reproduction* (1935–1939)

📖 *On the Concept of History* (1939)

Quotations in my work are like wayside robbers who leap out armed and relieve the stroller of his conviction.

––––––

To be happy is to be able to become aware of oneself without fright.

––––––

There is no document of civilization that is not at the same time a document of barbarism.

––––––

Every passion borders on the chaotic, but the collector's passion borders on the chaos of memories.

––––––

All human knowledge takes the form of interpretation.

––––––

Memory is not an instrument for surveying the past but its theater. It is the medium of past experience, just as the earth is the medium in which dead cities lie buried. He who seeks to approach his own buried past must conduct himself like a man digging.

––––––

Mechanical reproduction emancipates the work of art from its parasitical dependence on ritual.

––––––

Only a thoughtless observer can deny that correspondences come into play between the world of modern technology and the archaic symbol-world of mythology.

––––––

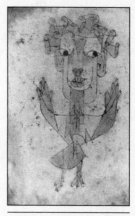

Not to find one's way around a city does not mean much. But to lose one's way in a city, as one loses one's way in a forest, requires some schooling. Street names must speak to the urban wanderer like the snapping of dry twigs, and little streets in the heart of the city must reflect the times of day, for him, as clearly as a mountain valley. This art I acquired rather late in life; it fulfilled a dream, of which the first traces were labyrinths on the blotting papers in my school notebooks.

––––––

In the fields with which we are concerned, knowledge exists only in lightning flashes. The text is the thunder rolling long afterwards.

Benjamin saw *Angelus Novus* by Paul Klee (Israel Museum, Jerusalem) as the embodiment of notions of history and progress.

A Klee painting named *Angelus Novus* shows an angel looking as though he is about to move away from something he is fixedly contemplating. His eyes are staring, his mouth is open, his wings are spread. This is how one pictures the angel of history. His face turned toward the past. Where we perceive a chain of events, he sees a single catastrophe which keeps piling wreckage upon wreckage and hurls it in front of his feet. The angel would like to stay, awaken the dead, and make whole what has been smashed. But a storm is blowing from Paradise; it has got caught in his wings with such violence that the angel can no longer close them. This storm irresistibly propels him into the future to which his back is turned, while the pile of debris before him grows skyward. This storm is what we call progress.

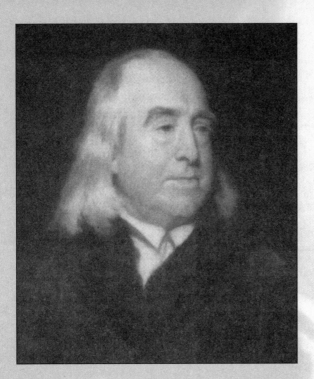

Jeremy Bentham
London, England, 1748–1832

Bentham was the father of the utilitarian school of philosophy. He was a child prodigy. By the age of three he was able to read and play the violin and began to study Latin at the age of five. He entered Oxford University at the age of twelve and at nineteen became a lawyer.

Early on he decided to devote himself to strictly intellectual pursuits and soon became a vital center of cultural exchange and the focal point of the utilitarian movement. James Mill and his son John Stuart Mill counted themselves as among his disciples.

At his death, according to his own wishes, his fully dressed body was displayed behind glass in a cabinet called the "Auto-icon" in the University College of London.

Recommended reading:

A Fragment on Government (1776)

Introduction to Principles of Morals and Legislation (1789)

A Treatise on Judicial Evidence (1827)

Nature has placed mankind under the governance of two sovereign masters, pain and pleasure. It is for them alone to point out what we ought to do, as well as to determine what we shall do. On the one hand the standard of right and wrong, on the other the chain of causes and effects, are fastened to their throne. They govern us in all we do, in all we say, in all we think: every effort we can make to throw off our subjection, will serve but to demonstrate and confirm it. In words a man may pretend to abjure their empire: but in reality he will remain subject to it all the while.

[The] fundamental axiom [of utilitarianism is] the greatest happiness of the greatest number that is the measure of right and wrong.

The question is not, Can [animals] reason? nor, Can they talk? But, Can they suffer?

Lawyers are the only persons in whom ignorance of the law is not punished.

Stretching his hand to reach the stars, man too often forgets the flowers at his feet.

Tyranny and anarchy are never far apart.

No power of government ought to be employed in the endeavor to establish any system or article of belief on the subject of religion.

Every law is an infraction of liberty.

What is the source of this premature anxiety to establish fundamental laws? It is the old conceit of being wiser than all posterity—wiser than those who will have had more experience,—the old desire of ruling over posterity—the old recipe for enabling the dead to chain down the living.

...in no instance has a system in regard to religion been ever established, but for the purpose, as well as with the effect of its being made an instrument of intimidation, corruption, and delusion, for the support of depredation and oppression in the hands of governments.

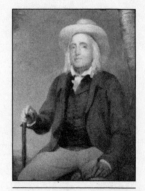

Jeremy Bentham was born to a well-to-do family and became a lawyer at the age of nineteen. He was extremely critical of the educational, judicial, and penal practices of his time. Throughout his life he developed ambitious schemes for social reform.

Constitutional Code

In every government, which has for its object and effect the pursuit of the happiness of the governors at the expense and by the correspondent sacrifice of the happiness of the governed, oppression at large will be the habitual and unintermitted practice of the government in all its ranks. The only species of government which has or can have for its object and effect the greatest happiness of the greatest number, is, as has been seen, a democracy.

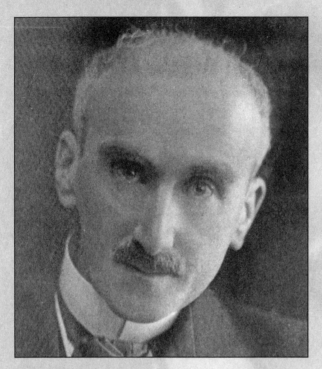

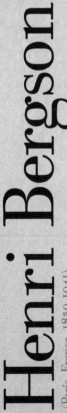

Henri Bergson
(París, France, 1859–1941)

Bergson was a representative of the Intuitionist School of French philosophy as well as a writer. He was awarded the Nobel Prize for Literature in 1927. During the Nazi Era, despite suffering from a serious illness, he voluntarily renounced all honors previously received in protest of anti-Semitic laws.

Opposed to the philosophical currents of positivism and mechanism, he sought to distance himself from scientific explanations of human behavior in favor of a philosophy that celebrated those values that constituted the "world of the spirit."

Forced to create his own philosophical approach, he cultivated awareness to direct his responses to the human condition.

Recommended reading:

Time and Free Will: An Essay on the Immediate Data of Consciousness (1910)
Matter and Memory (1911)
Laughter: An Essay on the Meaning of the Comic (1900)

Mind-energy (1920)

Philosophy is a battle against the spell language casts upon our intelligence.

———

I cannot escape the objection that there is no state of mind, however simple, that does not change every moment.

———

Religion is to mysticism what popularization is to science.

———

The open society is one which in principle embraces all of humanity.

———

Think like a man of action, act like a man of thought.

———

Man ought to put as much effort into simplifying his life as he does into complicating it.

———

Social cohesion is in a large part dependent on the necessity of defending itself against others.

———

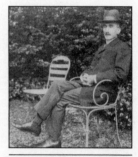

Men do not sufficiently realize that their future is in their own hands. Theirs is the task of determining first of all whether they want to go on living or not. Theirs the responsibility, then, for deciding if they want merely to live, or intend to make just the extra effort required for fulfilling, even on their refractory planet, the essential function of the universe, which is a machine for the making of gods.

———

The writer's art consists primarily in his ability to make us forget that he is using words.

———

To look ahead consists in projecting into the future what we have perceived in the past.

———

Comedy is much closer to reality than drama.

Bergson tried to clear a path separate from that defined by the scientific method. He sought other avenues toward esthetic and intellectual values that would lead to a world of spirit divorced from that delineated by the natural sciences.

Laughter: An Essay on the Meaning of the Comic

The first point to which attention should be called is that the comic does not exist outside the pale of what is strictly HUMAN....You may laugh at an animal, but only because you have detected in it some human attitude or expression. You may laugh at a hat, but what you are making fun of, in this case, is not the piece of felt or straw, but the shape that men have given it—the human caprice whose mould it has assumed. It is strange that so important a fact, and such a simple one too, has not attracted to a greater degree the attention of philosophers. Several have defined man as "an animal which laughs." They might equally well have defined him as an animal which is laughed at; for if any other animal, or some lifeless object, produces the same effect, it is always because of some resemblance to man, of the stamp he gives it or the use he puts it to.

39

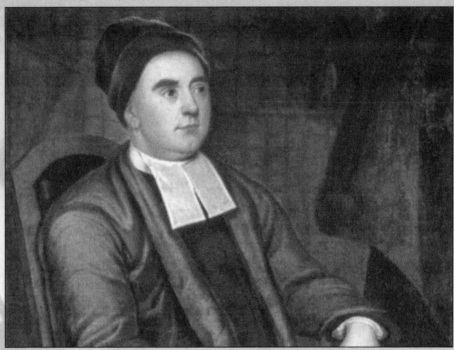

George Berkeley

(Dysert, Ireland, 1685–Oxford, England, 1753)

The principal achievement of the Irish philosopher George Berkeley, known also as Bishop Berkeley, having been invested with the See of Cloyne, was the development of the philosophical position known as subjective idealism, whose essence is expressed in the formulation "to exist is to be perceived."

According to this doctrine, man can only directly experience sensations and ideas of objects, but not abstractions.

One of Berkeley's main objectives was to counter materialism, the dominant theory of the time. Many ridiculed his theories, but others considered him a genius. He left Cloyne for England, residing in Oxford with his son until his death the following year.

Recommended reading:

A Treatise Concerning the Principles of Human Knowledge (1710)

Three Dialogues between Hylas and Philonus (1713)

The Analyst (1734)

It is indeed an opinion strangely prevailing amongst men, that houses, mountains, rivers, and in a word all sensible objects have an existence natural or real, distinct from their being perceived by the understanding. But with how great an assurance and acquiescence soever this principle may be entertained in the world; yet whoever shall find in his heart to call it in question, may, if I mistake not, perceive it to involve a manifest contradiction. For what are the forementioned objects but the things we perceive by sense, and what do we perceive besides our own ideas or sensations; and is it not plainly repugnant that any one of these or any combination of them should exist unperceived?

———

Esse est percipi: to exist is to be perceived.

———

Many things, for aught I know, may exist, whereof neither I nor any other man hath or can have any idea or notion whatsoever.

———

If a tree falls in a forest and no one is around to hear it, does it make a sound?

———

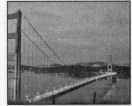

In vain do we extend our view into the heavens and pry into the entrails of the earth, in vain do we consult the writings of learned men and trace the dark footsteps of antiquity—we need only draw the curtain of words, to hold the fairest tree of knowledge, whose fruit is excellent, and within the reach of our hand.

———

From my own being, and from the dependency I find in myself and my ideas, I do, by an act of reason, necessarily infer the existence of a God, and of all created things in the mind of God.

———

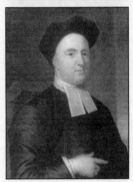

If we admit a thing so extraordinary as the creation of this world, it should seem that we admit something strange, and odd, and new to human apprehension, beyond any other miracle whatsoever.

———

Above: San Francisco's Golden Gate Bridge. The nearby town of Berkeley and its famous university are named after this philosopher.

The eye by long use comes to see even in the darkest cavern: and there is no subject so obscure but we may discern some glimpse of truth by long poring on it.

A Treatise Concerning the Principles of Human Knowledge

Philosophy being nothing else but the study of wisdom and truth, it may with reason be expected that those who have spent most time and pains in it should enjoy a greater calm and serenity of mind, a greater clearness and evidence of knowledge, and be less disturbed with doubts and difficulties than other men. Yet so it is, we see the illiterate bulk of mankind that walk the high-road of plain common sense, and are governed by the dictates of nature, for the most part easy and undisturbed. To them nothing that is familiar appears unaccountable or difficult to comprehend. They complain not of any want of evidence in their senses, and are out of all danger of becoming Sceptics. But no sooner do we depart from sense and instinct to follow the light of a superior principle, to reason, meditate, and reflect on the nature of things, but a thousand scruples spring up in our minds concerning those things which before we seemed fully to comprehend.

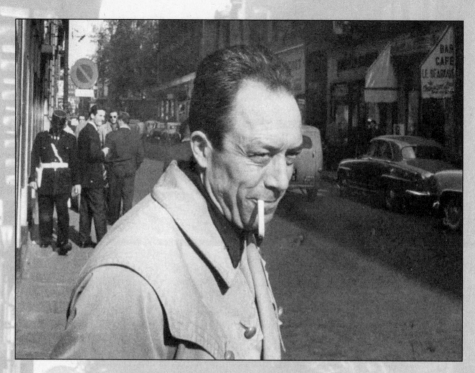

Albert Camus

(Mondovi, Algeria, 1913–Le Petit Villeblevin, France, 1960)

Camus was a writer and philosopher. His family was of Spanish origin and of humble circumstances. His father died at the First Battle of the Marne and the family moved to Algiers. There he attended university, completed his studies, and began to write.

In 1940 he moved to Paris where he worked for the French publishing house Gallimard. He fought for the resistance and displayed anarchist leanings. In 1952 he ended his friendship with Sartre. Breaking with existentialism, Marxism and Christianity, he elaborated his own reflections on the human condition.

In 1957 Camus was awarded the Nobel Prize for Literature. He died in a car accident in 1960. Found among his personal effects was an unpublished autobiography.

Recommended reading:

📖 📖 📖 *The Myth of Sisyphus 1942*

📖 📖 *The Rebel (1951)*

📖 *The Stranger (1942)*
The Plague (1947)

There is only one truly serious philosophical problem: suicide. To decide whether life is worth the trouble is to address philosophy's fundamental question. Everything else, whether the world exists in three dimensions, whether the mind has nine or twelve categories is secondary. These are games; first one must answer.

———

There can be no true goodness, nor true love, without the utmost clear-sightedness.

———

Can one be a saint without God? That's the problem, in fact the only problem, I'm up against today.

———

The slave begins by demanding justice and ends by wanting to wear a crown. He must dominate in his turn.

———

When the throne of God is overturned, the rebel realizes that it is now his own responsibility to create the justice, order, and unity that he sought in vain within his own condition, and in this way to justify the fall of God. Then begins the desperate effort to create, at the price of crime and murder if necessary, the dominion of man.

———

The aim of art, the aim of a life can only be to increase the sum of freedom and responsibility to be found in every man and in the world. It cannot, under any circumstances, be to reduce or suppress that freedom, even temporarily.

———

What, then, is that incalculable feeling that deprives the mind of the sleep necessary to life? A world that can be explained even with bad reasons is a familiar world. But, on the other hand, in a universe suddenly divested of illusions and lights, man feels an alien, a stranger. His exile is without remedy since he is deprived of the memory of a lost home or the hope of a promised land. This divorce between man and his life, the actor and his setting, is properly the feeling of absurdity.

———

The struggle itself toward the heights is enough to fill a man's heart. One must imagine Sisyphus happy.

———

There are causes worth dying for, but none worth killing for.

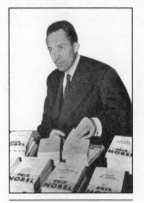

Nobel prize winner, Albert Camus was a passionate football fan. He abandoned communism in favor of anarchist and libertarian ideas.

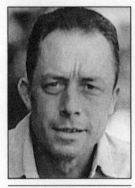

Wrestling with an absurd universe, Camus produced important reflections on the human condition, Christianity, and existentialism.

■ *Reflections on the Guillotine*

Capital punishment is the most premeditated of murders, to which no criminal's deed, however calculated, can be compared. For there to be an equivalency, the death penalty would have to punish a criminal who had warned his victim of the date on which he would inflict a horrible death on him and who, from that moment onward, had confined him at his mercy for months. Such a monster is not to be encountered in private life.

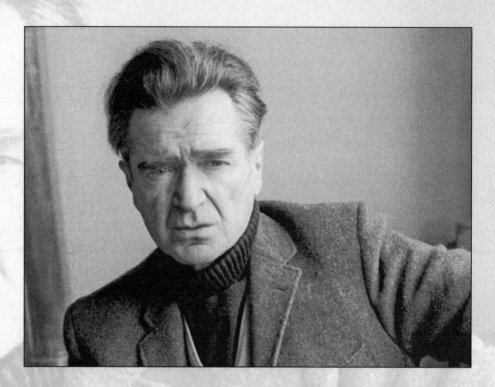

Emile Cioran
(Rasinari, Romania, 1911–Paris, France, 1995)

Emil Cioran was the son of an orthodox priest. He attended the University of Bucharest, where became acquainted with Eugene Ionesco and Mircea Eliade. In his youth he was a member of a fascist organization, something he repented of later on.

He moved to Paris in 1937 to continue his studies and remained there the greater part of his life. His first works were published in Romanian, but he soon began to write solely in French. His style is incisive, at times brutal, marked by deep pessimism. Fond of aphorisms and brief sayings, he explored themes of alienation, decadence, futility and the absurd.

Recommended reading:

📖 📖 📖 *All Gaul Is Divided* (1952)

📖 📖 *The Temptation to Exist* (1956)

📖 *The New Gods* (1969)

So long as man is protected by madness he functions and flourishes, but when he frees himself from the fruitful tyranny of fixed ideas, he is lost, ruined.

Lucidity's task: to attain a correct despair, an Olympian ferocity.

Without God, everything is nothingness; and with God? Supreme nothingness.

To hope is to contradict the future.

In every man sleeps a prophet, and when he wakes there is a little more evil in the world.

You are forgiven everything provided you have a trade, a subtitle to your name, a seal on your nothingness.

The pessimist has to invent new reasons to exist every day: he is a victim of the "meaning" of life.

Let us speak plainly: everything which keeps us from self-dissolution, every lie which protects us against our unbreathable certitudes is religious.

Without its assiduity to the ridiculous, would the human race have lasted more than a single generation?

What every man who loves his country hopes for in his inmost heart: the suppression of half his compatriots.

It is an understatement to say that in this society injustices abound: in truth, it is itself the quintessence of injustice.

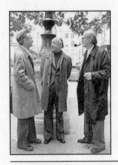

Photograph of Cioran, Ionesco and Eliade (1977).

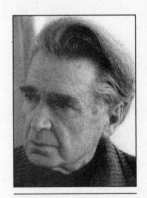

Cioran preaches the usefulness of despair in a hopeless world.

All Gaul Is Divided

However intimate we may be with the operations of the mind, we cannot think more than two or three minutes a day—unless, by taste or by profession, we practice, for hours on end, brutalizing words in order to extract ideas from them...The intellectual represents the major disgrace, the culminating failure of *Homo sapiens*.

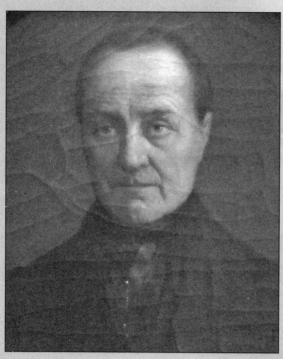

Auguste Comte

(Montpellier, France, 1798–Paris, France, 1857)

Comte was the creator of positivism, and according to many the founder of sociology as well. Having failed to retain an academic position he was force to rely on the financial help from friends. He was considered to be arrogant, irritable, even violent.

He entered into a mental institution in 1826 but left without finding a cure. After his divorce he began a tumultuous affair with a woman who, in 1848, would die of tuberculosis. She greatly influenced his later works, which emphasized the importance of women's role in society.

Recommended reading:

A General View of Positivism (1848)

Course in Positive Philosophy (1830–1842)

The Subjective Synthesis (1856)

The law is this:—that each of our leading conceptions—each branch of our knowledge—passes successively through three different theoretical conditions: the Theological, or fictitious; the Metaphysical, or abstract; and the Scientific, or positive.

If it is true that every theory must be based upon observed facts, it is equally true that facts can not be observed without the guidance of some theories. Without such guidance, our facts would be desultory and fruitless; we could not retain them: for the most part we could not even perceive them.

Mathematical Analysis is....the true rational basis of the whole system of our positive knowledge.

Indeed, every true science has for its object the determination of certain phenomena by means of others, in accordance with the relations which exist between them.

True positivism resides in the study of what is, to arrive at conclusions about what will be.

The dead govern the living.

To categorize intellectual development, each stage more perfect than the next, is the one of the most important tasks of positivist philosophy.

The only absolute maxim, is that there are no absolutes.

One cannot fully comprehend a science without knowing its history.

At each stage of our existence, whether individual or collective one needs always to apply the sacred formula of positivism: love as its principle, order as its base, and progress as its goal.

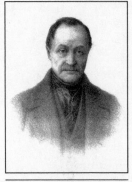

August Comte was a French mathematician and philosopher. He proposed that humanity and the individual as its constituent part go through three stages that correspond to distinct levels of intellectual development: the theological or fictional, the metaphysical or abstract, and the scientific or positivist. The transition from one stage to the next was a natural and necessary process, since it represented the natural unfolding of the human spirit.

A General View of Positivism

The object of all true philosophy is to frame a system which shall comprehend human life under every aspect, social as well as individual. It embraces therefore the three kinds of phenomena of which our life consists, Thoughts, Feelings, and Action. Under all of these aspects, the growth of Humanity is primarily spontaneous; and the basis upon which all wise attempts to modify it should proceed, can only be furnished by an exact acquaintance with the natural process.

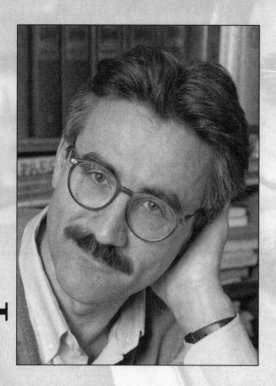

André Comte-Sponville

(Paris, France, 1952)

Comte-Sponville is currently one France's best known and most widely read philosophers. His work has the clear intent of making itself accessible to a wide audience, to make philosophy a possession common to all.

He has written a great deal over the perennial themes that philosophy has addressed since classical antiquity: happiness, freedom, and wisdom.

Whereas he recognizes himself as firmly within the tradition and history of Greco-Judeo-Christian values, he defines himself as a non-dogmatic atheist, finding a kind of rational and reasonable faith in wisdom, joy, love, and the eternity of the here and now.

Recommended reading:

📖 📖 📖 *Le Bonheur, désespérément* (2000)

📖 📖 *A Small Treatise on the Great Virtues* (2003)

📖 *The Book of Atheist Spirituality* (2009)

To live without God is possible, to live without spirituality impossible.

———

Schopenhauer expressed the essential in a phrase, which to me is the saddest formulation in all philosophy: "Our life oscillates like a pendulum from right to left, between suffering and boredom." Suffering when I want what I don't have, because I suffer from its absence; boredom because I have what I no longer desire.

———

The essential thing is not to lie, first of all not to oneself. Not to lie about life, ourselves and happiness.

———

To love some one who is absent is easy. It is much more difficult to love some who is present with whom we share our life.

———

If philosophy does not help us to be happy or at least less unhappy, what good is it?

———

Let us be resolutely optimistic and keep pessimism for better days.

———

To put the matter quite simply, the wisdom of despair that I refer to, the "gay despair" consists in hoping a bit less and loving a bit more.

———

One fears a thousand deaths, and experiences only one. All anxiety is imaginary; reality is its antidote.

———

Justice is not a virtue like other virtues. It is the horizon of all virtue and the law of their coexistence...All virtue is presupposed by it; all humanity requires it.

———

If you don't know how to live with yourself how can you live with someone else.

———

The sweet honey of poetry and the bitter absinthe of truth.

———

Wisdom is the destination, philosophy the path.

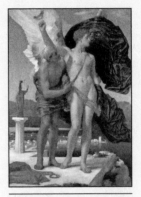

This philosopher is the author of *The Myth of Icarus*, a treatise on despair and unhappiness.

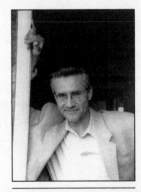

Comte-Sponville looks for spirituality without God, as he writes in *The Soul of Atheism*.

Le bonheur, désespérément

Happiness is the goal of philosophy but it is not its standard. The standard of philosophy is truth, at least the possible truth....It is not a matter of what makes me happy, but that which appears to be true to me. Only by trying to discover this by facing the truth be it sad or anguished, is the maximum amount of happiness possible. That means that if philosophy offers a choice between truth and happiness...only by choosing truth is philosophy worth its name. Better a true sadness than a false joy.

Arthur C. Danto

(Ann Arbor, Michigan, 1924–New York City, 2013)

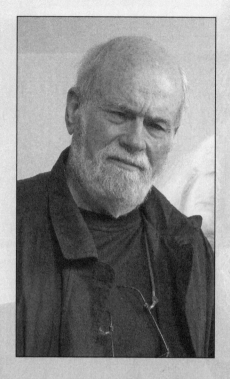

Danto was Professor of Philosophy at Columbia University for many years and a highly esteemed art critic. Following an analytic approach, he made significant contributions in many areas of philosophy, but his main work was on esthetics. His writings in this field are both provocative and elegantly conceived, treating both individual artists and artistic movements as well as the nature of art itself.

Danto examined the problems raised by the visual arts in today's world by looking at the grand masters, the great modernist painters, and contemporary artists as well.

Recommended reading:

The Transfiguration of the Commonplace (1981)

After the End of Art (1997)

The Madonna of the Future: Essays in a Pluralistic Art World (2000)

Hegel's early masterpiece, *The Phenomenology of Spirit,* has the form of a *bildungsroman,* in the sense that its hero, Geist, goes through a sequence of stages in order to achieve knowledge not merely of what it itself is, but that without the history of mishaps and misplaced enthusiasms, its knowledge would be empty.

―――――

Whether things really are the way the structure of our mind requires us to think they are is not something we can say. But neither does it greatly matter, since we have no alternative way of thinking about them.

―――――

A lot happens when the prince and princess live happily ever after— the king, his father, dies, so he is now ruler and she his queen, they have their children, she conducts discreet affairs with Sir Lancelot, there are border uprisings...but still the story ended when the love toward which their destinies drove them came to mutual consciousness when they knew, each knowing the other knew, that they were meant for each other.

―――――

My sense is that modernism does not follow romanticism in this way, or not merely: it is marked by an ascent to a new level of consciousness, which is reflected in painting as a kind of discontinuity, almost as if to emphasize that mimetic representation had become less important than some kind of reflection on the means and methods of representation.

―――――

Deconstruction, after all, is taken to be a method for demonstrating the way in which society has advanced and reinforced the interests of special groups—white, for example, and male; and, along a different coordinate, western or North-American.

―――――

...art is philosophically independent of aesthetics. That is a discovery that means something only to those concerned, as I was, with the philosophical definition of art, namely, what are the necessary and sufficient conditions for something being a work of art.

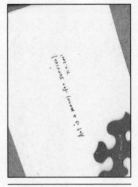

Work of Yoko Ono in the exhibition Art, Anti-Art, Non-Art Experimentations in the Public Sphere in Postwar Japan, 1950–1970. Getty Center, Los Angeles.

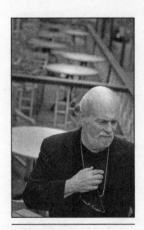

Danto's art criticism embraced philosopy.

■ *After the End of Art*

The sixties was a paroxysm of styles, in the course of whose contention...it gradually became clear...that there was no special way works of art had to look in contrast to what I have designated "mere real things"...nothing need mark the difference, outwardly, between Andy Warhol's Brillo Box and the Brillo boxes in the supermarket....It meant that as far as appearances were concerned, anything could be a work of art, and it meant that if you were going to find out what art was, you had to turn from sense experience to thought. You had, in brief, to turn to philosophy.

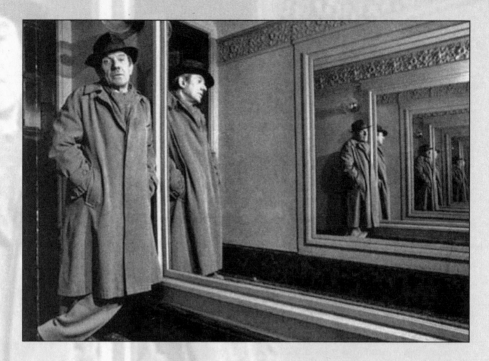

Deleuze studied philosophy at the Sorbonne. He began writing monographs, some touching on philosophy, but it wasn't until the end of the 1960s that he published works that testified to the uniqueness of his thinking.

In 1969 he met the psychoanalyst Félix Guattari and together they published two large volumes subsumed under the title *Capitalism and Schizophrenia*: *Anti-Oedipus* and *A Thousand Plateaus*.

In the last years of his life he suffered from a serious respiratory ailment that finally led to his taking his own life by jumping from the window of his apartment. Michel Foucault said on that occasion: "One day this will be called the Deleuzian century."

Recommended reading:

Difference and Repetition (1968)
The Logic of Sense (1969)

Anti-Oedipus (1972)

A Thousand Plateaus (1980)

There's no need to fear or hope, but only to look for new weapons.

We're tired of trees. We should stop believing in trees, roots, and radicles. They've made us suffer too much. All of arborescent culture is founded on them, from biology to linguistics. Nothing is beautiful or loving or political aside from underground stems and aerial root, adventitious growths and rhizomes.

Evaluations, in essence, are...ways of being, modes of existence of those who judge and evaluate.

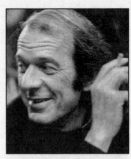

A book is a small cog in a much more complex, external machinery. Writing is a flow among others; it enjoys no special privilege and enters into relationships of current and counter-current, of back-wash with other flows—the flows of shit, sperm, speech, action, eroticism, money, politics, etc. Like Bloom, writing on the sand with one hand and masturbating with the other—two flows in what relationship?

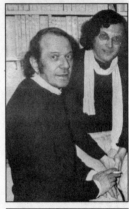

A concept is a brick. It can be used to build a courthouse of reason. Or it can be thrown through the window.

Bring something incomprehensible into the world!

It is not the slumber of reason that engenders monsters, but vigilant and insomniac rationality.

Christianity taught us to see the eye of the lord looking down upon us. Such forms of knowledge project an image of reality, at the expense of reality itself. They talk figures and icons and signs, but fail to perceive forces and flows. They bind us to other realities, and especially the reality of power as it subjugates us. Their function is to tame, and the result is the fabrication of docile and obedient subjects.

There's no democratic state that's not compromised to the very core by its part in generating human misery.

If you are a captive of another's dream, you're screwed.

Gilles Deleuze and Félix Guattari. According to Deleuze, "disciplined societies suffer a crisis in response to new forces that are gradually installing themselves as societies of control. In old societies sovereignty rested on simple machines, whereas disciplined societies equip themselves with energetic machines. Societies of control work through information machines. A technological evolution and a capitalist mutation."

Anti-Oedipus

Courage consists, however, in agreeing to flee rather than live tranquilly and hypocritically in false refuges. Values, morals, homelands, religions, and these private certitudes that our vanity and our complacency bestow generously on us, have many deceptive sojourns as the world arranges for those who think they are standing straight and at ease, among stable things.

Democritus of Abdera

(Abdera, Thrace c. 460–c. 360 BCE)

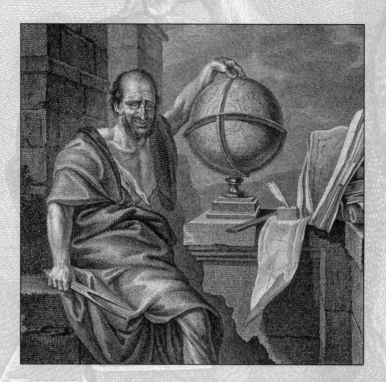

Democritus was the co-founder with his teacher, Leucippus, of the Atomist School. Little is known about his life, but all of the ancient writers that mention him concur that he lived to be over 100 years old. Hipparchus of Nicea following Diogenes averred that Democritus died at the age of 109. He was said to have lived extravagantly and considered the human condition to be essentially ridiculous.

According the atomist theory the universe is composed of tiny indivisible particles called atoms. Democritus held on this basis that all phenomena can be explained in strictly materialistic terms.

Recommended reading:

Guthrie, W.K.C., *History of Greek Philosophy* (1994)

Kirk, G.S. and J.E. Raven, *The Presocratic Philosophers* (1987)

Diogenes Laertius, *Lives of Eminent Philosophers* (1st century CE)

One has to recognize that human life is of short duration. That it is constantly disturbed by the shocks and difficulties of destiny. For that reason one should occupy oneself with accumulating possessions only to a moderate extent, and alleviate life's miseries as best as one can.

Medicine heals diseases of the body, wisdom frees the soul from passions.

Everything existing in the universe is the fruit of chance and necessity.

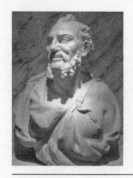

The best way for a man to lead his life is to have been as cheerful as possible and to have suffered as little as possible. This could happen if one did not seek one's pleasures in mortal things. The right-minded man is he who is not grieved by what he has not, but enjoys what he has. He is fortunate who is happy with moderate means, unfortunate who is unhappy with great possessions.

Democritus of Abdera was a contemporary of Socrates. It was said that he practiced meditation. He is credited with the authorship of over 70 works on topics ranging from ethics, physics, mathematics, music, and technology.

Raising children is an uncertain thing; success is reached only after a life of battle and worry.

Our sins are more easily remembered than our good deeds.

Nothing exists except atoms and empty space; everything else is opinion.

Everywhere man blames nature and fate. Yet his fate is mostly but the echo of his character and passions, his mistakes and weaknesses.

Many much-learned men have no intelligence.

If your desires are not great, a little will seem much to you; for small appetite makes poverty equivalent to wealth.

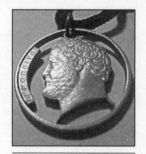

The animal needing something knows how much it needs, the man does not.

According to Democritus reality consisted of two elements: that which is, homogeneous and indivisible atoms, and that which is not, the vacuum.

Sextus Empíricus, *Adversus mathematicos*

It is said that Democritus refuted the reality of the appearance of our senses, saying that these to do not conform to the truth but rather to opinion, and that the truth behind all causes derives only from atoms and empty space. From convention comes sweetness, from convention bitterness, from convention heat, from convention cold, from convention all the different colors. In reality only atoms and empty space exist.

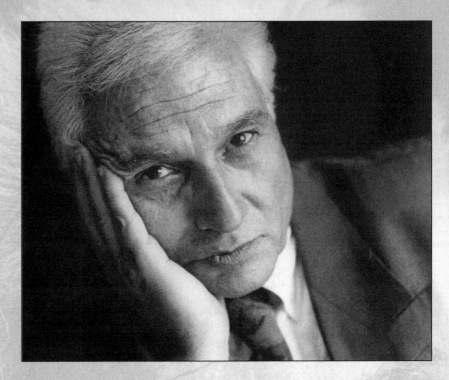

Jacques Derrida

(El-Bihar, Algeria, 1930–Paris, France, 2004)

Derrida was born to a Jewish family of Spanish origin. He studied philosophy in Paris and formed a lasting friendship with Louis Althusser. Other formative influences include Merleau-Ponty and Foucault. He was the first philosopher to develop the method of thought known as deconstruction.

In 1965 he obtained the position of Director of Studies at the École Normale Supérieure in the department of philosophy. He made many trips to the United States where his methods gained wide currency in academic circles. He was nominated for the Nobel Prize a number of times and was a notable political activist, defending progressive causes of all kinds, from the Prague Spring, to the fall of apartheid to the plight of the Palestinians. He died a victim of cancer.

Recommended reading:

📖 📖 📖 *Writing and Difference* (1967)

📖 📖 *Of Grammatology* (1967)

📖 *Margins of Philosophy* (1972)

What is called "objectivity," scientific for instance (in which I firmly believe, in a given situation) imposes itself only within a context which is extremely vast, old, firmly established, or rooted in a network of conventions...and yet which still remains a context.

Deconstruction never had meaning or interest, at least in my eyes, than as a radicalization, that is to say, also within the tradition of a certain Marxism, in a certain spirit of Marxism.

The only attitude (the only politics-judicial, medical, pedagogical and so forth) I would absolutely condemn is one which, directly or indirectly, cuts off the possibility of an essentially interminable questioning, that is, an effective and thus transforming questioning.

...consciousness offers itself to thought only as self-presence, as the perception of self in presence.

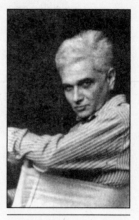

The work of Derrida is closely associated with poststructuralism and to some extent with postmodernism.

Learning to live ought to mean learning to die—to acknowledge, to accept, an absolute mortality—without positive outcome, or resurrection, or redemption, for oneself or for anyone else. That has been the old philosophical injunction since Plato: to be a philosopher is to learn how to die.

What is algebraically called "Europe" has to assume certain responsibilities, in the name of the future of humanity, in the name of international law—this is my faith and my religion.

There is no outside text.

If you read philosophical texts of the tradition, you'll notice they almost never said 'I,' and didn't speak in the first person. From Aristotle to Heidegger, they try to consider their own lives as something marginal or accidental. What was essential was their teaching and their thinking. Biography is something empirical and outside, and is considered an accident that isn't necessarily or essentially linked to the philosophical activity or system.

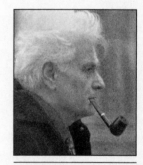

Derrida's creation, "deconstruction," continues to exercise considerable influence on other disciplines.

Interview

There is some negativity in deconstruction...You have to criticize, to ask questions, to challenge and sometimes to oppose. What I have said is that in the final instance, deconstruction is not negative although negativity is no doubt at work. Now, in order to criticize, to negate, to deny, you have first to say "yes". When you address the Other, even if it is to oppose the Other, you make a sort of promise—that is, to address the Other as Other, not to reduce the otherness of the Other, and to take into account the singularity of the Other. That's an irreducible affirmation, its the original ethics if you want. So from that point of view, there is an ethics of deconstruction. Not in the usual sense, but there is an affirmation.

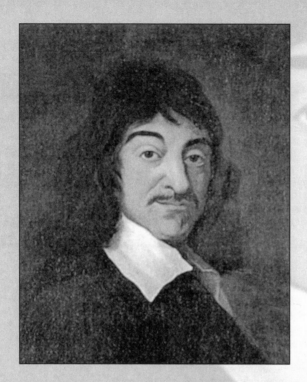

René Descartes

(Le Haye en Touranine, France, 1596–Stockholm, Sweden, 1650)

The modern age of philosophy begins with Descartes. As a child he received a thorough grounding in humanistic studies from his Jesuit teachers. Having embarked upon the study of medicine and law he moved to Holland in 1629 to devote himself to intellectual pursuits. His renown inspired Queen Christina of Sweden to invite him to act as her tutor. This honor may have cost him his life as the Queen's study regimen required that he rise at 5:00 AM, when he was accustomed to working in bed until noon. It is thought that he died of pneumonia brought on by exhaustion. His philosophical work challenged the authority of the scholastic tradition and combated prejudice. He promoted a methodical approach that prioritized evidence, analysis, syntheses, and empirical testing.

Recommended reading:

📖 📖 📖 *Discourse on Method* (1637)

📖 📖 *Metaphysical Meditations* (1641)
Rules for the Direction of Mind (1628)

📖 *The Passions of The Soul* (1649)

Cogito ergo sum (I think therefore I am).

On the one hand I have a clear and distinct idea of myself, in so far as I am a thinking, non-extended thing; and on the other hand I have a distinct idea of body, in so far a this is simply an extended, non-thinking thing. And, accordingly, it is certain that I am really distinct from my body, and exist without it

In my situation with one foot in one country and the other in another, I find myself quite happy.

If you would be a real seeker after truth, it is necessary that at least once in your life you doubt, as far as possible, all things.

The greatest minds, as they are capable of the highest excellencies, are open likewise to the greatest aberrations; and those who travel very slowly may yet make far greater progress, provided they keep always to the straight road, than those who, while they run, forsake it.

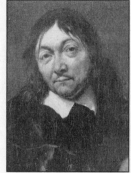

There is nothing so strange and unbelievable that has not been put forth by one philosopher or another.

I suppose therefore that all things I see are illusions; I believe that nothing has ever existed of everything my lying memory tells me. I think I have no senses. I believe that body, shape, extension, motion, location are functions. What is there then that can be taken as true? Perhaps only this one thing, that nothing at all is certain.

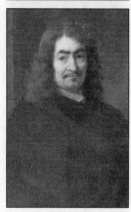

One always needs to guard against self-deceit. What I take to be gold or diamonds may be nothing other than copper or glass. I know how much room there is for error in matters that are close to us and how greatly the judgments of our friends are suspect in what pertains to us.

It's not enough to have a good mind. One needs to apply it in the right way.

In my opinion mathematics governs nature.

Descartes offered an ontological proof of God, based upon deduction rather than the proof of the senses.

Discourse on Method

I have spent much time in study of languages and reading ancient books, their histories and their fables. This is a way of conversing with other centuries and traveling. It is good to know the customs of diverse peoples; in this way we can better judge our own and realize that those which are different from ours are neither ridiculous or unreasonable....But when one spends to much time traveling one becomes a stranger in his own country; and when one is too curious about the way things were in the past, one usually remains ignorant about what is going on in the present.

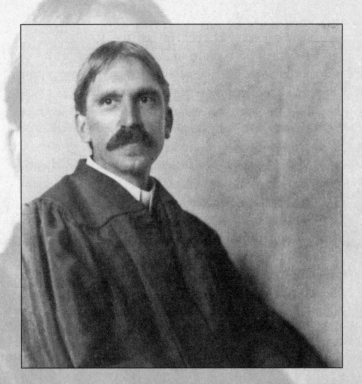

John Dewey

(Burlington, Vermont, 1859–New York City, 1952)x

John Dewey was the leading figure in nineteenth and early twentieth-century philosophical discourse in the United States and the most important representative of the philosophy of pragmatism. In addition, he was an educator and actively engaged in the promotion of an informed populace, which he felt essential for a democracy. Soon after the turn of the century he became a professor at the University of Chicago, where he pioneered functional psychology, which emphasized the influence of the social environment on the individual. This idea was carried over in his writings on education. Dewey held that the school was an institution through which society itself could be reformed.

Recommended reading:

Experience and Nature (1925)

The School and Society (1899)
Logic: Theory of Inquiry (1938)
Democracy and Education (1916)

Liberalism and Social Action (1935)

Persons do not become a society by living in physical proximity any more than a man ceases to be socially influenced by being so many feet or miles removed from others.

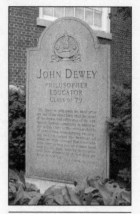

The teacher is not in the school to impose certain ideas or to form certain habits in the child, but is there as a member of the community to select the influences which shall affect the child and to assist him in properly responding to these. Thus the teacher becomes a partner in the learning process, guiding students to independently discover meaning within the subject area. This philosophy has become an increasingly popular idea within present-day teacher preparatory programs.

Every one has experienced how learning an appropriate name for what was dim and vague cleared up and crystallized the whole matter. Some meaning seems distinct almost within reach, but is elusive; it refuses to condense into definite form; the attaching of a word somehow (just how, it is almost impossible to say) puts limits around the meaning, draws it out from the void, makes it stand out as an entity on its own account.

Grave of John Dewey on the campus of the University of Vermont, Burlington.

What Humanism means to me is an expansion, not a contraction, of human life, *an expansion in which nature and the science of nature are made the willing servants of human good.*

Education is a social process; education is growth; education is not preparation for life but is life itself.

The self is not something ready-made, but something in continuous formation through choice of action.

A problem well put is half solved.

A philosophy has no private store of knowledge or methods for attaining truth, so it has no private access to good. As it accepts knowledge and principles from those competent in science and inquiry, it accepts the goods that are diffused in human experience. It has no Mosaic or Pauline authority of revelation entrusted to it. But it has the authority of intelligence, of criticism of these common and natural goods.

Experience and Nature

An empirical philosophy is in any case a kind of intellectual disrobing. We cannot permanently divest ourselves of the intellectual habits we take on and wear when we assimilate the culture of our own time and place. But intelligent furthering of culture demands that we take some of them off, that we inspect them critically to see what they are made of and what wearing them does to us. We cannot achieve recovery of primitive naïveté. But there is attainable a cultivated naïveté of eye, ear and thought.

Wilhelm Dilthey

(Biebrich, Germany, 1833–Tyrol, Austria, 1911)

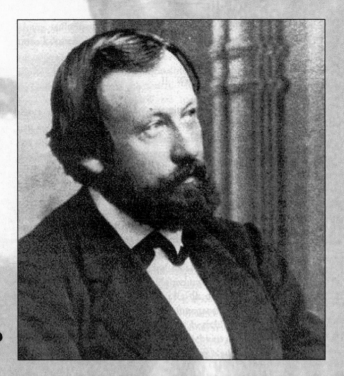

Son of a Protestant pastor, Dilthey set out to study theology but soon found that his interests lay in philosophy, philology and history. He studied in Heidelberg and Berlin.

In 1866 he took a post as Professor in Basel, and in 1882, as the culmination of his academic career, he was awarded a professorship in Berlin. It was then that his first works were published.

Dilthey proposed a model of study that emphasized what he called "human sciences" or "sciences of the mind" in contradistinction to the epistemological approach of the natural sciences. He died suddenly while on vacation in the Tyrolean Alps, in 1911. He is considered to be one of the most important voices in hermeneutics and historicism.

Recommended reading:

Introduction to the Human Sciences (1883)

The Essence of Philosophy (1907)

Poetry and Experience (1906)

While time advances, we remain surrounded with the ruins of Rome, its cathedrals and castles.

―――――

The ship of our life is carried forward on a constantly moving stream, and the present is always wherever we enter these waves with whatever we suffer, remember, and hope, that is, whenever we live in the fullness of our reality. We constantly sail into this stream, and the moment the future becomes the present, it also begins to sink into the past.

―――――

Lived experience can never be fully resolved into concepts, but its dark, deep tonality accompanies, even if merely marginally, all conceptual thought in the human sciences.

―――――

Psychic Life is something unfathomable. Whoever is concerned with the human sciences simply must, at some point, have strained to plumb this inexhaustible source.

―――――

All science is experiential; but all experience must be related back to and derives its validity from the conditions and context of consciousness in which it arises, i.e., the totality of our nature.

―――――

We explain by means of purely intellectual processes, but we understand by means of the cooperation of all the powers of the mind in comprehension. In understanding we start from the connection of the given, living whole, in order to make the past comprehensible in terms of it.

―――――

What man is, only history tells.

―――――

What is experienced within cannot be categorized in concepts that have been developed for the external world of the senses.

―――――

In light of this state of the human sciences I have undertaken to provide a philosophical foundation for the principle of the Historical School and for those modes of research into society currently dominated by that school; this should settle the conflict between the Historical School and abstract theories.

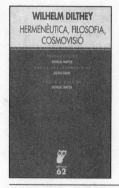

Wilhelm Dilthey was a sociologist and historian, as well as a student of psychology and hermeneutics.

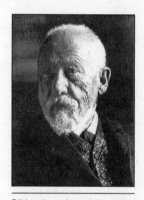

Dilthey investigated the historical dimension of human experience.

Introduction to the Human Sciences

Thus there arose in me both a need and a plan for the foundation of the human sciences. The answers given to these questions by Comte and the positivists and by J. S. Mill and the empiricists seemed to me to truncate and mutilate historical reality in order to assimilate it to the concepts and methods of the natural sciences....Only in inner experience, in facts of consciousness, have I found a firm anchor for my thinking, and I trust that my reader will be convinced by my proof of this.

Diogenes of Sinope

(Sinope, Ionia, c.413; Corinth, 324 BCE)

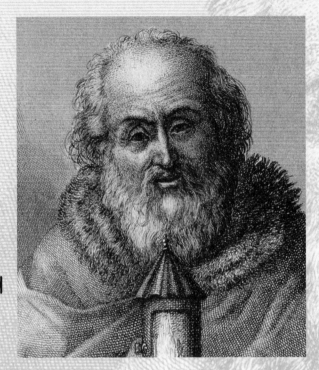

Diogenes, known as Diogenes the Cynic as well as Diogenes the dog, belonged to the school of the Cynics. He was a provocateur and often criticized by the society in which he lived in a marginal fashion. It is said that he lived in a barrel or a large ceramic jar.

None of his writings have been preserved. Most of what we know about him comes from Diogenes Laertius's Lives of Eminent Philosophers. However, the anecdotes that he transmitted about Diogenes have turned him into a legend. Plato wrote that Diogenes said that Socrates was a madman.

When he was exiled from his native city, he riposted: "They have condemned me to leave; I have condemned them to stay."

Recommended reading:

Diogenes Laertius, *Lives of Eminent Philosophers* (1st century BCE)

Luis E. Navia, *Diogenes the Cynic* (2005)

The Cynic Philosophers from Diogenes to Julian (trans. and ed. By Robert Dobbin, 2013)

Anecdotes about Diogenes the Cynic, from Diogenes Laertius:

The question was put to him what countryman he was, and he replied, "A citizen of the world."

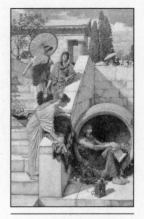

Once when Alexander the Great came and stood by him, and said, "I am Alexander, the great king." "And I," said he, "am Diogenes the dog." And when he was asked to what actions of his it was owing that he was called a dog, he said, "Because I fawn upon those who give me anything, and bark at those who give me nothing, and bite the rogues."

When asked why people give to beggars but not philosophers, he said, "Because they think it possible that they themselves may become lame and blind, but they do not expect ever to turn into philosophers."

When the question was put to him, what beast inflicts the worst bite, he said, "Of wild beasts the sycophant, and of the tame animals the flatterer."

J. W. Waterhouse, *Diogenes and the Barrel.*

He used to say that men were wrong for complaining of fortune; for they ask of the Gods what appear to be good things, not what are really so. And to those who were alarmed at dreams he said, that they did not regard what they do while they are awake, but made a great fuss about what they fancy when they are asleep.

A man once asked him what was the proper time for supper, and he made answer, "if you are a rich man, whenever you please, and if you are a poor man, whenever you can."

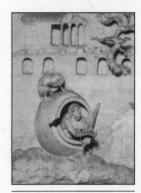

Once, when he was sitting in the sun in the Craneum, Alexander was standing by, and said to him, "Ask any favor you choose of me." And he replied, "Cease to shade me from the sun."

Diogenes in his dwelling. It was said in a play on words that cynics (*kynikos*) were doglike (in Greek *kyon* means dog).

One of his frequent sayings was, "That men contended with one another in punching and kicking, but no one showed any emulation in the pursuit of virtue." He also used to say, "that musicians fitted the strings to the lyre properly, but left all the habits of their soul ill-arranged." And, "that mathematicians kept their eyes fixed on the sun and moon, and overlooked what was under their feet."

■ **Diógenes Laertius,** *Lives of Eminent Philosophers*

On one occasion he saw a child drinking out of his hands, and so he threw away the cup which belonged to his wallet, saying, "This child has beaten me in simplicity." He also threw away his spoon, after seeing a boy, when he had broken his vessel, take up his lentils with a crust of bread. And he used to argue thus: "Everything belongs to the gods; and wise men are friends of the gods. All things are in common among friends; therefore everything belongs to wise men."

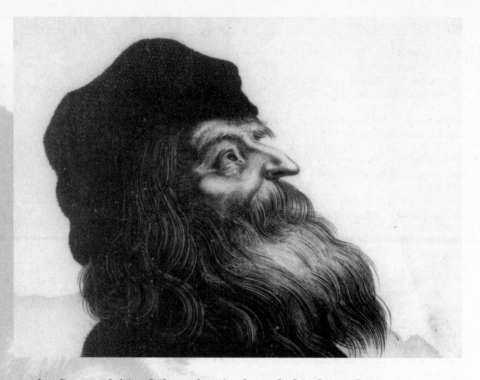

Empedocles

(Agrigento, Sicily 495-435 BCE)

The figure of this philosopher is shrouded in legend. He was known for the practice of medicine and magic. Miracles were attributed him and some considered him to be a god.

In response to the question of origins he referred to the four elements: earth, water, fire and air, and that they transform themselves through their intermixture into all phenomena. The union and separation of these elements is caused by the cosmic forces Love and Strife.

In regard to his divine status, Diogenes Laertius reports that some claimed that he jumped into Mount Etna's crater of fire and disappeared from the earth.

Recommended reading:

Diogenes Laertius, *Lives of Eminent Philosophers* (1st century BCE)

Barnes, Jonathan: *The Presocratic Philosophers* (1992)

Guthrie, W.K.C., *History of Greek Philosophy* (1994)

Friends who inhabit the mighty town by tawny Acragas which crowns
the citadel, caring for good deeds, greetings; I, an immortal God, no
longer mortal, wander among you, honored by all, adorned with holy
diadems and blooming garlands. To whatever illustrious towns I go, I
am praised by men and women, and accompanied by thousands, who
thirst for deliverance, some ask for prophecies, and some entreat, for
remedies against all kinds of disease.

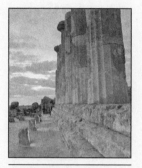

For before this I was born once a boy, and a maiden, and a plant, and a
bird, and a darting fish in the sea.

But come, examine by every means each thing how it is clear, neither
putting greater faith in anything seen than in what is heard, nor in a
thundering sound more than in the clear assertions of the tongue, nor
keep from trusting any of the other members in which there lies means
of knowledge, but know each thing in the way in which it is clear.

Columns from the Greek
temple at Agrigentum.

Fools! for they have no far-reaching studious thoughts who think that
what was not before comes into being or that anything dies and perishes
utterly.

No mortal thing has a beginning, nor does it end in death and
obliteration; there is only a mixing and then separating of what was
mixed, but by mortal men these processes are named "beginnings."

No wise man dreams such folly in his heart, That only whilst we live
what men call life, We have our being and take our good and ill, And
ere as mortals we compacted be. And when as mortals we be loosed
apart, We are as nothing.

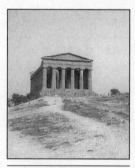

God is a circle whose center is everywhere, and its circumference
nowhere.

These [elements] never cease changing place continually, now being all
united by Love into one, now each borne apart by the hatred
engendered of Strife, until they are brought together in the unity of the
all, and become subject to it.

Empedocles lived in
Agrigentum where he
formulated his theory of the
four elements: earth, water,
fire and air.

Hear first the four roots of all things: bright Zeus, life-giving Hera (air),
and Aidoneus (earth), and Nestis who moistens the springs of men with
her tears.

Diogenes Laertius, *Lives of Eminent Philosophers*

And when a pestilence attacked the people of Selinus, by reason of the bad smells
arising from the adjacent river, so that men died and the women bore dead children, Empedocles contrived a plan, and brought into the same channel two other
rivers at his own expense; and so, by mixing their waters with that of the other
river, he sweetened the stream...the people of Selinus were on one occasion holding a festival on the bank of the river, Empedocles appeared among them; and they
rising up, offered him adoration, and prayed to him as to a God. And he wishing to
confirm this idea which they had adopted of him, leaped into the fire.

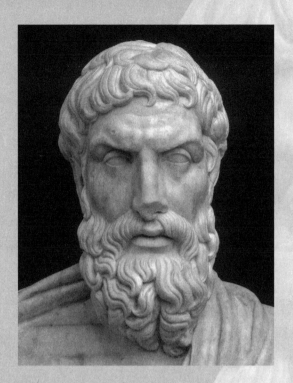

Epicurus was probably born on the island of Samos; however, he spent his early childhood in Athens. He dedicated much of his youth to the study of philosophy, looking for practical knowledge that would be useful in life and lead to greater happiness.

He founded a school on the island of Lesbos called "The Garden," a small estate where he lived in retirement with a small number of students and acquaintances, and devoted his time to the study of philosophy and the pursuit of friendship. Unlike Plato's Academy and Aristotle's Lyceum, the Garden was open to women. An inscription on the gate leading to the garden read: "Stranger, here you will do well to tarry; here our highest good is pleasure."

Epicurus

Samos, Greece, 341–Athens, Greece, 270 BCE)

Recommended reading:

📖 📖 📖 *Letter to Menoeceus*

📖 📖 *Letter to Herodotus*

📖 *Letter to Idomeneus*

Brief quotations

Let no one be slow to seek wisdom when he is young nor weary in the search of it when he has grown old. For no age is too early or too late for the health of the soul. And to say that the season for studying philosophy has not yet come, or that it is past and gone, is like saying that the season for happiness is not yet or that it is now no more. Therefore, both old and young alike ought to seek wisdom, the former in order that, as age comes over him, he may be young in good things because of the grace of what has been, and the latter in order that, while he is young, he may at the same time be old, because he has no fear of the things which are to come. So we must exercise ourselves in the things which bring happiness, since, if that be present, we have everything, and, if that be absent, all our actions are directed towards attaining it.

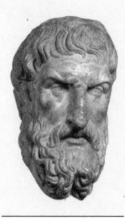

He who is not satisfied with a little, is satisfied with nothing.

The wealth required by nature is limited and is easy to procure; but the wealth required by vain ideals extends to infinity.

---

300 manuscripts and 37 treatises have been attributed to Epicurus. Unhappily none remain extant. Three letters and quotations from other writers are all that are left.

Of all the means which wisdom acquires to ensure happiness throughout the whole of life, by far the most important is friendship.

Pleasure is the principle and end to a happy life.

By pleasure we mean the absence of pain in the body and of trouble in the soul.

While therefore all pleasure is good, because it is naturally akin, not all pleasure is worthy of choice, just as all pain is an evil and yet not all pain is equally to be shunned.

To begin with, nothing comes into being out of what is non-existent.

I have never wished to cater to the crowd; for what I know they do not approve, and what they approve I do not know.

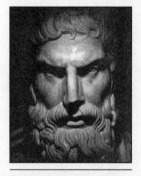

It is impossible to live a pleasant life without living wisely and well and justly. And it is impossible to live wisely and well and justly without living a pleasant life.

Letter to Menoeceus

Death, therefore, the most awful of evils, is nothing to us, seeing that, when we are death is not come, and when death is come, we are not. It is nothing, then, either to the living or the dead, for with the living it is not and the dead exist no longer. But in the world, at one time people shun death as the greatest of all evils and at another time choose it as a respite from the evils in life. The wise person does not deprecate life nor does he fear the cessation of life.

Erasmus of Rotterdam

(Rotterdam, Holland, 1469–Basel, Switzerland, 1536)

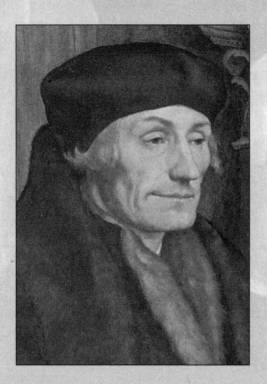

Erasmus was a Dutch philosopher and theologian. The illegitimate son of a priest, he was one of the leading lights of the incipient movement of humanism and a force for reformation of the Church.

He studied at the University of Paris, which was greatly influenced by the thinkers of the Italian Renaissance. In 1521 he moved to Basel, Switzerland. He was inevitably drawn into the controversy surrounding Luther and the Reformation, despite his best efforts at conciliation.

In the end his work was banned by the Church, despite the fact that it was neither anti-Catholic nor anti-clerical, but rather sought the purification of Church doctrine and the liberalization of its institutions.

Recommended reading:

In Praise of Folly (1509)

Adagia (Collection of Latin Proverbs (1508)

Sileni Alcibiadis (1515)

But counsel, you'll say, is not of least concern in matters of war. In a general I grant it; but this thing of warring is not part of philosophy, but managed by parasites, panders, thieves, cut-throats, plowmen, sots, spendthrifts, and such other dregs of mankind, not philosophers; who how unapt they are even for common converse, let Socrates, whom the oracle of Apollo, though not so wisely, judged "the wisest of all men living," be witness; who stepping up to speak somewhat, I know not what, in public was forced to come down again well laughed at for his pains.

And how great a happiness is this, think you? While, as if Holy Writ were a nose of wax, they fashion and refashion it according to their pleasure; while they require that their own conclusions, subscribed by two or three Schoolmen, be accounted greater than Solon's laws and preferred before the papal decretals; while, as censors of the world, they force everyone to a recantation that differs but a hair's breadth from the least of their explicit or implicit determinations.

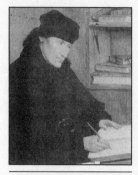

Many well-known sayings and adages are attributed to Erasmus, among them: "Prevention is better than cure;" "Crocodile tears;" "Rara avis."

The grass is always greener in the next field.

In the land of the blind the one-eyed man is king.

The most disadvantageous peace is better than the most just war.

I have given my heart and soul to Greek literature. If I come into money first I purchase books of Greek authors, then clothing.

For what is life but a play in which everyone acts a part until the curtain comes down?

This type of man who is devoted to the study of wisdom is always most unlucky in everything, and particularly when it comes to procreating children; I imagine this is because Nature wants to ensure that the evils of wisdom shall not spread further throughout mankind.

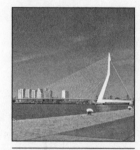

The Erasmus Bridge in Rotterdam. The relation between Luther and Erasmus was intense, but even though he criticized the Catholic Church and called for reform, he did not leave it.

In Praise of Folly

At what rate soever the world talks of me (for I am not ignorant what an ill report Folly has got, even among the most foolish), yet that I am that she, that only she, whose deity recreates both gods and men, even this is a sufficient argument, that I no sooner stepped up to speak to this full assembly than all your faces put on a kind of new and unwonted pleasantness. So suddenly have you cleared your brows, and with so frolic and hearty a laughter given me your applause, that in truth as many of you as I behold on every side of me seem to me no less than Homer's gods drunk with nectar and nepenthe; whereas before, you sat as lumpish and pensive as if you had come from consulting an oracle.

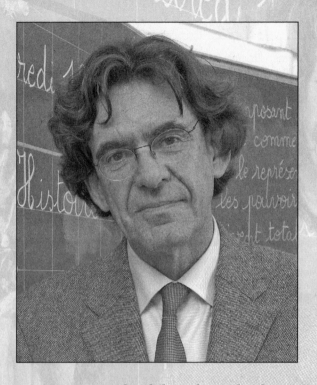

Luc Ferry

(París, France 1951)

Luc Ferry taught philosophy at the the Institute of Political Studies in Lyon and at the University of Caen. Between 2002 and 2004 he served as French Minister of Youth, National Education and Research. As such he was in charge of measures banning the display of religious symbols in schools.

His work, *The New Ecological Order*, won the Prix Médicis and provoked controversy between environmentalists and the more radical deep ecology movement. In recent years Ferry has become increasingly popular in France. Some of his books have sold over 100,000 copies and have been published in translation in over 25 countries. According to Ferry the revolution in education of the 1970s was immensely helpful to students, freeing them to be creative in new unregimented ways.

Recommended reading:

The New Ecological Order (1992)

Learning to Live (2006)

Man Made God: The Meaning of Life (1996)

We have the impression that economic forces, financial markets, new technologies, transform our everyday lives far more than ministers or legislators.

Consumption is an addiction.

Philosophy assists us in overcoming the fear of death. The fear of death is the source of all of our fears.

Human action can be summed up in the well-known Christian precept: "Do unto others as you would have done to you." This should be in the forefront of contemporary philosophic thinking, leading us to place the experience of others at the center of our moral awareness.

Human beings are capable of escaping the program of nature. They can act in ways not governed by self interest, that is to say fundamentally unnatural. They can also torture and kill. No other animal tortures or murders; they are none of them sadists.

Cartesian philosophy has led to the devaluation of nature in general and animals in particular.

It is clear that the highly vaunted "liberal values" lead in actuality to an abasement of every value and that capitalist society is *par excellence* that which believes in nothing, since domination of the world has no object other than itself.

Pure science is a myth. In its research science is never disinterested. There are always hidden interest: economic, political...

We live between memories and projects, between nostalgia and hope.

Man's increasing power over the world has become a process that is totally automatic, uncontrollable, even blind.

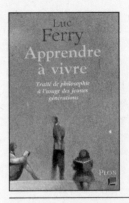

French edition of one of Ferry's books, Apprendre à vivre (Learning to Live).

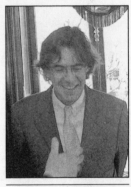

According to Ferry, it is a mistake to think that the classroom can substitute work for play, just as it is a lie that youth is happiness and growing old misery. "The dominance of a culture that preaches the easy way ruins the culture of interesting ways."

Learning to Live

If philosophy, like religion, finds its deepest source in the reflection on human finitude, on the fact that as mortal beings, our time is counted, and that we are the only beings in this world fully aware of that fact, then the question of what we are going to do with the limited time at our disposal cannot be avoided.

Ludwig A. Feuerbach

(Landshut, Germany, 1804–Rechenberg, Germany, 1872)

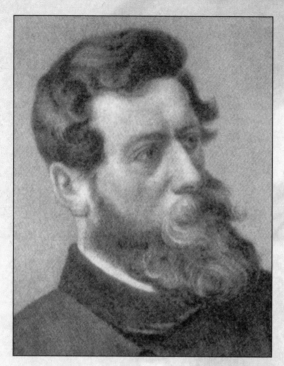

Feuerbach studied theology and philosophy in Berlin. He was a disciple of Hegel. At first he was greatly influenced by his teacher, but soon he began to criticize the ideas of the master. The two axes upon which he constituted his philosophy were the materialist critique of all speculative systems and an anthropological conception of religion.

In contrast to Hegel's idealism, which elevated the notion of spirit over reason, Feuerbach affirmed corporeal and sensible reality of the human person. He held that man was not created by God in God's image, but rather that man creates God, projecting onto him an idealized image.

Recommended reading:

Principles of the Philosophy of the Future (1843)

The Essence of Christianity (1841)

Thoughts about Death and Immortality (1830)

Philosophy is the recognition of that which is. To think and conceive the causes and the natures of things as they are is the supreme law and task of the philosopher.

The new philosophy requires the complete and absolute dissolution of any contradictions between theology and anthropology.

The new philosophy bases itself on the truth of love, on the truth of feeling. In love, in feeling in general, every human being confesses to the truth of the new philosophy.

If the old philosophy avers: that which is not thought does not exist; the new philosophy in contrast says that which is not loved, that which cannot be loved, does not exist.

We become conscious and certain of truth only through the other, even if not through this or that accidental other. That which is true belongs neither to me nor exclusively to you, but is common to all...

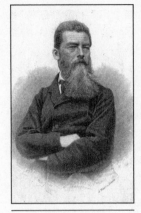

Engraving of Ludwig A. Feuerbach.

Feelings, everyday feelings, contain the deepest and highest truths.

God did not, as the Bible says, make man in His image; on the contrary man, as I have shown in *The Essence of Christianity,* made God in his image.

Taken in its reality or regarded as real, the real is the object of the senses—the sensuous. Truth, reality, and sensuousness are one and the same thing. Only a sensuous being is a true and real being. Only through the senses is an object given in the true sense, not through thought for itself. The object given by and identical with ideation is merely thought.

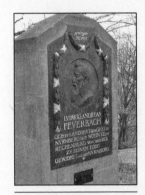

The new philosophy looks upon being-being as given to us not only as thinking, but also as really existing being—as the object of being, as its own object. Being as the object of being—and this alone is truly, and deserves the name of, being—is sensuous being; that is, the being involved in sense perception, feeling, and love. Or in other words, being is a secret underlying sense perception, feeling, and love.

Monument to Feuerbach in Nuremberg, Germany.

Principles of the Philosophy of the Future

Desire not to be a philosopher if being a philosopher means being different to man; do not be anything more than a thinking man; think not as a thinker, that is, not as one confined to a faculty which is isolated in so far as it is torn away from the totality of the real being of man; think as a living, real being, in which capacity you are exposed to the vivifying and refreshing waves of the ocean of the world; think as one who exists, as one who is in the world and is part of the world...only then can you be sure that being and thought are united in all your thinking.

Johann Gottlieb Fichte

(Rammenau, Germany, 1762–Berlin, Germany, 1814)

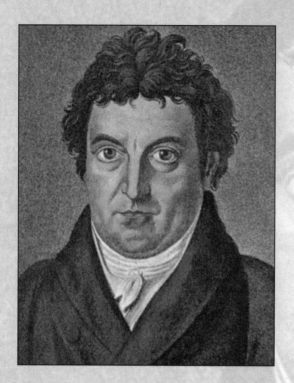

Fichte is considered to be one of the fathers of German idealism. He followed in the footsteps of Kant and was a precursor to Hegel. He came from a very poor family, and it was only due to the generosity of a noble patron that he was able to pursue his education.

Fichte studied theology in Leipzig and traveled to Königsberg to meet Kant, who, impressed with his writing, introduced him to his own publisher, thereby starting Fichte on his career in philosophy.

In 1813 at the height of the Napoleonic War he enlisted in the militia. His wife, who worked as a volunteer nurse tending the wounded, contracted typhus. Although she eventually recovered, she infected Fichte, who died of the disease at the age of 51.

Recommended reading:

📖 📖 📖 *Foundation of the Entire Science of Knowledge* (1794)

📖 📖 *Attempt at a Critique of All Revelation* (1792)

📖 *Addresses to the German Nation* (1807)

The type of philosophy one favors depends upon the kind of man he is.

———

Authentic freedom of thought can provoke an adverse reaction from some individuals, but it is without exception of benefit to the totality of human existence on earth.

———

No, your majesty, you are not our God. From God we hope for happiness, from you the defense of our rights. You do not owe us kindness; you owe us justice.

———

Man can do what he should; if he says he cannot, it is because he will not.

———

My mind can take no hold on the present world, nor rest in it a moment, but my whole nature rushes with irresistible force towards a future and better state of being.

———

The prince says that we cannot know what will make us happy. He knows the secret and will guide us and we should follow him blindly. He places a noose around the neck of humanity crying, "Calm down, calm down; all will be well."

———

In its recognition of marriage, the state abandons all pretense of considering the woman as a legal person. Her husband occupies this position for her. Matrimony annuls her personhood.

———

Order the hurricane to be calm, and after that give the same order to our subversive opinions.

———

A man cannot be inherited or purchased or ruled; he cannot be the property of anyone else, since he is his own property. In the depths of his heart there is a divine spark that elevates him above the rest of the animal kingdom and that he possesses in God's world: his conscience.

———

By philosophy the mind of man comes to itself, and from henceforth rests on itself without foreign aid, and is completely master of itself, as the dancer of his feet, or the boxer of his hands.

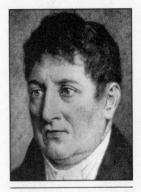

Johann Gottlieb Fichte's idealism posited that reality is a product of the thinking subject, in contrast to realism, which affirms that objects exist independently of our perception of them.

Fichte also established that self-consciousness is a social phenomenon. He stated that a rational being reaches the fullness of awareness when he realizes that other people's awareness is the same as his own.

Attempt at a Critique of All Revelation

So long as finite beings remain finite, they will continue to stand—for that is the concept of finitude in morality—under other laws than those of reason. Consequently, they will never be able to produce by themselves the complete congruency of happiness with morality. The moral law, however, requires this quite unconditionally. Therefore, this law can never cease to be valid, since it will never be achieved; its claim can never end, since it will never be fulfilled. It is valid for eternity.

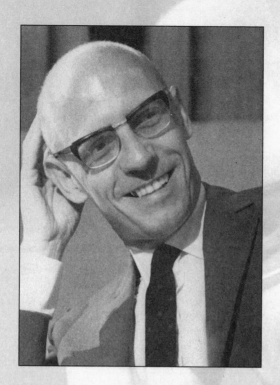

Michel Foucault

(Poitiers, France, 1926–Paris, 1984)

The work of this French philosopher has had a wide influence upon the social sciences and humanities in Europe and the United States. His writings call into question modern theories of knowledge, power, and subjectivity, defying conventional thinking on such relevant issues as mental institutions, sexuality, and prisons.

In 1970 Foucault was elected to the most prestigious academic society in France, La Collège de France, assuming a chair he created for himself in the "history of systems of thought." By the late 1970s he became disillusioned with activism and hopes of real political change. He traveled much of the world in his later years, gaining an extraordinary international reputation. He died of AIDS in 1984.

Recommended reading:

Madness and Civilization (1960)
Archaeology of Knowledge (1969)

Discipline and Punish: The Birth of the Prison (1975)

History of Sexuality (3 vols. 1976-1984)

Schools serve the same social functions as prisons and mental institutions—to define, classify, control, and regulate people.

———

The soul is the prison of the body.

———

I don't feel that it is necessary to know exactly what I am. The main interest in life and work is to become someone else that you were not in the beginning. If you knew when you began a book what you would say at the end, do you think that you would have the courage to write it? What is true for writing and for a love relationship is true also for life. The game is worthwhile insofar as we don't know what will be the end.

———

Madness is the absolute break with the work of art; it forms the constitutive moment of abolition, which dissolves in time the truth of the work of art.

———

As the archaeology of our thought easily shows, man is an invention of recent date. And one perhaps nearing its end.

———

Justice is an idea that has been invented and can function in different types of societies as a tool to assert political and economic power, or as a weapon against that power.

———

Nietzsche was a revelation to me. I felt that there was someone quite different from what I had been taught. I read him with a great passion and broke with my life, left my job in the asylum, left France: I had the feeling I had been trapped. Through Nietzsche, I had become a stranger to all that.

———

...if you are not like everybody else, then you are abnormal, if you are abnormal , then you are sick. These three categories, not being like everybody else, not being normal and being sick are in fact very different but have been reduced to the same thing.

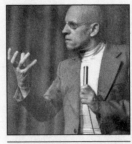

"Furious activist," as his friend the ultra-Maoist Defert called him, Foucault denounced the micro-structures of power in industrialized societies. In politics he formulated a declaration decriminalizing all relations between consenting adults, in which category he included those over fifteen years old.

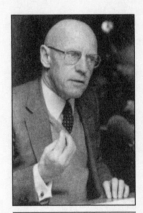

"Don't ask me who I am or that I stay the same."

Madness and Civilization

In the serene world of mental illness, modern man no longer communicates with the madman...The constitution of madness as a mental illness, at the end of the eighteenth century, affords the evidence of a broken dialogue, posits the separation as already effected, and thrusts into oblivion all those stammered, imperfect words without fixed syntax in which the exchange between madness and reason was made. The language of psychiatry, which is a monologue of reason about madness, has been established only on the basis of such a silence.

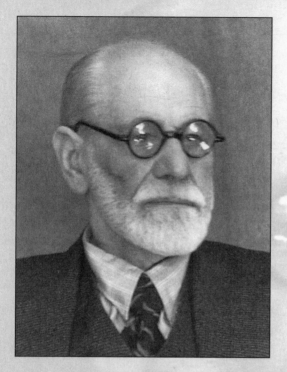

Sigmund Freud

(Freiburg, Moravia, 1856–London, England, 1939)

Freud's family moved to Vienna when he was still a child, and he lived there almost the rest of his life. Philosopher, doctor, and neurologist, Sigmund Schlomo Freud was the creator of the method and theory of psychoanalysis. Early in his career his colleague, Josef Breuer, interested him in the therapeutic benefit of hypnosis. During a three-year residence in a Parisian hospital he came to view hysteria as problem worthy of serious investigation. On his return to Vienna he opened a private practice. He utilized free association and dream analysis to develop what he termed the "talking cure," thereby establishing the beginning of the discipline of psychoanalysis.

His theories and methods of treatment caused consternation in the Vienna of his time and continue to spark controversy.

Recommended reading:

The Interpretation of Dreams (1899)
The Ego and the Id (1923)

The Psychopathology of Everyday Life (1904)

The Future of an Illusion (1930)
Civilization and Its Discontents (1930)

Modern medicine has not produced any tranquilizing medication as effective as a few kind words.

I have been most fortunate in life. Nothing has been easy for me.

What progress we are making. In the Middle Ages they would have burned me. Now they are content with burning my books.

The first individual to hurl an insult rather than a stone at his enemy was the founder of civilization.

If two people are always in agreement with each, then it is certain that one of them thinks for both.

The great question that has never been answered, and which I have not yet been able to answer, despite my thirty years of research into the feminine soul, is "What does a woman want?"

The poor ego has a still harder time of it; it has to serve three harsh masters, and it has to do its best to reconcile the claims and demands of all three....The three tyrants are the external world, the superego, and the id.

Most people do not really want freedom, because freedom involves responsibility, and most people are frightened of responsibility.

Dreams are the royal road to the unconscious.

It is impossible to overlook the extent to which civilization is built up upon a renunciation of instinct.

Man has, as it were, become a kind of prosthetic God.

Religion is a system of wishful illusions together with a disavowal of reality, such as we find nowhere else but in a state of blissful hallucinatory confusion. Religion's eleventh commandment is "Thou shalt not question."

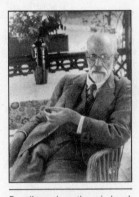

Freud's work on the mind and human behavior has had tremendous impact on the social sciences, philosophy, and medicine. His interest in neurology led to the development of a theory and practice that have been replaced by the empirical discoveries of recent decades; psychiatry and psychology today have rejected many of the intuitions of its founder. Nonetheless his emphasis on the study of dreams and the importance of "Freudian slips", remains invaluable as do his ideas on the ego and the unconscious and the informing presence of the sexual drive in people's lives.

The Future of an Illusion

Thus I must contradict you when you go on to argue that men are completely unable to do without the consolation of the religious illusion....That is true, certainly, of the men into whom you have instilled the sweet—or bitter-sweet—poison from childhood onwards. But what of the other men...who do not suffer from the neurosis. They will, it is true, find themselves in a difficult situation....They will be in the same position as a child who has left the parental house where he was so warm and comfortable. But surely infantilism is destined to be surmounted. Men cannot remain children for ever; they must in the end go out into 'hostile life'. We may call this education to reality. Need I confess to you that the whole purpose of my book is to point out the necessity for this forward step?

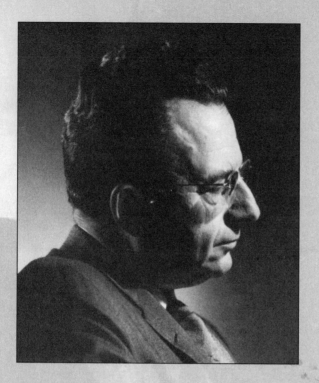

Erich Fromm

(Frankfurt, Germany, 1900–Muralto, Switzerland, 1980)

Fromm studied in Heidelberg and was an active participant in the Frankfurt School. Afterwards he was marginalized on account of his heterodox interpretation of psychoanalytic theory and his divergences with other members, especially Marcuse and Adorno.

In 1934 after National Socialism's assumption of power, he emigrated to the United States. In 1950 he moved to Mexico and taught at the Universidad Nacional. He also lectured in psychology at Michigan State University and later at New York University.

He retired in 1965 and devoted himself to travel. He took up residence in Muralto, Switzerland in 1974, where he lived until his death shortly before his eightieth birthday. Fromm is considered to be one of principle renovators of psychoanalytic theory and practice.

Recommended reading:

Escape from Freedom (1941)
The Art of Loving (1956)

To Have or to Be (1966)

The Sane Society (1955)

To love one person productively means to be related to his human core, to him as representing mankind. Love for one individual, in so far as it is divorced from love for man, can refer only to the superficial and to the accidental; of necessity it remains shallow.

Society must be organized in such a way that man's social, loving nature is not separated from his social existence, but becomes one with it. If it is true, as I have tried to show, that love is the only sane and satisfactory answer to the problem of human existence, then any society which excludes, relatively, the development of love, must in the long run perish of its own contradiction with the basic necessities of human nature.

To have faith in the possibility of love as a social and not only exceptional-individual phenomenon, is a rational faith based on the insight into the very nature of man.

Man is the only animal for whom his own existence is a problem which he has to solve. One cannot be deeply responsive to the world without being saddened very often.

The whole life of the individual is nothing but the process of giving birth to himself; we should be fully born when we die—although it is the tragic fate of most individuals to die before they are born.

If I am what I have, and if I lose what I have, who then am I?

Human beings had two basic orientations: HAVING and BEING. HAVING: seeks to acquire, possess things even people. BEING: focuses on the experience; exchanging, engaging, sharing with other people.

The quest for certainty blocks the search for meaning. Uncertainty is the very condition to impel man to unfold his powers.

Care and responsibility are constituent elements of love, but without respect for and knowledge of the beloved person, love deteriorates into domination and possessiveness.

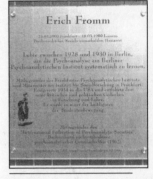

Memorial plaque to Erich Fromm in Berlin.

In his work Fromm accuses contemporary man of passivity and over-identification with commercial values. This has resulted in his transformation into a kind of commodity and his perception of himself as an investment.

The Art of Loving

Modern man has transformed himself into a commodity; he experiences his life energy as an investment with which he should make the highest profit, considering his position and the situation on the personality market. He is alienated from himself, from his fellow men and from nature. His main aim is profitable exchange of his skills, knowledge, and of himself, his "personality package" with others who are equally intent on a fair and profitable exchange. Life has no goal except the one to move, no principle except the one of fair exchange, no satisfaction except the one to consume.

Hans-Georg Gadamer

(Marburg, Germany, 1900–Heidelberg, Germany, 2002)

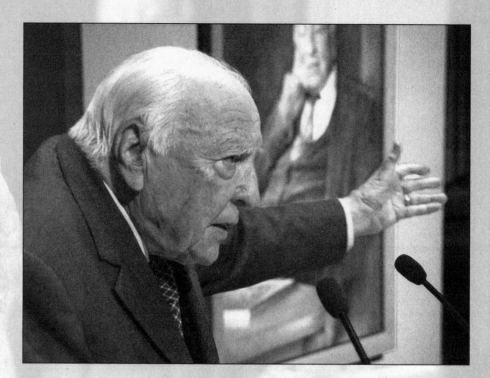

Gadamer was the son of a professor of pharmacology at the University of Marburg who later became that university's rector. His son followed the path of the humanities. He was a student of Husserl and friend of Hannah Arendt, but Heidegger exercised the most influence on his thought.

Unlike Heidegger, Gadamer opposed the Nazi regime and distanced himself from academia until after the war, when he was appointed rector of the University of Leipzig. He left that post when Leipzig became a part of East Germany and moved first to the University of Frankfurt, finally settling at the University of Heidelberg. He engaged in a fruitful debate with Jürgen Habermas over the possibility of historical-cultural transcendence in light of the contemporary social milieu.

Recommended reading:

Truth and Method (1960)

Philosophical Hermeneutics (1986)

The Relevance of the Beautiful (1977)

The more language is a living operation, the less we are aware of it. Thus it follows that from the forgetfulness of language that its real being consists in what is said in it. What is said in it constitutes the common world in which we live....The real being of language is that into which we are taken up when we hear it—what is said.

Someone who speaks in an idiom that no one understands, doesn't speak at all. To speak is to speak to another.

What man needs is not just the persistent posing of ultimate questions, but the sense of what is feasible, what is possible, what is correct, here and now. The philosopher, of all people, must, I think, be aware of the tension between what he claims to achieve and the reality in which he finds himself.

The work of art that says something confronts us itself. That is, it expresses something in such a way that what is said is like a discovery, a disclosure of something previously concealed.

Being that can be understood is language.

Human civilization differs essentially from nature in that it is only simply a place where capacities and power work themselves out; man becomes what he is through what he does and how he behaves—i.e., he behaves in a certain way because of what he has become.

In fact history does not belong to us but rather we to it.

Life itself, flowing temporality, is ordered toward the formation of enduring units of significance. Life interprets itself. Life itself has a hermeneutic structure. Thus life constitutes the real ground of the human sciences. Hermeneutics is not a romantic heritage of Dilthey's thinking, but follows from the fact that philosophy is grounded in "life."

The individual case does not serve only to confirm a law from which practical predictions can be made. Its ideal is rather to understand the phenomenon itself in its unique and historical concreteness.

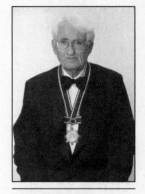

Photograph of Jürgen Habermas, opponent of Gadamer in a celebrated philosophical debate.

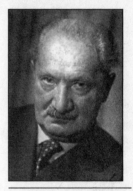

Heidegger was a key figure in the development of Gadamer's thinking.

Truth and Method

The hermeneutic task becomes of itself a questioning of things and is always in part so defined...A person trying to understand something will not resign himself from the start to relying on his own accidental fore-meanings, ignoring as consistently and stubbornly as possible the actual meaning of the text until the latter becomes so persistently audible that it breaks through what the interpreter imagines it to be...a person trying to understand a text is prepared for it to tell him something.

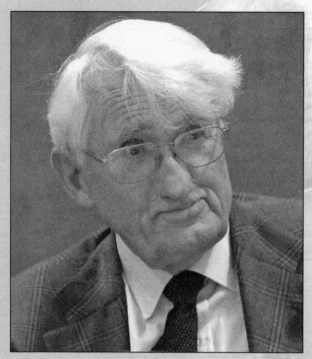

Jürgen Habermas

(Düsseldorf, Germany, 1929)

After completing his doctoral thesis on Schelling, Habermas studied with Adorno and Horkheimer at the Johann Wolfgang Goethe University Frankfurt am Main Institute for Social Research. He went on to teach in Frankfurt and Heidelberg.

Sociologist and philosopher, he is the most important heir to the luminaries of the Frankfurt school. His interest in the theories of communicative action and practical philosophy have led to fertile debates with contemporary philosophers such as Gadamer, Lyotard, and Sloterdijk.

Habermas has received numerous awards including The Prince of Asturias Award in Social Sciences and the Gottfried Wilhelm Leibniz Prize for research.

Recommended reading:

The Theory of Communicative Action (1981)

The Inclusion of the Other (1996)

Legitimation Crisis (1975)

I shall develop the thesis that anyone acting communicatively must, in performing any speech act, raise universal validity claims and suppose that they can be vindicated.

———

Reaching and understanding is the process of bringing about an agreement on the presupposed basis of validity claims that are mutually recognized.

———

Since moral principles are always already immersed in concrete historical contexts of action, there can be no justification or assessment of norms according to a universal procedure that ensures impartiality.

———

The state is in danger of falling into disrepute due to the evidence of its inadequate resources.

———

The difference between political terror and ordinary crime becomes clear during the change of regimes, in which former terrorists become well-regarded representatives of their country.

———

Only one who takes over his own life history can see in it the realization of his self. Responsibility to take over one's own biography means to get clear about who one wants to be.

———

I cannot imagine a context that would some day, in some manner, make the monstrous crime of September 11 an understandable or comprehensible political act.

———

...we understand a speech act when we know the kinds of reasons that a speaker could provide in order to convince a hearer that he is entitled in the given circumstances to claim validity for his utterance—in short, when we know what makes it acceptable.

———

The task of universal pragmatics is to identify and reconstruct universal conditions of possible mutual understanding.

———

Each murder is one too many.

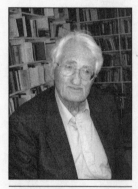

Habermas has received wide academic recognition. As professor at the University of Frankfurt from 1964 to 1971 he emerged as one of the leading proponents of critical theory.

For the normative self-understanding of modernity, Christianity has functioned as more than just a precursor or catalyst. Universalistic egalitarianism, from which sprang the ideals of freedom and a collective life in solidarity, the autonomous conduct of life and emancipation, the individual morality of conscience, human rights and democracy, is the direct legacy of the Judaic ethic of justice and the Christian ethic of love....Up to this very day there is no alternative to it. And in light of the current challenges of a post-national constellation, we must draw sustenance now, as in the past, from this substance. Everything else is idle postmodern talk.

Georg W. F. Hegel

(Stuttgart, Germany, 1770–1831)

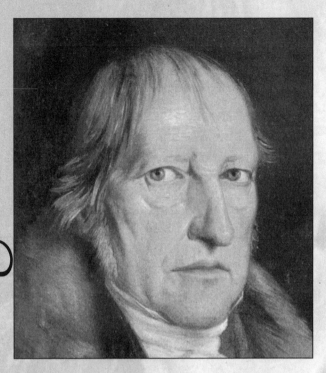

The German philosopher Georg Wilhelm Friedrich Hegel is one of the most influential figures in the history of Western thought and the greatest representative of idealism. He studied at the University of Tubingen. There he met Holderin and Schelling and the three collaborated on a critical study of the philosophical idealism of Kant and his successor, Fichte. This work preceded the development of the dialectic. He observed: "Thought is where true freedom resides."

Other powerful influences on Hegel's thought were Spinoza, Rousseau, and the French Revolution. After his death his followers divided into two opposing groups: the Hegelians of the right with a conservative bent, and those of the Left, such as Marx, whose theory of historical materialism owes much to Hegel's dialectic.

Recommended reading:

📖 📖 📖 *Phenomenology of Spirit* (1806)

📖 📖 *Science of Logic* (1816)

📖 *Elements of the Philosophy of Right* (1819)

In its works of art the people have deposited their most intimate thoughts and fertile intuitions. Often art is the only key permitting us to penetrate the secrets of wisdom and the mysteries of religion. The world of art is truer than that of nature or history.

———

Nothing great is produced in this world without great passion.

———

Genuine tragedies in the world arise not out of the conflict between right and wrong, but between two rights.

———

Drama is not a choice between good and evil, but between two goods.

———

Men of great talent are those who recognize the spirit of the people and know how to guide them toward that end. Exceptional men guide the people to conform to the universal spirit.

———

Reading the newspaper is the realist's morning prayer.

———

When we sense or when we feel we are determined, not free. We are only free when we gain awareness of these sensations.

———

The essence of the modern state is the union of the universal with the full freedom of the particular, and with the welfare of individuals.

———

The History of the world is none other than the progress of the consciousness of Freedom; a progress whose development according to the necessity of its nature, it is our business to investigate.

———

Not curiosity, not vanity, not the consideration of expediency, not duty and conscientiousness, but an unquenchable, unhappy thirst that brooks no compromise leads us to truth.

———

What experience and history teach is this—that nations and governments have never learned anything from history, or acted upon any lessons they might have drawn from it.

———

The History of the world is none other than the progress of the consciousness of Freedom; a progress whose development according to he necessity of its nature, it is our business to investigate.

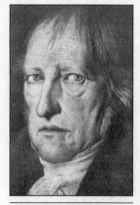

Thesis, antithesis and synthesis: Hegel was responsible for a new dialectical approach and a vast and complex philosophical system. He also engaged in a profound study of logic. ("Reality is the unity of essence and existence. Essence is neither subordinate or superior to phenomena...essence concretizes phenomena.")

His approach to questions of aesthetics evinced disquietude before the phenomenon of beauty and explored the character of arts' relationship to freedom and the spirit.

Upon his death his followers divided into two opposing camps. Among the left-leaning Hegelians his most famous offspring is Karl Marx.

Phenomenology of Spirit

The life of God—the life which the mind apprehends and enjoys as it rises to the absolute unity of all things—may be described as a play of love with itself; but this idea sinks to an edifying truism, or even to a platitude, when it does not embrace in it the earnestness, the pain, the patience, and labor, involved in the negative aspect of things.

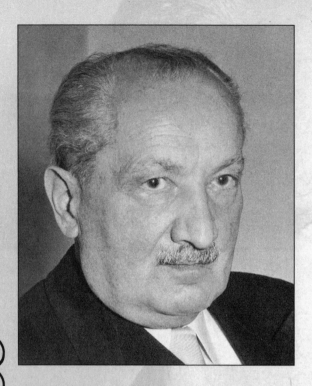

Martin Heidegger

(Messkirch, Germany, 1889–Freiburg, Germany, 1976)

Many consider Heidegger to be the father of existentialism. He was a student of Husserl and took from him the phenomenological method, which he used in a unique way in his masterful work, *Being and Time*, to articulate an exhaustive analysis of humanity and its place in the world.

His fame as professor at the University of Freiburg quickly spread throughout Germany. In 1933 the National Socialist government named him rector of the university. His acceptance of this post under the Nazis resulted in his condemnation by many of his peers. Later on he renounced his position, although he continued to teach.

Recommended reading:

Being and Time (1927)

Origin of the Work of Art (1936)
What Is Metaphysics (1929)

The Principle of Reason (1955)

Everywhere we remain unfree and chained to technology, whether we passionately affirm or deny it. But we are delivered over to it in the worst possible way when we regard it as something neutral; for this conception of it, to which today we particularly like to do homage, makes us utterly blind to the essence of technology.

———

If I take death into my life, acknowledge it, and face it squarely, I will free myself from the anxiety of death and the pettiness of life—and only then will I be free to become myself.

———

Nevertheless, the ultimate business of philosophy is to preserve the force of the most elemental words in which Being expresses itself, and to keep the common understanding from leveling them off to that unintelligibility which functions in turn as a source of pseudo-problems.

———

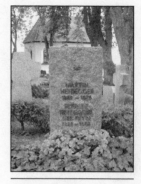

Heidegger's tomb.

Man acts as though he were the shaper and master of language, while in fact language remains the master of man.

———

Man is not the lord of beings. Man is the shepherd of Being.

———

Language is the house of the truth of Being.

———

Thinking only begins at the point where we have come to know that Reason, glorified for centuries, is the most obstinate adversary of thinking.

———

What seems natural to us is probably just something familiar in a long tradition that has forgotten the unfamiliar source from which it arose. And yet this unfamiliar source once struck man as strange and caused him to think and to wonder.

———

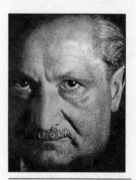

We name time when we say: every thing has its time. This means: everything which actually is, every being comes and goes at the right time and remains for a time during the time allotted to it. Every thing has its time.

———

Heidegger's *Being and Time* left an indelible impression on twentieth-century philosophical thought.

Truth is that which makes a people certain, clear, and strong.

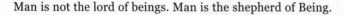

■ *Being and Time*

Why are there beings at all instead of nothing? That is the question. Presumably it is not an arbitrary question, "Why are there beings at all instead of nothing"—this is obviously the first of all questions. Of course it is not the first question in the chronological sense....And yet, we are each touched once, maybe even every now and then, by the concealed power of this question, without properly grasping what is happening to us. In great despair, for example, when all weight tends to dwindle away from things and the sense of things grows dark, the question looms.

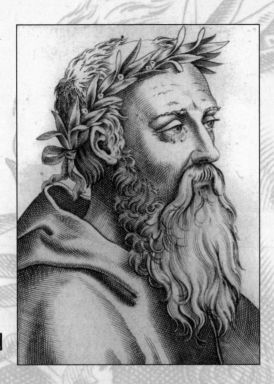

Heraclitus of Ephesus

(Ephesus, Ionia c. 544–c.484 BCE)

Little is known about the life of Heraclitus. He is said to have come from a well-to-do family and lived all of his life in Ephesus, a city on the coast of Ionia. To judge by the testimony of ancient writers he had little to do with his fellow citizens.

Of his work only fragments survive, which have been preserved in the writings of other philosophers. He employed an aphoristic style, which often expressed itself in paradoxes reminiscent of the Oracle of Delphi. He maintained that the foundation of all phenomena is constant change. Change is the only permanent reality, and this was governed by a law he named *logos*. Everything is transformed in a continuous process of being born and dying.

Recommended reading:

Diogenes Laertius, *Lives of Eminent Philosophers* (1st century CE)

Martin Heidegger, *Heraclitus* (1967)

Jean Brun, *Heraclitus* (1965)

For what sense or understanding have they? They follow minstrels and take the multitude for a teacher, not knowing that many are bad and few good. For the best men choose one thing above all—immortal glory among mortals; but the masses stuff themselves like cattle.

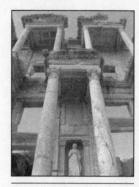

Everything flows, and nothing stands still.

He called change a pathway up and down and this determines the birth of the world (Diogenes Laertius)

Eternity is a child playing checkers; the kingdom belongs to a child.

This universe, which is the same for all, has not been made by any god or man, but it always has been, is, and will be an ever-living fire, kindling itself by regular measures and going out by regular measures.

Ruins of the Library of Celsus in Ephesus.

Nature loves to hide itself.

The road up and the road down is one and the same.

God is day and night, winter and summer, war and peace, surfeit and hunger.

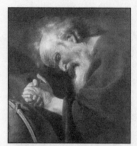

Character is destiny.

Much learning does not teach understanding.

One cannot step into the same river twice.

All things are in flux; the flux is subject to a unifying measure or rational principle. This principle (logos, the hidden harmony behind all change) bound opposites together in a unified tension, which is like that of a lyre, where a stable harmonious sound emerges from the tension of the opposing forces that arise from the bow bound together by the string.

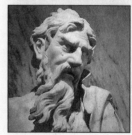

Images of Heraclitus.

Fragment

As in nighttime a man kindles for himself (*haptetai*) a light, so when a living man lies down in death with his vision extinguished, he attaches himself (*haptetai*) to the state of death; even as one who has been awake lies down with his vision extinguished and attaches himself to the state of sleep.

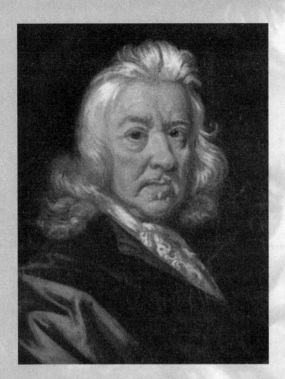

Thomas Hobbes

(Malmesbury, England, 1688–Derbyshire, England, 1679)

Hobbes can claim to be not only the founder of moral and political philosophy in England, but in Europe as a whole. His works range widely: logic, language, law, religion, aesthetics, and human nature. He was secretary to Francis Bacon, knew Galileo personally, corresponded with Descartes, and engaged in bitter arguments with church authorities and Oxford dons.

Hobbes was born prematurely, which he credited to his mother's fear of the imminent invasion of the Spanish Armada. This early insecurity is evident in many of his ideas. He often confessed himself fearful and said that he was the first to leave England at the start of the English Civil War. His work signals a clean break with the Middle Ages, occurring at a key moment in history when the two branches of government, the monarchy and the parliament, fought for supremacy.

Recommended reading:

Leviathan (1651)

De corpore (1655)

De homine (1658)

My mother gave birth to twins: myself and fear.

And the life of man, solitary, poor, nasty, brutish, and short.

The condition of man...is a condition of war of everyone against everyone.

The right of nature...is the liberty each man hath to use his own power, as he will himself, for the preservation of his own nature; that is to say, of his own life.

The obligation of subjects to the sovereign is understood to last as long, and no longer, than the power lasteth by which he is able to protect them.

I put for the general inclination of all mankind, a perpetual and restless desire of power after power, that ceaseth only in death.

I am about to take my last voyage, a great leap in the dark.

There is no such thing as perpetual tranquility of mind while we live here; because life itself is but motion, and can never be without desire, nor without fear, no more than without sense.

Science is the knowledge of Consequences, and dependence of one fact upon another: by which, out of that we can presently do, we know how to do something else when we will, or the like, another time.

For the Laws of Nature (as Justice, Equity, Modesty, Mercy, and, in sum, doing to others, as we would be done to) of themselves, without the terror of some Power, to cause them to be observed, are contrary to our natural Passions, that carry us to Partiality, Pride, Revenge, and the like. And Covenants, without the Sword, are but Words, and of no strength to secure a man at all.

But if one Subject giveth Counsel to another, to do anything contrary to the Laws, whether that Counsel proceed from evil intention, or from ignorance only, it is punishable by the Commonwealth; because ignorance of the Law, is no good excuse, where every man is bound to take notice of the Laws to which he is subject.

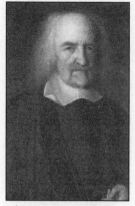

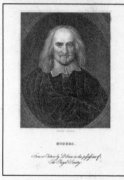

HOBBES.

In Leviathan Hobbes formally signals the transition from the doctrine of natural law to the theory of rights as arising from the social contract.

■ *Leviathan*

The right of nature, which Writers commonly call Jus Naturale, is the Liberty each man hath, to use his own power, as he will himself, for the preservation of his own Nature; that is to say, of his own Life; and consequently, of doing any thing, which in his own Judgement, and Reason, he shall conceive to be the aptest means thereunto.

By liberty is understood, according to the proper signification of the word, the absence of external impediments; which impediments may oft take away part of man's power to do what he would, but cannot hinder him from using the power left him according as his judgement and reason shall dictate to him.

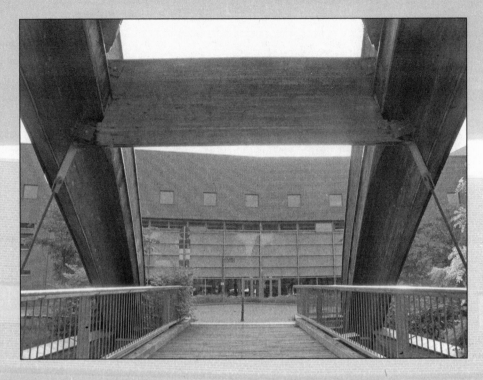

Max Horkheimer

(Stuttgart, Germany, 1895–Nuremberg, Germany, 1973)

Son of a Jewish factory owner, Horkeimer abandoned his studies to work in his father's factory. He fought in World War I and when it was over returned to university where he studied psychology and philosophy.

When the Nazis took over Germany, he emigrated to Switzerland and then to New York where he collaborated with other emigré thinkers of the Frankfurt School.

Along with Theodor Adorno, he was one of the founders of critical theory, and assimilating certain currents of Marxist thought, he elaborated a theory of capitalist culture, which sought to provide an interpretative basis for a free society.

Recommended reading:

Critique of Instrumental Reason (1967)

Eclipse of Reason (1947)

Dialectic of Enlightenment (1947, with Theodor Adorno)

The complexity of the connection between the world of perception and the world of physics does not preclude that such a connection can be shown to exist at any time.

————

At present, when the prevailing forms of society have become hindrances to the free expression of human powers, it is precisely the abstract branches of science, mathematics and theoretical physics, which...offer a less distorted form of knowledge than other branches of science which are interwoven with the pattern of daily life, and the practicality of which seemingly testifies to their realistic character.

————

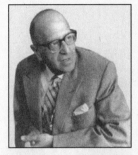

When even the dictators of today appeal to reason, they mean that they possess the most tanks. They were rational enough to build them; others should be rational enough to yield to them.

————

Whoever desires to live among men has to obey their laws—this is what the secular morality of Western civilization comes down to...Rationality in the form of such obedience swallows up everything, even the freedom to think.

————

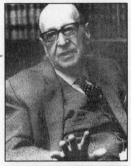

The new order contradicts reason so fundamentally that reason does not dare to doubt it. Even the consciousness of oppression fades. The more incommensurate become the concentration of power and the helplessness of the individual, the more difficult for him to penetrate the human origin of his misery.

————

Reason as an organ for perceiving the true nature of reality and determining the guiding principles of our lives has come to be regarded as obsolete.

————

Reason has never really directed social reality, but now reason has been so thoroughly purged of any specific trend or preference that it has finally renounced even the task of passing judgment on man's actions and way of life. Reason has turned them over for ultimate sanction to the conflicting interests to which our world actually seems abandoned.

Two images of Max Horkheimer, one of the leading figures of the Frankfurt School.

Preceding page: Photograph of Johann Wolfgang Goethe University Frankfurt am Main Institute for Social Research

■ *The Latest Attack on Metaphysics*

A man discovers what he is actually worth in this world when he faces society as a man, without money, name, or powerful connections, stripped of all but his native potentialities. He soon finds that nothing has less weight than his human qualities. They are prized so low that the market does not even list them. Strict science, which acknowledges man only as a biological concept, reflects man's lot in the actual world; in himself, man is nothing more than a member of a species. In the eyes of the world, the quality of humanity confers no title to existence, nay, not even a right of sojourn. Such title must be certified by special social circumstances stipulated in documents to be presented on demand.

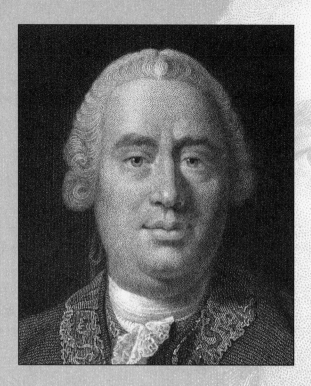

David Hume

(Edinburgh, Scotland, 1711–1776)

avid Hume was admitted to the University of Edinburgh at the age of twelve. His father slated him for a career in law, but his only interest was philosophy. A true autodidact, Hume had little time for his professors, insisting that he could learn everything that he needed to know from books.

His theory of causality—following which our ideas about cause and effect are not derived from the nature of things but rather from habit, custom, and sentiment—called into question the belief in unchanging laws of nature.

His theory of knowledge ascribed a preponderant role to sensation, in contradistinction to Descartes' elevation of reason. Hume's philosophy is the one of the most important expressions of empiricism.

Recommended reading:

A Treatise on Human Nature (1739)

An Enquiry Concerning Human Understanding (1748)

An Enquiry Concerning the Principles of Morals (1751)

Reason is, and ought only to be, the slave of the passions, and can never pretend to any other office than to serve and obey them.

———

A wise man's kingdom is his own breast: or, if he ever looks farther, it will only be to the judgment of a select few, who are free from prejudices, and capable of examining his work. Nothing indeed can be a stronger presumption of falsehood than the approbation of the multitude.

———

Methinks I am like a man, who having struck on many shoals, and having narrowly escap'd shipwreck in passing a small frith, has yet the temerity to put out to sea in the same leaky weather-beaten vessel, and even carries his ambition so far as to think of compassing the globe under these disadvantageous circumstances.

———

For my part, when I enter most intimately into what I call myself, I always stumble on some particular perception or other, of heat or cold, light or shade, love or hatred, pain or pleasure. I never can catch myself at any time without a perception, and never can observe any thing but the perception.

———

Beauty in things exists in the mind which contemplates them.

———

There is a very remarkable inclination in human nature to bestow on external objects the same emotions which it observes in itself, and to find everywhere those ideas which are most present to it.

———

It is not reason which is the guide of life, but custom.

———

It is not contrary to reason to prefer the destruction of the whole world to the scratching of my finger.

———

That the sun will not rise tomorrow is no less intelligible a proposition, and implies no more contradiction, than the affirmation, that it will rise.

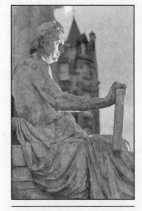

Statue honoring the Scottish philosopher, economist, and historian, David Hume. His work constituted a deepened articulation of skepticism and empiricism.

Hume argued that ideas derive solely from sensory experience, which is the foundation of all knowledge.

An Enquiry Concerning the Principles of Morals

DISPUTES with men, pertinaciously obstinate in their principles, are, of all others, the most irksome; except, perhaps, those with persons, entirely disingenuous, who really do not believe the opinions they defend, but engage in the controversy, from affectation, from a spirit of opposition, or from a desire of showing wit and ingenuity, superior to the rest of mankind....And as reasoning is not the source, whence either disputant derives his tenets; it is in vain to expect, that any logic, which speaks not to the affections, will ever engage him to embrace sounder principles.

Edmund Husserl

(Prostejov, Moravia, 1859–Friburg, Germany, 1938)

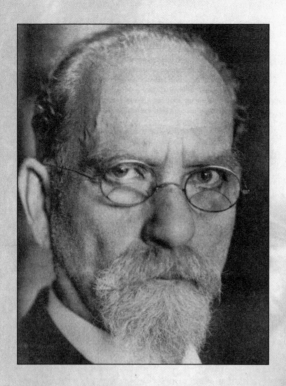

Husserl came from a Jewish Family. He studied in Berlin and then in Vienna. As his thought developed he broke with the positivism of Comte, which sought to provide a scientific basis for philosophy.

By the beginning of the twentieth century he had begun to articulate the foundations of the phenomenological approach, a method of philosophical analysis that had enormous influence on thinkers such as Heidegger and later, Sartre, Ortega y Gasset and Lacan.

From 1916 he held the Chair of Philosophy at the University of Friburg, until the National Socialist takeover in 1933 ended his teaching career. Nonetheless, phenomenology endured as one of the most fertile trends in contemporary philosophy.

Recommended reading:

📖 📖 📖 *Logical Investigations* (1900)

📖 📖 *Ideas: General Introduction to Pure Phenomenology* (1913)

📖 *Cartesian Meditations* (1931)

A new fundamental science, pure phenomenology, has developed within philosophy: This is a science of a thoroughly new type and endless scope. It is inferior in methodological rigor to none of the modern sciences. All philosophical disciplines are rooted in pure phenomenology, through whose development, and through it alone, they obtain their proper force.

First, anyone who seriously intends to become a philosopher must "once in his life" withdraw into himself and attempt, within himself, to overthrow and build anew all the sciences that, up to then, he has been accepting.

The method of phenomenology is to go back to things themselves.

Natural objects, for example, must be experienced before any theorizing about them can occur.

I seek not to instruct but only to lead, to point out and describe what I see. I claim no other right than that of speaking according to my best lights, principally before myself but in the same manner also before others, as one who has lived in all its seriousness the fate of a philosophical existence.

Phenomenology is by no means psychology. It is found in a new dimension and demands an essentially different attitude from that of psychology as well as of any science of spatial–temporal existence.

...pure phenomenology is the science of pure consciousness.

What phenomenology wants, in all these investigations, is to establish what admits of being stated with the universal validity of theory.

Philosophers, as things now stand, are all too fond of offering criticism from on high instead of studying and understanding things from within.

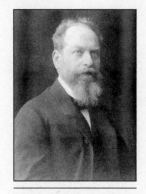

Edmund Husserl, founder of the phenomenological method, considered that the fundamental characteristic of consciousness was intentionality. Husserl's discoveries led him to affirm that by studying the structure of consciousness, we ought to be able to distinguish between the act of awareness and the phenomena to which we direct our attention, the objects of consciousness. Furthermore, the awareness of what is essential can only be realized by eliminating all preconceived ideas about the external world.

The Idea of Phenomenology

It is to this world that our judgments refer. We make statements—sometimes singular, sometimes general—about things: their relations, their alterations, their functional dependencies and laws of transformation. Thus we find expression for what presents itself in direct experience. Following up on motives provided by experience itself, we infer from what is directly experienced in perception and memory to what is not experienced; we generalize; we apply in turn general knowledge to particular cases, or, in analytical thought, deduce new generalizations from general knowledge. Pieces of knowledge do not follow upon one another as a matter of mere succession. Rather, they enter into logical relations with each other, they follow from each other, they "agree" with each other, they confirm each other, thereby strengthening their logical power.

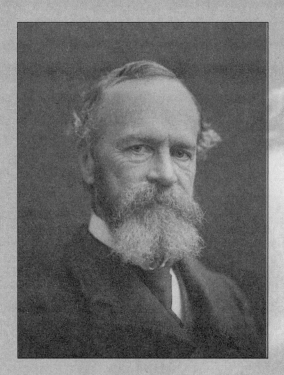

William James

(New York City, 1842–Tamworth, New Hampshire, 1910)x

William James came from a prominent New York family. He was brother to the distinguished novelist, Henry, and his sister Alice was a famous diarist. William graduated from Harvard with a degree in medicine. He was correspondent and friend to many of the most important intellectual figures of his time, including Louis Agassiz, Ralph Waldo Emerson, Mark Twain, Henri Bergson, and Sigmund Freud.

James was associated with the Pragmatist School of American thought, which included Charles Peirce and John Dewey. He was also responsible for the development of radical empiricism. He is best known today for his work *The Varieties of Religious Experience*.

Recommended reading:

The Varieties of Religious Experience (1902)

Principles of Psychology (1890)

Essays in Radical Empiricism (1912)

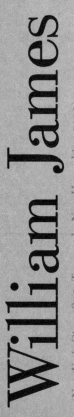

The art of being wise is knowing what to overlook.

A great many people think they are thinking when they are merely rearranging their prejudices.

Whenever two people meet, there are really six people present. There is each man as he sees himself, each man as the other person sees him, and each man as he really is.

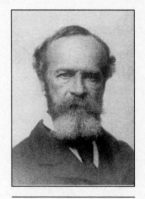

I am done with great things and big things, great institutions and big success, and I am for those tiny, invisible molecular moral forces that work from individual to individual, creeping through the crannies of the world like so many rootlets, or like the capillary oozing of water, yet which if you give them time, will rend the hardest monuments of man's pride.

To change one's life: 1. Start immediately, 2. Do it flamboyantly, 3. No exceptions.

William James came from a brilliant family that included both the novelist Henry James and the diarist Alice James.

Religion...is a man's total reaction upon life.

Take the happiest man, the one most envied by the world, and in nine cases out of ten his inmost consciousness is one of failure. Either his ideals in the line of his achievements are pitched far higher than the achievements themselves, or else he has secret ideals of which the world knows nothing, and in regard to which he inwardly knows himself to be found wanting.

Religion, therefore, as I now ask you arbitrarily to take it, shall mean for us the feelings, acts, and experiences of individual men in their solitude, so far as they apprehend themselves to stand in relation to whatever they may consider the divine. Since the relation may be either moral, physical, or ritual, it is evident that out of religion in the sense in which we take it, theologies, philosophies, and ecclesiastical organizations may secondarily grow.

Varieties of Religious Experience

There are moments of sentimental and mystical experience...that carry an enormous sense of inner authority and illumination with them when they come. But they come seldom, and they do not come to everyone; and the rest of life makes either no connection with them, or tends to contradict them more than it confirms them. Some persons follow more the voice of the moment in these cases, some prefer to be guided by the average results. Hence the sad discordancy of so many of the spiritual judgments of human beings.

Vladimir Jankélévitch

(Bourges, France, 1903–Paris, 1985)

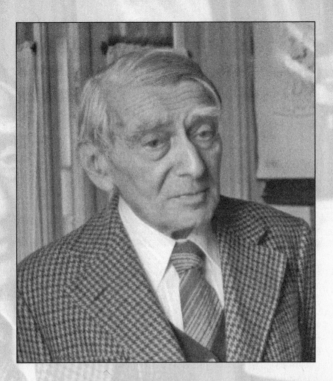

Jankélévitch was a disciple of Henri Bergson and devoted his first book to the study of that philosopher's work. In 1943 he joined the Popular Front and was active with the resistance. He was wounded during the war. In 1951 he was appointed Professor of Moral Philosophy at the Sorbonne.

He produced an extensive body of work centering on problems concerning the experience of day-to-day life, as well as writing extensively on music and modern composers.

Perhaps his most emblematic study was a beautifully written book entitled *Death*. About this he remarked, "the philosophy of death is a meditation on life."

Recommended reading:

📖 📖 📖 *Death* (1966)

📖 📖 *The Moral Paradox* (1981)

📖 *The Pure and the Impure* (1960)

Life is not a novel that we read and reread, nor is it a record that we know we will hear from the first to the last note. Real life is a like a book that we read for the first time.

In falling leaves man has a vague premonition of new buds, just as in the melancholy of night, he senses the nearness of dawn.

Nature in spring does not count its daisies or preoccupy itself with whether there are more or less budding flowers. Similarly the person who has a notion of eternity before him does not economize moments of time or worries about one hour more or less. But for the condemned man, to whom there remain only few hours of life, each minute is like the drops of water at the bottom of the bottle to a man in the desert.

When the tragic light of evidence and overwhelming certainty counsel us to renunciation and capitulation, crazy hope says to the impossible it is possible and to the irrational it is reasonable.

Existence is here in order to exist, not to reflect upon existence, just as breathing is the act of breathing, not the act of regarding the breath.

For me there is no death that is really mine; it belongs to others. I only die through others never through myself. In the same way that I can only know the death of others, so others cannot know their own deaths.

While waiting for the beautiful day on which tolerance becomes love, we say that tolerance, that prosaic virtue, is the best thing possible. Tolerance—however little the word is esteemed—is an adequate response. In waiting for better things to come, that is, for men to love one another, or at least to understand and recognize one another, we consider it a good thing to be able to bear with each other.

When one considers how familiar death is and how total is our ignorance of it, and that there is not escape from it, we have to admit that it is a well-guarded secret.

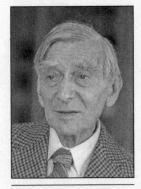

Born in France, Vladimir Jankélévitch was the son of Russian immigrants. His work, centered upon daily life in the world, emphasized the moral imperative as a passageway leading to an entirely different order of things. His affirmation of liberty sustains his ethics, which reveals the scope of his axiology (the philosophical study of values).

Moral Philosophy

In [Rembrandt's] *The Night Watch*, at the bottom right of the canvas, coming out of the shadows in which almost the entire work is shrouded, there is a man dressed in yellow. What is the significance of this man of gold? We can't be sure. But it is nice to think that he is the principle of adventure. In the obscurity of night, man introduces light. Can we not say that chiaroscuro is the ambiguous illumination of the journey of adventure? Drawn forward by the certain uncertainty of future death, adventure, is in a manner of speaking, open and closed, ajar, this unformed form that we call human life.

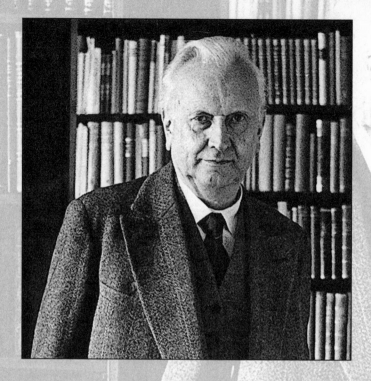

Karl Jaspers

(Oldenburg, Germany, 1883–Basel, Switzerland, 1969)

Before occupying the Chair of Philosophy at the University of Heidelberg, Jaspers studied medicine and worked as a doctor in a psychiatric hospital in that same city. There he found himself in stark disagreement with the way in which the medical community approached mental illness.

Jaspers was one of the founders of Christian existentialism. He was the author of over thirty books and extremely influential in twentieth-century theology, philosophy, and psychology.

Since his wife was Jewish he was forced out of his academic position by the Nazi regime and was unable to teach while it was in power. In 1948 he accepted the Chair of Philosophy in Basel, Switzerland, a post he held until shortly before his death.

Recommended reading:

Way to Wisdom: An Introduction to Philosophy (1951)

The Question of German Guilt (1946)

Reason and Existenz (1955)

Man, if he is to remain man, must advance by way of consciousness. There is no road leading backward....We can no longer veil reality from ourselves by renouncing self-consciousness without simultaneously excluding ourselves from the historical course of human existence.

When language is used without true significance, it loses its purpose as a means of communication and becomes an end in itself.

But each one of us is guilty insofar as he remained inactive. The guilt of passivity is different. Impotence excuses; no moral law demands a spectacular death. Plato already deemed it a matter of course to go into hiding in desperate times of calamity, and to survive. But passivity knows itself morally guilty of every failure, every neglect to act whenever possible, to shield the imperiled, to relieve wrong, to countervail. Impotent submission always left a margin of activity which, though not without risk, could still be cautiously effective. Its anxious omission weighs upon the individual as moral guilt. Blindness for the misfortune of others, lack of imagination of the heart, inner differences toward the witnessed evil—that is moral guilt.

The only satisfaction which man derives from a radical commitment to knowledge is the hope of advancing the frontier of knowledge to a point beyond which he cannot advance except by transcending knowledge itself.

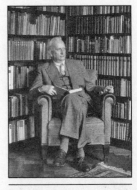

With the disintegration of all that he had revered, existence, to him, had become a desert in which only one thing remained, namely that which had relentlessly forced him into this path: truthfulness that knows no limits and is not subject to any condition.

The German philosopher and psychiatrist Karl Jaspers. Like Heidegger, he sought to comprehend the meaning of existence. His reflections on Nietzsche are key to his existentialist position.

Philosophy as practice does not mean its restriction to utility or applicability, that is, to what serves morality or produces serenity of soul.

We cannot avoid conflict, conflict with society, other individuals and with oneself. Conflicts may be the sources of defeat, lost life and a limitation of our potentiality but they may also lead to greater depth of living and the birth of more far-reaching unities, which flourish in the tensions that engender them.

■ *Philosophy*

The Greek word for philosopher (*philosophos*) connotes a distinction from *sophos*. It signifies the lover of wisdom (knowledge) as distinguished from the one who considers himself wise in the possession of knowledge. This meaning of the word still endures: the essence of philosophy is not the possession of the truth but the search for truth....Philosophy means to be on the way. Its questions are more essential than its answers, and every answer becomes a new question.

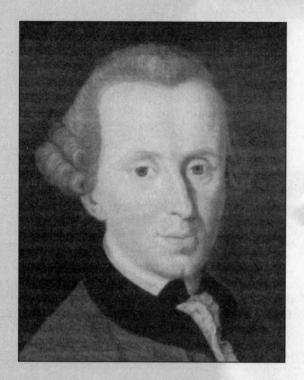

Immanuel Kant

(Köningsberg, Prussia, 1724–1804)

Kant spent his entire life in Köningsberg. He was the most admired and influential German philosopher of his day and also gained fame as a man who regulated his life according to a methodical and unvarying routine. For example, it was said that his neighbors set their clocks to his daily walks. The only time he changed his regimen was to attend a reading of *Émile* by Rousseau.

Kant's writings led to a veritable revolution in philosophy, proposing a new solution to the problem of consciousness and shattering the limitations of empiricism and rationalism.

Recommended reading:

📖 📖 📖 *Critique of Pure Reason* (1781)

📖 📖 *Critique of Practical Reason* (1788)
Groundwork of the Metaphysics of Morals (1785)

📖 *Critique of Judgement* (1790)

Freedom is the sole unoriginated birthright of man, and belongs to him by force of his humanity; and is independent of the will and co-action of every other in so far as this consists with every other person's freedom.

Out of the crooked timber of humanity, no straight thing was ever made.

By a lie a man throws away and, as it were, annihilates his dignity as a man. A man who himself does not believe what he tells another...has even less worth than if he were a mere thing...makes himself a mere deceptive appearance of man, not man himself.

Through laziness and cowardice a large part of mankind, even after nature has freed them from alien guidance, gladly remain immature. It is because of laziness and cowardice that it is so easy for others to usurp the role of guardians. It is so comfortable to be a minor!

Nature has willed that man should, by himself, produce everything that goes beyond the mechanical ordering of his animal existence, and that he should partake of no other happiness or perfection than that which he himself, independently of instinct, has created by his own reason.

Act only on that maxim which you can at the same time will that it should become a universal law. [Kant's categorical imperative]

All the interests of my reason, speculative as well as practical, combine in the three following questions: 1. What can I know? 2. What ought I to do? 3. What may I hope?

Only the descent into the hell of self-knowledge can pave the way to godliness.

Human reason has this peculiar fate that in one species of its knowledge it is burdened by questions which, as prescribed by the very nature of reason itself, it is not able to ignore, but which, as transcending all its powers, it is also not able to answer.

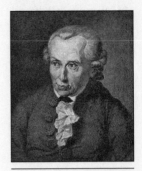

Kant is considered to be the culminating thinker of Enlightenment philosophy. He was a man of tremendous erudition and left an indelible mark on theories of justice, ethics and aesthetics. He sought to ground his philosophy in the realities of human life.

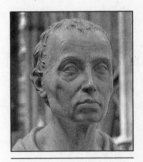

As a philosopher Kant examined consciousness, the phenomenological representations of self, as it relates to the external and internal worlds.

Idea for a Universal History

One cannot suppress a certain indignation when one sees men's actions on the great world stage and finds, beside the wisdom that appears here and there among individuals, everything in the large woven together from folly, childish vanity, even from childish malice and destructiveness. In the end, one does not know what to think of the human race, so conceited in its gifts.

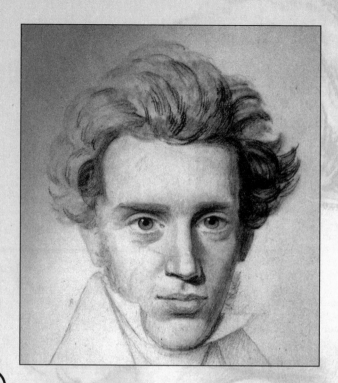

Soren Kierkegaard

(Copenhagen, Denmark, 1813–1855)

The religious obsessions of Kierkegaard's father, a Lutheran minister, consumed by a sense of guilt, deeply affected his son's philosophical approach, which grappled with the problem of emotions in the confrontation with life. He studied theology and philosophy in Copenhagen where he became acquainted with the work of Hegel, concerning which he developed a notable critique.

Kierkegaard's life, especially his painful experiences, such as his ill-fated love with Regine Olsen, colored his philosophical works, which display great dramatic and poetic power. They are full of parables, aphorisms, fictitious letters and diaries as well as pseudonymous and fictitious characters. His wrestling with religious questions acted as a potent stimulus on contemporary thinkers and writers.

Recommended reading:

Either/Or (1843)

Repetition (1843)
Fear and Trembling (1843)

The Concept of Dread (1844)

Brief quotations

I am convinced that God is love, this thought has for me a primitive lyrical validity. When it is present to me, I am unspeakably blissful, when it is absent, I long for it more vehemently than does the lover for his object.

———

Life is not a problem to be solved, but a reality to be experienced.

———

Life can only be understood backwards; but it must be lived forwards.

———

The highest and most beautiful things in life are not to be heard about, nor read about, nor seen but, if one will, are to be lived.

———

Most men pursue pleasure with such breathless haste that they hurry past it.

———

Purity of heart is to will one thing.

———

Love is all, it gives all, and it takes all.

———

Don't you know that a midnight hour comes when everyone has to take off his mask? Do you think life always lets itself be trifled with? Do you think you can sneak off a little before midnight to escape this?

———

Anxiety is the dizziness of freedom.

———

What we call worldliness simply consists of such people who, if one may so express it, pawn themselves to the world.

———

The Bible is very easy to understand. But we Christians are a bunch of scheming swindlers. We pretend to be unable to understand it because we know very well that the minute we understand, we are obliged to act accordingly.

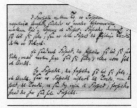

Manuscript of Kierkegaard's *Philosophical Fragments*. The philosopher left it for the reader to discover the significance of his writings, since according to his parable, "the task needs to be difficult, since only through difficulty is the nobility of the heart revealed." His philosophical work has greatly influenced existentialism, humanism, postmodernism, among other currents of thought.

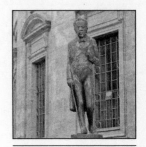

Soren Aabye Kiekegaard.

Fear and Trembling

If at the bottom consciousness of the eternal were not implanted in man; if the basis of all that exists were but a confusedly fermenting element which, convulsed by obscure passions, produced all, both the great and the insignificant; if under everything there lay a bottomless void never to be filled, what else were life but despair? If there were no sacred bonds between man and man; if one generation arose after another, as in the forest the leaves of one season succeed the leaves of another...if the generations of man passed through the world like a ship passing through the sea and the wind over the desert—a fruitless and a vain thing; if eternal oblivion ever greedily watching for its prey and there existed no power strong enough to wrest it from its clutches—how empty were life then, and how dismal!

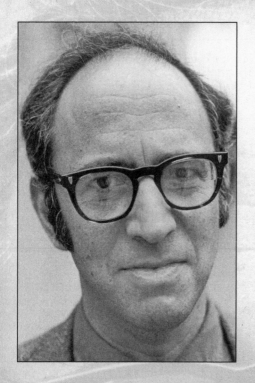

Thomas Kuhn

(Cincinnati, Ohio, 1922–Boston, Massachusetts, 1996)

Kuhn received his doctorate in physics from Harvard University and taught philosophy and the history of science at Harvard as well as at Berkeley, Princeton, and MIT.

Acclaimed for his contributions to the philosophy of science in the 1960s, he examined and popularized the concept of "paradigm."

In contrast to the ideas of Popper, Kuhn argued that the development of the sciences consists of quiet and conservative periods interrupted by violent revolutions that transform their conceptual bases.

Recommended reading:

📖 📖 📖 *The Structure of Scientific Revolutions* (1962)

📖 📖 *The Essential Tension* (1977)

📖 *The Copernican Revolution* (1957)

Why should a change in paradigm be called a revolution? In the face of the vast and essential differences between political and scientific development, what parallelism can justify the metaphor that finds revolutions in both?

When paradigms enter, as they must, into a debate about paradigm choice, their role is necessarily circular. Each group uses its own paradigm to argue in that paradigm's defense.

Looking at a bubble-chamber photograph, the student sees confused and broken lines, the physicist a record of familiar subnuclear events. Only after a number of transformations of vision does the student become an inhabitant of the scientist's world, seeing what the scientist sees and responding as the scientist does.

In both political and scientific development the sense of malfunction that can lead to crisis is prerequisite to revolution.

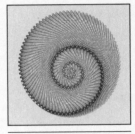

But for men like Kelvin, Crookes, and Roentgen, whose research dealt with radiation theory or with cathode ray tubes, the emergence of X-rays necessarily violated one paradigm as it created another. That is why these rays were discovered only through something's first going wrong with normal research.

In its approach to the entire field of science Kuhn's work proposed a major reenvisioning. It demonstrated that it is not sufficient to regard science as finding its sole justification within itself, just as it is impossible to posit a neutral observer.

Like the choice between competing political institutions, that between competing paradigms proves to be a choice between incompatible modes of community life.

Scientific revolutions...need seem revolutionary only to those whose paradigms are affected by them. To outsiders they may, like the Balkan revolutions of the early twentieth century, seem normal parts of the developmental process.

Normal science, the activity in which most scientists inevitably spend most all their time, is predicated on the assumption that the scientific community knows what the world is like. Normal science often suppresses fundamental novelties because they are necessarily subversive of its basic commitments. As a puzzle-solving activity, normal science does not aim at novelties of fact or theory and, when successful, finds none.

█ *Structure of Scientific Revolutions*

...during revolutions scientists see new and different things when looking with familiar instruments in places they have looked before. It is rather as if the professional community had been suddenly transported to another planet where familiar objects are seen in a different light and are joined by unfamiliar ones as well. Of course nothing of quite that sort does occur; there is no geographical transplantation; outside the laboratory everyday affairs usually continue as before. Nevertheless, paradigm changes do cause scientists to see the world of their research-engagement differently.

Gottfried Wilhelm von Leibniz

(Leipzig, Germany, 1644–Hanover, Germany, 1716)

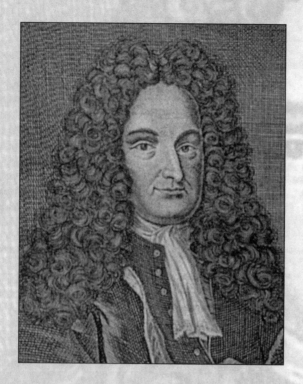

Orphaned at the age of six, Leibniz was self taught. He won a place at the court of the Duke of Hanover, working there as jurist, counselor, diplomat, librarian, and historian. He was the first great German philosopher and one of the most important thinkers of the seventeenth and eighteenth centuries.

He passed his free time reflecting not only on philosophical questions, but on mathematics, geology, linguistics, and historiography as well. Although almost all of his works were published posthumously, he was honored and renowned during his lifetime. There was a lively debate as to whether it was he or Isaac Newton who was the first to discover the foundations of calculus (in fact their discoveries were made independently of each other at around the same time).

Recommended reading:

📖 📖 📖 *New Essays on Human Understanding* (1765, published posthumously)
📖 📖 *Monadology* (1720)

📖 *Théodicée* (1710)

Every substance is as a world apart, independent of everything else except God.

———

I am convinced that the unwritten knowledge scattered among men of different callings surpasses in quantity and in importance anything we find in books, and that the greater part of our wealth has yet to be recorded.

———

Our reasonings are grounded upon two great principles, that of contradiction, in virtue of which we judge false that which involves a contradiction, and true that which is opposed or contradictory to the false; And that of sufficient reason, in virtue of which we hold that there can be no fact real or existing, no statement true, unless these be a sufficient reason, why it should be so and not otherwise, although these reasons usually cannot be known by us.

———

Love consists in looking upon the happiness of the other as our own.

———

Why is there anything at all rather than nothing whatsoever?

———

This is the best of all possible worlds.

———

Nothing is without reason.

———

There are also two kinds of truths, those of reasoning and those of fact. Truths of reasoning are necessary and their opposite is impossible: truths of fact are contingent and their opposite is possible. When a truth is necessary, its reason can be found by analysis, resolving it into more simple ideas and truths, until we come to those which are primary.

———

Now, as in the Ideas of God there is an infinite number of possible universes, and as only one of them can be actual, there must be a sufficient reason for the choice of God, which leads Him to decide upon one rather than another.

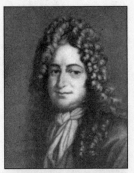

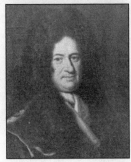

Concerning Gottfried Wilhem von Leibniz, even someone as opposed to him as the encyclopedist and atheist Diderot was reported as saying: "There has perhaps never been a man who read as widely, studied as much, meditated as much and written as much as Leibniz…If his ideas had been expressed in the style of Plato, the philosopher of Leipzig would have ceded nothing to the philosopher of Athens.

■ *Monadology*

Thus the organic body of each living being is a kind of divine machine or natural automaton, which infinitely surpasses all artificial automata. For a machine made by the skill of man is not a machine in each of its parts. For instance the tooth of a brass wheel has parts or fragments which for us are not artificial products, and which do not have the special characteristics of the machine, for they give no indication of the use for which the wheel was intended. But the machines of nature, namely, living bodies, are still machines in their smallest parts ad infinitum. It is this that constitutes the difference between nature and art, that is to say, between the divine art and ours.

Gilles Lipovetsky

(París, France 1944)

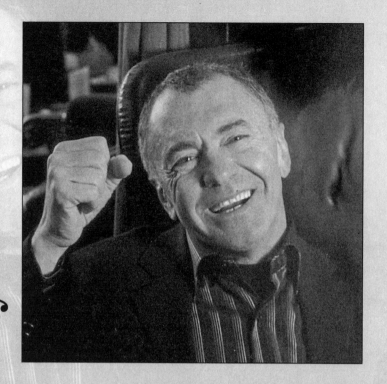

Lipovetsky is a French philosopher of Polish extraction. He is Professor of Philosophy at the University of Grenoble, as well as a member of the *Conseil d'analyse de la société* of the French government.

His 1983 book, *The Empty Era*, provoked heated debate. The work of this intellectual attempts to find a new perspective on the analysis of the individual within contemporary society, placing emphasis on mass culture and the ephemerality of its movements.

With a clear, accessible prose style, Lipovetsky argues that in contemporary society, the principle of fashion (being up-to-date) has replaced tradition and exacerbated narcissism and apathy.

Recommended reading:

The Empty Era (1983)

The Third Woman (1997)

The Empire of the Ephemeral (1987)

Only idiots never change opinion.

———

I don't believe in postmodernism, but in hypermodernism, which is a kind of perpetual flight, in which everything is excess.

———

No one still believes in the radiant power of revolution and progress. Most people living in the here and now, prefer to hold on to youth, rather than attempt to forge a new man.

———

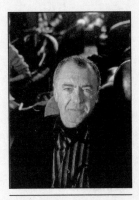

We are all analysts, simultaneously interpreting and being interpreted. Don Juan is dead, a new, more disquieting figure has taken his place: Narcissus, existing for himself, in his crystal capsule.

———

In the era of the fabulous, difficult antinomies, those between truth and falsehood, beauty and ugliness, reality and illusion, sense and nonsense, all vanish.

———

Lipovetsky's principal thesis is that traditional philosophy is out of step with time, caught up with unreal forms and ideas. It is a prisoner to Platonic notions and is divorced from the interests of a society defined by mass culture. In opposition to this escapist tendency, Lipovetsky focuses on concrete reality, the study of the popular and ephemeral phenomena that characterize contemporary culture.

Hedonism, the promised consumption of pleasures, propels society stimulating the quest for happiness in its referentials, but in actuality multiplying anxieties, depression, disquietude, and daily dissatisfaction.

———

Publicity which used to be about a product and its benefits, has become a campaign to disseminate values and a vision emphasizing the spectacular, directed toward signifiers.

———

It is excitation and sensation that is being purchased. All consumers resemble to some extent collectors of experience, looking for some immediate gratification.

———

The ideal is no longer to lose oneself in an intoxicating iconoclasm, but to find happiness in balance, to achieve an inner harmony, to live a peaceful, measured, sane existence.

In addition to his work on the ephemeral and frivolous, Lipovetsky has produced important historical studies over the fluctuations in style and taste.

■ *The Empty Era*

There is a general agreement among psychologists: over the last twenty or thirty years, narcissistic disorders constitute the majority of psychic problems treated by therapists, rather than the classic neuroses of the nineteenth century—hysteria, phobias, obsessions—on which psychoanalysis dwelled. Narcissistic disorders do not present themselves in well-defined symptoms, but are characterized by a diffuse malaise that penetrates everything, a feeling of interior emptiness, an inability to care about things and other people.

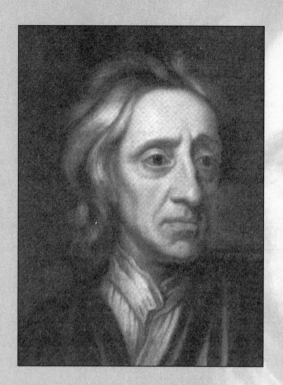

John Locke

(Somerset, England, 1632–Essex, England, 1704)

This empirical philosopher is considered to be the father of political liberalism. He rejected the notion of innate ideas and determinism, maintaining the sensory origin of thought and insisting that the human mind was a *tabula rasa* (blank slate). Locke considered religion to be a private matter, one that should not affect human relations.

Locke studied at Oxford but did not subscribe to the reigning philosophical currents. Insofar as politics was concerned he affirmed that sovereignty emanated from the governed and that the State was established for the protection of private property.

Recommended reading:

📖 📖 📖 *An Essay Concerning Human Understanding* (1690)

📖 📖 *Two Treatises of Government* (1689)

📖 *A Letter Concerning Toleration* (1667)

The reason why men enter into society is the preservation of their property.

Let us then suppose the mind to be, as we say, white paper void of all characters, without any ideas. How comes it to be furnished? Whence comes it by that vast store which the busy and boundless fancy of man has painted on it with an almost endless variety? Whence has it all the materials of reason and knowledge? To this I answer, in one word, from experience.

The end of law is not to abolish or restrain, but to preserve and enlarge freedom. For in all the states of created beings capable of law, where there is no law, there is no freedom.

The state of nature has a law of nature to govern it, which obliges every one: and reason, which is that law, teaches all mankind, who will but consult it, that being all equal and independent, no one ought to harm another in his life, health, liberty, or possessions.

No one is by nature bound to any particular church or sect; everyone voluntarily joins the society in which he thinks he has found the creed and mode of worship that is truly acceptable to God.

The natural liberty of man is to be free from any superior power on earth, and not to be under the will or legislative authority of man, but to have only the law of nature for his rule.

Government has no other end, but the preservation of property.

We are like chameleons, we take our hue and the color of our moral character, from those who are around us.

Locke's epitaph: "Stop Traveller! Near this place lieth John Locke. If you ask what kind of a man he was, he answers that he lived content with his own small fortune. Bred a scholar, he made his learning subservient only to the cause of truth."

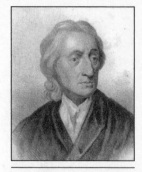

As a philosopher Locke affirmed that the mind of a person at the moment of birth is a *tabula rasa,* a sheet of white paper, upon which experience imprints ideas. These are not derived from intuition or innate concepts. At the same time he maintained that all individuals are born free, independent, and equal. According to Locke experience is the source of all ideas.

In politics, the "father of modern liberalism" stated that sovereignty derives from the people, that private property is a basic right, prior to the establishment of government, and that the primary raison d'etre for government is the protection of private property and the rights of its individual citizens.

Two Treatises of Government

...for no man, or society of men, having a power to deliver up their preservation, or consequently the means of it, to the absolute will and arbitrary dominion of another; whenever any one shall go about to bring them into such a slavish condition, they will always have a right to preserve what they have not a power to part with; and to rid themselves of those who invade this fundamental, sacred, and unalterable law of self-preservation, for which they entered into society. And thus the community may be said in this respect to be always the supreme power...

Jean François Lyotard

(Versailles, France, 1924–Paris, 1998)

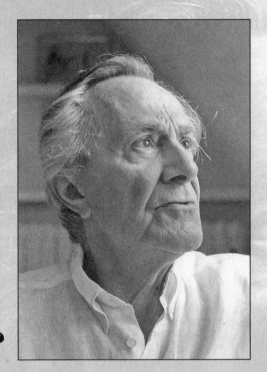

Lyotard was a member of the group "Socialism or Barbarism," a group of French intellectuals on the Left that opposed the Stalinism of Soviet communism.

He was president of the International College of Philosophy and Professor emeritus at the University of Paris. From 1973 he distanced himself from both Marxism and psychoanalysis. Many consider him to be the father of postmodernism.

According to Lyotard, postmodernism holds that there is a change in mentality in relation to the problem of meaning. His best-known thesis is that we have left behind the epoch of grand explanations, that we can no longer attempt to discover the meaning behind the march of history.

Recommended reading:

📖 📖 📖 *The Postmodern Condition: A Report on Knowledge* (1979)

📖 📖 *Libidinal Economy* (1974)

📖 *The Differend: Phrases in Dispute* (1983)

The task of thought is to think.

A self does not amount to much, but no self is an island; each exists in a fabric of relations that is now more complex and mobile than ever before.

What is new in all of this is that the old poles of attraction represented by nation-states, parties, professions, institutions, and historical traditions are losing their attraction.

Knowledge is and will be produced in order to be sold, it is and will be consumed in order to be valorized in a new production: in both cases, the goal is exchange. Knowledge ceases to be an end in itself, it loses its use-value.

Knowledge in the form of an informational commodity indispensable to productive power is already, and will continue to be, a major—perhaps the major—stake in the worldwide competition for power. It is conceivable that the nation-states will one day fight for control of information, just as they battled in the past for control over territory, and afterwards for control over access to and exploitation of raw materials and cheap labor.Our working hypothesis is that the status of knowledge is altered as societies enter what is known as the postindustrial age and cultures enter what is known as the postmodern age.

Scientific knowledge requires that one language game, denotative, be retained and all others excluded....Scientific knowledge is in this way set apart from the language games that combine to form the social bond.

In contemporary society and culture—postindustrial society, postmodern culture—... the grand narrative has lost its credibility, regardless of what mode of unification it uses, regardless of whether it is a speculative narrative or a narrative of emancipation.

One can decide that the principal role of knowledge is as an indispensable element in the functioning of society, and act in accordance with that decision, only if one has already decided that society is a giant machine.

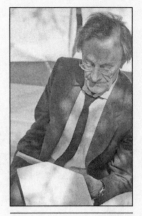

"Sooner or later it all comes down to money..." Lyotard distrusts all grand narratives: idealism, Christianity, Marxism, liberalism, none of these can lead to liberation.

According to Lyotard, postmodern culture is characterized by incredulity in respect to grand ideas, which are invalid in their practical effects. Rather than propose an alternative system, he seeks a climate permitting many different approaches to promoting concrete change. The operative criteria are technological not judgment over what is true versus what is false. He defends cultural plurality and the richness of diversity.

Postmodernism for Children

Eclecticism is the degree zero of contemporary general culture: one listens to reggae, watches a western, eats McDonald's food for lunch and local cuisine for dinner, wears Paris perfume in Tokyo and "retro" clothes in Hong Kong; knowledge is a matter for TV games. It is easy to find a public for eclectic works.

Niccolò Machiavelli

(Florence, Italy, 1469–1527)

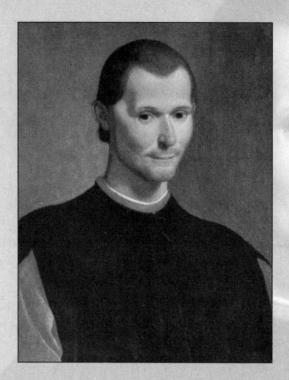

Not only did Machiavelli's thought have great impact on Renaissance Italy, but he can be seen as the most important political theorist of his time. As a diplomat serving the Republic of Florence he became acquainted with the leading political and ecclesiastical figures of Italy and France. After the fall of the Republic in 1512 he retired from politics, producing works that established him as the founder of modern political philosophy.

Machiavelli affirmed the autonomy of political power: that it was not derived from the natural order, but rather was the result of human actions. He observed that all communities are riven by competing interests, those of the people and those of the ruling class.

Recommended reading:

📖 📖 📖 *The Prince* (1513)

📖 📖 *The Art of War* (1519-1520)

📖 *Discourses on Livy* (1512-1517)

Upon this, one has to remark that men ought either to be well treated or crushed, because they can avenge themselves of lighter injuries, of more serious ones they cannot; therefore the injury that is to be done to a man ought to be of such a kind that one does not stand in fear of revenge.

A prince ought to have no other aim or thought, nor select anything else for his study, than war and its rules and discipline; for this is the sole art that belongs to him who rules, and it is of such force that it not only upholds those who are born princes, but it often enables men to rise from a private station to that rank.

The question arises whether it is better to be loved more than feared, or feared more than loved. The reply is, that one ought to be both feared and loved, but as it is difficult for the two to go together, it is much safer to be feared than loved, if one of the two has to be wanting.

Never attempt to win by force what can be won by deception.

The best fortress which a prince can possess is the affection of his people.

Men never do good unless necessity drives them to it; but when they are free to choose and can do just as they please, confusion and disorder become rampant.

So in all human affairs one notices, if one examines them closely, that it is impossible to remove one inconvenience without another emerging.

Men are driven by two principal impulses, either by love or by fear.

There is nothing more important than appearing to be religious.

The ends justify the means.

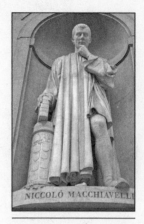

Statue of Machiavelli in Florence. On the preceding page he wears the dress of a political functionary of the Florentine Republic.

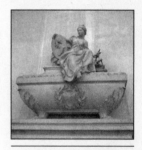

Tomb of Niccolò Machiavelli. He can justly be considered as the first political theorist.

The Prince

You must know, then, that there are two methods of fighting, the one by law, the other by force: the first method is that of men, the second of beasts; but as the first method is often insufficient, one must have recourse to the second. It is therefore necessary to know well how to use both the beast and the man....A prince being thus obliged to know well how to act as a beast must imitate the fox and the lion, for the lion cannot protect himself from snares, and the fox cannot defend himself from wolves. One must therefore be a fox to recognize snares, and a lion to frighten wolves. Those that wish to be only lions do not understand this.

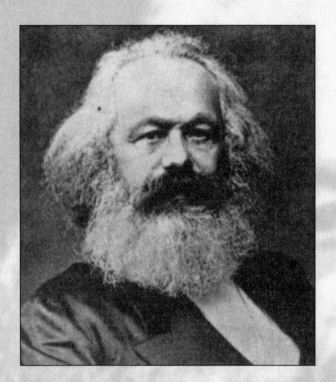

Karl Marx

(Trier, Prussia, 1818–London, England, 1883)

Father of the theory of scientific socialism, Marx was a philosopher, sociologist, historian, and economist. His writings changed the course of modern history. He studied philosophy in Berlin and soon involved himself in work directed to the social realities of his day. He founded a journal, which was censored by the authorities. He was exiled in 1843 and moved to Paris where he met and became friends with his collaborator, Friedrich Engels.

Expelled from France for his inflammatory writings and his fame as a revolutionary, he left for Brussels where he spearheaded The League of the Just, a socialist-utopian organization.

Forced to leave Paris, he relocated to London. There he organized the First International and wrote his masterwork: *Das Kapital*.

Recommended reading:

📖 📖 📖 *Das Kapital* (1864-1877)

📖 📖 *The Communist Manifesto* (1848, written with Engels)

📖 *The German Ideology* (1932, written with Engels, published posthumously)

124

From each according to his abilities, to each according to his needs.

———

The history of all hitherto existing society is the history of class struggles.

———

...a class of laborers, who live only so long as they find work, and who find work only so long as their labor increase capital. These laborers, who must sell themselves piecemeal, are a commodity, like every other article of commerce, and are consequently exposed to all the vicissitudes of competition, to all the fluctuations of the market.

———

In place of the bourgeois society, with its classes and class antagonisms, shall we have an association, in which the free development of each is the condition for the free development of all.

———

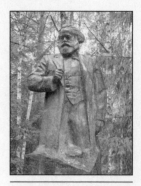

Statue of Karl Marx in a forest in Lithuania.

In every stock-jobbing swindle everyone knows that some time or other the crash must come, but every one hopes that it may fall on the head of his neighbor, after he himself has caught the shower of gold and placed it in safety.

———

In its beginnings, the credit system sneaks in as a modest helper of accumulation and draws by invisible threads the money resources scattered all over the surface of society into the hands of individual or associated capitalists. But soon it becomes a new and formidable weapon in the competitive struggle, and finally it transforms itself into an immense social mechanism for the centralization of capital.

———

The Irish famine of 1846 killed more than 1,000,000 people, but it killed poor devils only. To the wealthy of the country it did not the slightest damage.

———

In the social production of their life, men enter into definite relations that are indispensable and independent of their will; these relations of production correspond to a definite stage of development of their material forces of production. The sum total of these relations of production constitutes the economic structure of society—the real foundation, on which rises a legal and political superstructure and to which correspond definite forms of social consciousness. The mode of production of material life determines the social, political and intellectual life process in general. It is not the consciousness of men that determines their being, but, on the contrary, their social being that determines their consciousness.

Das Kapital.

Kritik der politischen Oekonomie.

Von

Karl Marx.

Erster Band.
Buch 1: Der Produktionsprocess des Kapitals.

Hamburg
Verlag von Otto Meissner.
1867.

Title page from the first edition of *Das Kapital*. Inspired by the first great crisis in industrial capitalism (1830), Marx sought to develop an economic theory adequate to explain the crisis and at the same time motivate the proletariat toward revolutionary action.

■ *The Communist Manifesto*

The Communists disdain to conceal their views and aims. They openly declare that their ends can be attained only by the forcible overthrow of all existing social conditions. Let the ruling classes tremble at a Communistic revolution. The proletarians have nothing to lose but their chains. They have a world to win.

WORKING MEN OF ALL COUNTRIES, UNITE!

Maurice Merleau-Ponty

(Rochefort-sur-Mer, France, 1908–Paris, 1961)

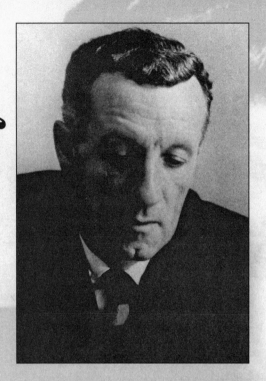

Continuing on the path laid out by Husserl, Merleau-Ponty investigated the importance of the physical body in perception and the relationship between the individual and society. He was a classmate at university with Sartre and is considered alongside him as one of the founding thinkers of the existentialist movement.

At the end of the Second World War he was named Professor of Philosophy at the University of Lyons and the College of France. He also lectured on child psychology at the Sorbonne.

He played an important role in *Les Temps Moderne*, the journal founded by Sartre and Simone de Beauvoir, until he broke with them over political differences.

Recommended reading:

Phenomenology of Perception (1945)

Sense and Non-Sense (1948)

The Visible and the Invisible (1960)

All consciousness is perceptual consciousness.

———

Insofar as I have hands, feet, a body, I sustain around me intentions which are not dependent on my decisions and which affect my surroundings in a way that I do not choose.—

———

The world is...the natural setting of, and field for, all my thoughts and all my explicit perceptions. Truth does not inhabit only the inner man, or more accurately, there is no inner man, man is in the world, and we must therefore rediscover, after the natural world, the social world, not as an object or sum of objects, but as a permanent field or dimension of existence.

———

Our view of man will remain superficial so long as we fail to go back to that origin [of silence], so long as we fail to find, beneath the chatter of words, the primordial silence, and as long as we do not describe the action which breaks this silence. The spoken word is a gesture, and its meaning, a world.

———

Visible and mobile, my body is a thing among things; it's caught in the fabric of the world, and its cohesion is that of a thing. But, because it moves itself and sees, it holds things in a circle around itself.

———

Science manipulates things and gives up living in them. It makes its own limited models of things; operating upon these indices or variables to effect whatever transformations are permitted by their definition, it comes face to face with the real world only at rare intervals. Science is and always will be that admirably active, ingenious, and bold way of thinking whose fundamental bias is to treat everything as though it were an object-in-general—as though it meant nothing to us and yet was predestined for our own use.

———

The flesh is at the heart of the world.

———

Discover vision, not as a "thinking about seeing," to use Descartes expression, but as a gaze at grips with a visible world, and that is why for me there can be another's gaze.

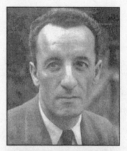

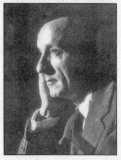

According to Merleau-Ponty perception possesses an active dimension in that it provides the basic window upon the life of the world. The primary status of perception, which assumes such importance in this work, is a legacy of his study of Husserl.

Distancing himself from the more materialist approach of Sartre, Merleau-Ponty conceived of consciousness as intentional corporality.

■ *Phenomenology of Perception*

Being established in my life, buttressed by my thinking nature, fastened down in this transcendental field which was opened for me by my first perception, and in which all absence is merely the obverse of a presence, all silence a modality of the being of sound, I enjoy a sort of ubiquity and theoretical eternity. I feel destined to move in a flow of endless life, neither the beginning nor the end of which I can experience in thought, since it is my living self who thinks of them, and since thus my life always precedes and survives itself.

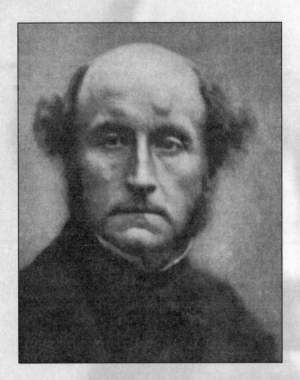

John Stuart Mill

(London, England, 1806–Avignon, France, 1873)

Son of Scottish economist James Mill and godson of Jeremy Bentham, John Stuart Mill became the most important figure in British philosophical thinking in the Victorian era.

An economist and politician, Mill was elected to parliament where he dedicated himself to radical causes such as women's rights and the abolition of slavery.

Mill was influenced by Enlightenment thinkers and German romanticism. He deepened the concept of utilitarianism developed by Bentham, placing primary emphasis on the intellect and the imagination, and promoting education as the key to happiness.

Recommended reading:

📖 📖 📖 *Utilitarianism* (1861)

📖 📖 *On Liberty* (1859)

📖 *The Subjection of Women* (1869)

128

It is better to be a human dissatisfied than a pig satisfied; better to be Socrates dissatisfied than a fool satisfied. And if the fool, or the pig, are of a different opinion, it is because they only know their own side of the question. The other party to the comparison knows both sides.

———

The best state for human nature is that in which, while no one is poor, no one desires to be richer, nor has any reason to fear being thrust back by the efforts of others to push themselves forward.

———

Capacity for nobler feelings is in most natures a very tender plant, easily killed, not only by hostile influences, but my mere want of sustenance.

———

In the golden rule of Jesus of Nazareth, we read the complete spirit of the ethics of utility. To do as one would be done by, and to love one's neighbour as oneself, constitute the ideal perfection of utilitarian morality.

———

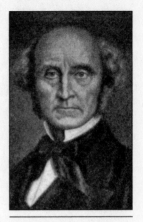

According to Mill, experience is the sole corrective for the false customs that militate against the individual and the fulfillment of his potential. In order for him to correct his errors, his ideas must hew closely to his experience.

That principle is, that the sole end for which mankind are warranted, individually or collectively, in interfering with the liberty of action of any of their number, is self-protection. That the only purpose for which power can be rightfully exercised over any member of a civilized community, against his will, is to prevent harm to others.

———

What, in unenlightened societies, colour, race, religion, or in the case of a conquered country, nationality, are to some men, sex is to all women; a peremptory exclusion from almost all honourable occupations, but either such as cannot be fulfilled by others, or such as those others do not think worthy of their acceptance.

———

Whenever the general disposition of the people is such, that each individual regards those only of his interests which are selfish, and does not dwell on, or concern himself for, his share of the general interest, in such a state of things, good government is impossible.

■ *The Subjection of Women*

The law of servitude in marriage is a monstrous contradiction to all the principles of the modern world, and to all the experience through which those principles have been slowly and painfully worked out. It is the sole case, now that negro slavery has been abolished, in which a human being in the plenitude of every faculty is delivered up to the tender mercies of another human being, in the hope forsooth that this other will use the power solely for the good of the person subjected to it. Marriage is the only actual bondage known to our law. There remain no legal slaves, except the mistress of every house.

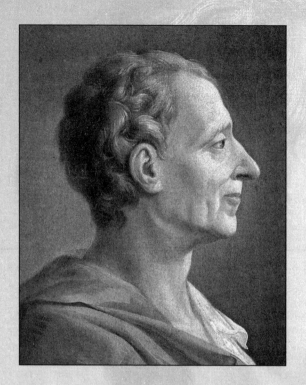

Montesquieu

(Bordeaux, France, 1680–1755)

Charles-Louis de Secondat, Baron de la Brède and de Montesquieu, was a politician, sociologist, historian, philosopher, and above all, a brilliant writer. In his work he undertook the difficult task of describing the social reality of his day with an analytic method.

Having resigned his position as parliamentarian in Bordeaux, Montesquieu moved to Paris. He visited London and found there a prosperous country whose government was open to criticism. On his return to Bordeaux he wrote *The Spirit of the Laws* a work that was highly praised but at the same time condemned by the Catholic Church and placed on the Index of Prohibited Books.

An important aspect of his thought is the doctrine of "separation of powers" in government, a principle that is recognized by constitutions the world over.

Recommended reading:

The Spirit of Laws (1734)

The Persian Letters (1721)

Defense of the Spirit of the Laws (1750)

...zeal for the advancement of religion is different from a due attachment to it; and that in order to love it and fulfill its behests, it is not necessary to hate and persecute those who are opposed to it.

———

No kingdom has shed more blood than the kingdom of Christ.

———

I have never known any distress that an hour's reading did not relieve.

———

Better it is to say that the government most comfortable to nature is that which best agrees with the humor and disposition of the people in whose favor it is established.

———

...constant experience shows us that every man invested with power is apt to abuse it, and to carry his authority as far as it will go. Is it not strange, though true, to say that virtue itself has need of limits? To prevent this abuse, it is necessary from the very nature of things that power should be a check to power. A government may be so constituted, as no man shall be compelled to do things to which the law does not oblige him, nor forced to abstain from things which the law permits.

———

Mankind by their industry, and by the influence of good laws, have rendered the earth more proper for their abode.

———

The alms given to a naked man in the street do not fulfill the obligations of the state, which owes to every citizen a certain subsistence, a proper nourishment, convenient clothing, and a kind of life not incompatible with health.

———

There is no greater tyranny than that which is perpetrated under the shield of the law and in the name of justice.

———

The Tyranny of a prince in an oligarchy is not so dangerous to the public welfare as the apathy of a citizen in a democracy.

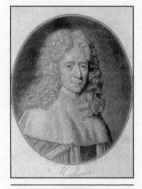

Precursor of liberalism, Montesquieu undertook the groundbreaking task of describing social realities in an analytic fashion. Not contenting himself with a simple recital of facts, he sought to organize and reduce the apparent diversity of social arrangements to well-defined categories.

In other words he sought to give a sociological account with the assumption that an order or causality existed susceptible to rational interpretation.

The Spirit of the Laws

Slavery, properly so called, is the establishment of a right which gives to one man such a power over another as renders him absolute master of his life and fortune. The state of slavery is in its own nature bad. It is neither useful to the master nor to the slave; not to the slave, because he can do nothing through a motive of virtue; nor to the master, because by having an unlimited authority over his slaves he insensibly accustoms himself to the want of all moral virtues, and thence becomes fierce, hasty, severe, choleric, voluptuous, and cruel...where it is of the utmost importance that human nature should not be debased or dispirited, there ought to be no slavery.

Friedrich Nietzsche

(Röcken, Germany, 1844–Weimar, Germany, 1900)

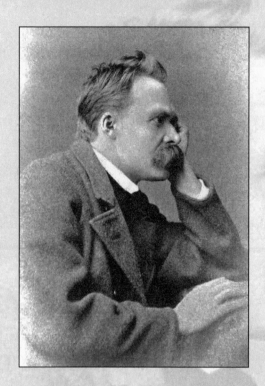

Nietzsche was the son of a Protestant minister who died when he was just four years old. He was a very well-behaved boy, earning the nickname "the little pastor." At age seventeen he began his studies in theology, but soon abandoned it for philosophy, a subject he was later to teach at the University of Basel.

Nietzsche suffered from frequent migraine attacks, which ended his teaching career. He resigned his post in 1879 and resolved to dedicate himself entirely to his philosophical labors. In 1889 he suffered a mental collapse from which he never recovered. Nietzache's work is of great beauty and profundity. It has been immensely and sometimes notoriously influential on theology, as well on existentialism, phenomenology, poststructuralism and postmodernism.

Recommended reading:

Thus Spake Zarathustra (1885)

Human, All Too Human(1878)
Beyond Good and Evil (1886)

The Birth of Tragedy (1872)

There are no facts, only interpretations.

It is a matter of honor with me to be absolutely clean and unequivocal in relation to anti-Semitism, namely, opposed to it, as I am in my writings.

He who fights with monsters should look to it that he himself does not become a monster. And when you gaze long into an abyss the abyss also gazes into you.

Underneath this reality in which we live and have our being, another and altogether different reality lies concealed.

"I have done that", says my memory. "I cannot have done that"—says my pride, and remains adamant. At last—memory yields.

There are no beautiful surfaces without a terrible depth.

Be careful, lest in casting out your demon you exorcise the best thing in you.

We have art in order not to die of the truth.

That which does not kill us makes us stronger.

You must have chaos within you to give birth to a dancing star.

In heaven, all the interesting people are missing.

The individual has always had to struggle to keep from being overwhelmed by the tribe. If you try it, you will be lonely often, and sometimes frightened. But no price is too high to pay for the privilege of owning yourself.

One is punished most for one's virtues.

The thought of suicide is a powerful solace: by means of it one gets through many a bad night.

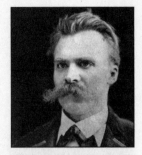

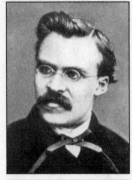

Paul Ricoeur called Freud, Marx and Nietzsche "the school of suspicion" in that they challenged conventional notions of meaning and experience.

Nietzsche's meditations over the triumph of secularism in the wake of the Enlightenment, encapsulated in his observation "God is dead," established a paradigm that many of the most celebrated intellectuals since have worked within.

Thus Spake Zarathustra

God is dead. God remains dead. And we have killed him. How shall we comfort ourselves, the murderers of all murderers? What was holiest and mightiest of all that the world has yet owned has bled to death under our knives: who will wipe this blood off us? What water is there for us to clean ourselves? What festivals of atonement, what sacred games shall we have to invent? Is not the greatness of this deed too great for us? Must we ourselves not become gods simply to appear worthy of it?

José Ortega y Gasset

(Madrid, Spain, 1883–1955)

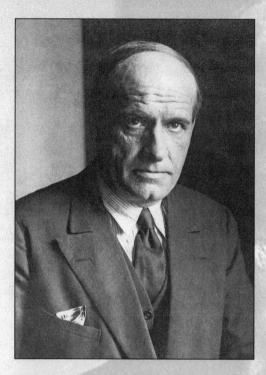

Born into a wealthy family, Ortega y Gasset studied at a Jesuit college and grew up in a cultured environment, associating with journalists and political figures. After receiving a doctorate in philosophy in Madrid, he continued his studies in Germany. Upon his return to Spain he began his teaching career, receiving a position as Professor of Metaphysics.

In 1923 he founded the *Revista de Occidente*, a journal that dealt with the most important philosophical ideas of the time. In 1936 he opposed Franco's rise to power. He spent years of exile first in Argentina then in Paris, Holland and finally Lisbon.He returned to Spain in 1945 and founded the Institute of Humanities, although he did not regain his teaching position. His writings have been widely influential.

Recommended reading:

The Revolt of the Masses (1930)

Meditations on Quixote (1914)

Invertebrate Spain (1921)

134

I am I and my circumstance; and, if I do not save it, I do not save myself.

...falling in love is a state of mental misery which has a restricting, impoverishing, and paralyzing effect upon the development of our consciousness.

By speaking, by thinking, we undertake to clarify things, and that forces us to exacerbate them, dislocate them, schematize them. Every concept is in itself an exaggeration.

Scientific truth is characterized by its exactness and the certainty of its predictions. But these admirable qualities are contrived by science at the cost of remaining on a plane of secondary problems, leaving intact the ultimate and decisive questions....Yet science is but a small part of the human mind and organism. Where it stops, man does not stop.

Life is a series of collisions with the future; it is not the sum of what we have been, but what we yearn to be.

Man is that unique animal for whom superfluity is a necessity.

Living is a constant process of deciding what we are going to do.

Tell me to what you pay attention and I will tell you who you are.

We cannot put off living until we are ready. The most salient characteristic of life is its coerciveness: it is always urgent, "here and now," without any possible postponement. Life is fired at us point-blank.

We have need of history in its entirety, not to fall back into it, but to see if we can escape from it.

Effort is only effort when it begins to hurt.

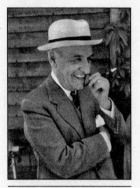

In the 1930s, Ortega y Gasset organized along with other intellectuals of the time the Group at the Service of the Republic Not linked to a specific political party, it was dedicated to the promotion of republican values.

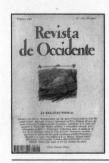

The journal, *Revista de Occidente*, was founded in 1923 by Ortega y Gasset and continues in print over 90 years after its first issue. It is devoted to philosophy and the arts.

Revolt of the Masses

Liberalism—it is well to recall this today—is the supreme form of generosity; it is the right which the majority concedes to minorities and hence it is the noblest cry that has ever resounded in this planet. It announces the determination to share existence with the enemy; more than that, with an enemy which is weak. It was incredible that the human species should have arrived at so noble an attitude, so paradoxical, so refined, so acrobatic, so anti-natural. Hence, it is not to be wondered at that this same humanity should soon appear anxious to get rid of it. It is a discipline too difficult and complex to take firm root on earth.

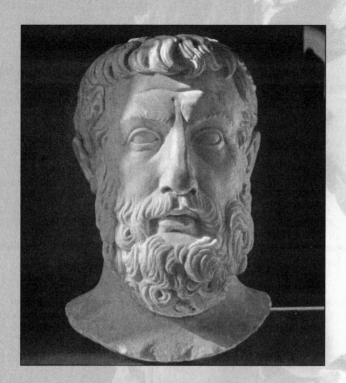

Parmenides

(Elea, Magna Graecia, c. 548–470 BCE)

It is thought that Parmenides abandoned Pythagoreanism to found his own school. Many consider him to be the most important of all the Presocratic philosophers. Plato called him the "great," and Heidegger saw his philosophy as the beginning of the history of metaphysics, the question of being.

He composed a philosophical treatise in verse, *On Nature,* the greater part of which can be found in Simplicius. Parmenides argued that the exercise of reason was essential for the pursuit of truth, to the extent that he argued one must put aside the evidence of one's senses and rely solely on reason to arrive at the true nature of things.

Recommended reading:

Diogenes Laertius, *Lives of Eminent Philosophers* (1st century BCE)

Kirk, G.S. and J.E. Raven, *The Presocratic Philosophers* (1987)

Jonathan Barnes, *The Presocratic Philosophers* (1992)

Brief quotations

Thinking and the thought that it is are the same; for you will not find thinking apart from what is, in relation to which it is uttered.

For to be aware and to be are the same.

It is necessary to speak and to think what is; for being is, but nothing is not.

Helplessness guides the wandering thought in their breasts; they are carried along deaf and blind alike, dazed, beasts without judgment, convinced that to be and not to be are the same and not the same, and that the road of all things is a backward-turning one.

[What exists] is now, all at once, one and continuous....Nor is it divisible, since it is all alike; nor is there any more or less of it in one place which might prevent it from holding together, but all is full of what is.

For this view, that That Which Is Not exists, can never predominate. You must debar your thought from this way of search, nor let ordinary experience in its variety force you along this way, (namely, that of allowing) the eye, sightless as it is, and the ear, full of sound, and the tongue, to rule; but (you must) judge by means of the Reason the much-contested proof which is expounded by me.

There is one story left, one road: that it is. And on this road there are very many signs that, being, is uncreated and imperishable, whole, unique, unwavering, and complete.

We can speak and think only of what exists. And what exists is uncreated and imperishable for it is whole and unchanging and complete. It was not or nor shall be different since it is now, all at once, one and continuous.

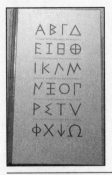

Extract from the *Fragments of Parmenides*, which comprises phrases and reflections of the philosopher.

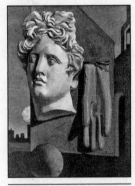

Parmenides was one of the first metaphysicians. The painting above entitled *The Metaphysical School* is by Giorgio de Chirico.

Proem

The steeds that bear me carried me as far as ever my heart desired, since they brought me and set me on the renowned Way of the goddess, who with her own hands conducts the man who knows through all things. On what way was I borne along; for on it did the wise steeds carry me, drawing my car, and maidens showed the way. And the axle, glowing in the socket—for it was urged round by the whirling wheels at each end—gave forth a sound as of a pipe, when the daughters of the Sun, hasting to convey me into the light, threw back their veils from off their faces and left the abode of Night.

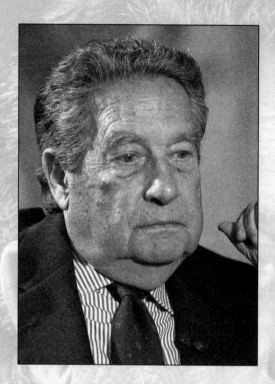

Octavio Paz

(Mexico City, Mexico, 1914–1998)

Awarded the Nobel Prize for Literature in 1990, Octavio Paz Lozano was one of the great poets, essayists, and thinkers in the Spanish language. Son of a father who fought alongside of Emiliano Zapata, he soon immersed himself in poetry and politics.

Time spent in Spain during the Civil War was a decisive factor in the formation of his character and opinions. It brought him into contact with movements of international solidarity as well as with the horrors of totalitarianism.

His association with the surrealist movement in Paris in the 1940s was another determining influence in his philosophical vision of modern literature, liberty, pre-modern cultures, and the roots of the contemporary world.

Recommended reading:

The Labyrinth of Solitude (1950)
The Children of the Mire (1974)

Alternating Current (1973)

Configuration (1971)

138

There can be no society without poetry, but society can never be realized as poetry, it is never poetic. Sometimes the two terms seek to break apart. They cannot.

To fight evil is to fight ourselves.

The modern age is one of acceleration of historical time. Acceleration is fusion: all time and space flow together into the here and now.

Modern literature is a passionate negation of the modern era.

Modern tradition is the tradition of rupture.

Modern man likes to pretend that his thinking is wide-awake. But this wide-awake thinking has led us into the mazes of a nightmare in which the torture chambers are endlessly repeated in the mirrors of reason.

It is always difficult to give oneself up; few persons anywhere ever succeed in doing so, and even fewer transcend the possessive stage to know love for what it actually is: a perpetual discovery, and immersion in the waters of reality, an unending re-creation.

Literature is the expression of a feeling of deprivation, a recourse against a sense of something missing. But the contrary is also true: language is what makes us human. It is a recourse against the meaningless noise and silence of nature and history.

Love reveals to us the highest form of freedom.

When we learn to speak, we learn to translate.

Eroticism is first and foremost a thirst for otherness. And the supernatural is the supreme otherness. This is perhaps the most noble aim of poetry, to attach ourselves to the world around us, to turn desire into love, to embrace, finally what always evades us, what is beyond, but what is always there—the unspoken, the spirit, the soul.

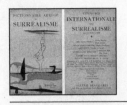

In Paris Paz came into contact with surrealism. For the Mexican writer and thinker, surrealism was not merely the expression of a dream state, it held the revolutionary power to effect new realities.

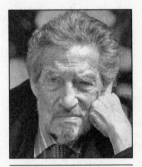

As a thinker Paz was fully committed to his political ideas. In 1968 he renounced his diplomatic career in protest of the Mexican government's brutal repression of student demonstrations.

The Labyrinth of Solitude

Solitude is the profoundest fact of the human condition. Man is the only being who knows he is alone, and the only one who seeks out another. His nature—if that word can be used in reference to man, who has 'invented' himself by saying 'no' to nature—consists in his longing to realize himself in another. Man is nostalgia and a search for communion. Therefore, when he is aware of himself he is aware of his lack of another, that is, of his solitude.

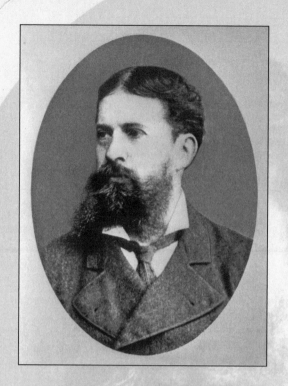

Charles S. Peirce

(Cambridge, Massachusetts, 1839–Milford, Pennsylvania, 1914)

Charles Sanders Peirce is considered to be the founder of semiotics. A Boston Brahmin and son of a Harvard professor, Peirce graduated from Harvard. He suffered from a neurological disorder that made him irascible and isolated him. Although he taught for a time at Johns Hopkins, he was dismissed from that position on account of certain irregularities in his personal life. He retired to Pennsylvania and lived much of his later life in penury. Assistance from his friend William James, relieved some of his financial hardship, but he died bankrupt. Peirce published only one book in his lifetime. After his death almost 1650 unpublished manuscripts were discovered that continue to be edited and brought into print.

Recommended reading:

Chance, Love and Logic: Philosophical Essays (1923)

Semiotics and Signifiers (1977)

Reasoning and the Logic of Things (1992)

Few persons care to study logic, because everybody conceives himself to be proficient enough in the art of reasoning already. But I observe that this satisfaction is limited to one's own ratiocination and does not extend to that of other men. We come to the full possession of our power of drawing inferences the last of all our faculties, for it is not so much a natural gift as a long and difficult art.

———

Our idea of anything is our idea of its sensible effects; and if we fancy that we have any other we deceive ourselves, and mistake a mere sensation accompanying the thought for a part of the thought itself.

———

I define a Sign as anything which is so determined by something else, called its Object, and so determines an effect upon a person, which effect I call its Interpretant, that the latter is thereby mediately determined by the former.

———

The entire universe is perfused with signs, if it is not composed exclusively of signs.

———

Of the fifty or hundred systems of philosophy that have been advanced at different times of the world's history, perhaps the larger number have been, not so much results of historical evolution, as happy thoughts which have accidently occurred to their authors.

———

The only possible way of accounting for the laws of nature and for uniformity in general is to suppose them results of evolution. This supposes them not to be absolute, not to be obeyed precisely.

———

Three conceptions are perpetually turning up at every point in every theory of logic, and in the most rounded systems they occur in connection with one another. They are conceptions so very broad and consequently indefinite that they are hard to seize and may be easily overlooked....First is the conception of being or existing independent of anything else. Second is the conception of being relative to, the conception of reaction with, something else. Third is the conception of mediation, whereby a first and second are brought into relation.

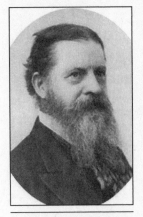

Peirce's life was marked by professional disappointment, and poverty. He left behind an enormous body of work, most of which was unpublished in his lifetime.

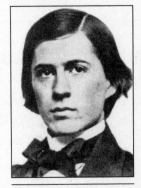

Charles Sander Peirce in 1859.

The Algebra of Logic

If the sign were not related to its object except by the mind thinking of them separately, it would not fulfill the function of a sign at all. Supposing, then, the relation of the sign to its object does not lie in a mental association, there must be a direct dual relation of the sign to its object independent of the mind using the sign. In the second of the three cases just spoken of, this dual relation is not degenerate, and the sign signifies its object solely by virtue of being really connected with it. Of this nature are all natural signs and physical symptoms. I call such a sign an index, a pointing finger being the type of the class.

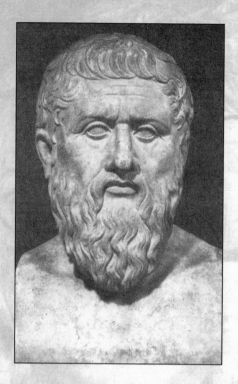

Plato was a student of Socrates and teacher of Aristotle. His real name was Aristocles; he was dubbed Plato, meaning "broad", because of his stature or the breadth of his eloquence. Plato founded the celebrated Academy in Athens. On its front an inscription read: "No one may enter here with knowing geometry." Geometry was considered preparation for dialectics, the highest form of pedagogy.

Most of Plato's works are written in the form of dialogues. They are not dated, and scholars have yet to agree on their chronology.

Plato's writings have been so influential that Alfred North Whitehead remarked that the entire Western philosophical tradition consists in a series of footnotes to his work.

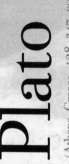

Plato
(Athens, Greece, 428–347, BCE)

Recommended reading:

📖 📖 📖 *The Republic, The Symposium, Phaedo, Phaedrus* (Classed as middle dialogues)

📖 📖 *Parmenides, Timaeus, Sophist, Laws* (Classed as late dialogues)

No evil can happen to a good man, neither in life nor after death.

And all knowledge, when separated from justice and virtue, is seen to be cunning and not wisdom; wherefore make this your first and last and constant and all-absorbing aim, to exceed, if possible, not only us but all your ancestors in virtue;...the madness of love is the greatest of heaven's blessings...

Until philosophers are kings, or the kings and princes of this world have the spirit and power of philosophy, and political greatness and wisdom meet in one, and those commoner natures who pursue either to the exclusion of the other are compelled to stand aside, cities will never have rest from their evils—no, nor the human race, as I believe—and then only will this our State have a possibility of life and behold the light of day.

No human thing is of serious importance.

Ignorance, the root and stem of all evil.

For a man to conquer himself is the first and noblest of all victories.

Wise men speak because they have something to say; fools because they have to say something.

Music gives a soul to the universe, wings to the mind, flight to the imagination and life to everything.

We can easily forgive a child who is afraid of the dark; the real tragedy of life is when men are afraid of the light.

According to Greek mythology, humans were originally created with four arms, four legs and a head with two faces. Fearing their power, Zeus split them into two separate parts, condemning them to spend their lives in search of their other halves.

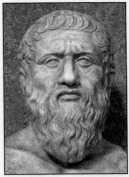

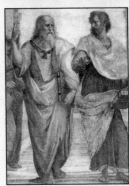

Plato (left) and Aristotle from Raphael's *School of Athens*. The author of *The Republic* and other dialogues has been of incalculable importance in the history of philosophy. It has often been said that the entire discipline of philosophy would not have existed without his works.

■ *The Laws*

The ruler of the universe has ordered all things with a view to the preservation and perfection of the whole, and each part has an appointed state of action and passion; and the smallest action or passion of any part affecting the minutest fraction has a presiding minister. And one of these portions of the universe is thine own, stubborn man, which, however little, has the whole in view; and you do not seem to be aware that this and every other creation is for the sake of the whole, and in order that the life of the whole may be blessed; and that you are created for the sake of the whole, and not the whole for the sake of you...And you are annoyed because you do not see how that which is best for you is, as far as the laws of the creation admit of this, best also for the universe.

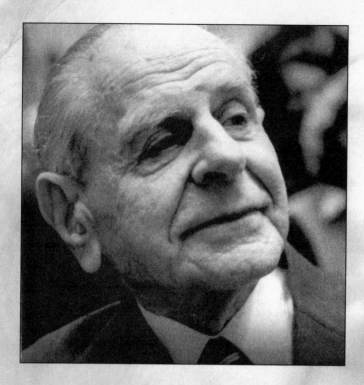

Karl R. Popper

(Vienna, Austria, 1902–London, England, 1994)

Popper traveled to England in 1935 where he spent two years before emigrating to New Zealand, where he obtained a position as Lecturer in Philosophy at the University of New Zealand. He returned to England in 1945 and taught at the London School of Economics. His work, *Conjectures and Refutations* took issue on some points with the philosophical positions of the Vienna Circle. He rejected the criterion of verification and proposed in its stead the standard of falsification to distinguish between scientific and non-scientific disciplines. In other words, the fundamental characteristic of a scientific theory is that it can be proved false. His system is referred to as critical rationalism. Popper was knighted by Queen Elizabeth in 1969.

Recommended reading:

Conjectures and Refutations (1963)

The Open Society and Its Enemies (1945)

The Logic of Scientific Discovery (1934)
The Poverty of Historicism (1945)

You can choose whatever name you like for the two types of government. I personally call the type of government which can be removed without violence "democracy," and the other "tyranny".

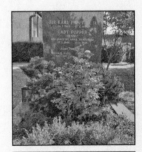

Manuscript page from Karl Popper, 1992. Popper's conjectures about scientific thought and method can be seen as sustaining the entire structure of his philosophical ideas. His work enjoyed enormous popularity, though less within the scientific community. His theory of falsification has generally been accepted as a valid criterion for determining scientific discourse.

If we are uncritical we shall always find what we want: we shall look for, and find, confirmations, and we shall look away from, and not see, whatever might be dangerous to our pet theories. In this way it is only too easy to obtain what appears to be overwhelming evidence in favor of a theory which, if approached critically, would have been refuted.

For it was my master who taught me not only how very little I knew but also that any wisdom to which I might ever aspire could consist only in realizing more fully the infinity of my ignorance.

The genuine rationalist does not think that he or anyone else is in possession of the truth; nor does he think that mere criticism as such helps us achieve new ideas. But he does think that, in the sphere of ideas, only critical discussion can help us sort the wheat from the chaff. He is well aware that acceptance or rejection of an idea is never a purely rational matter; but he thinks that only critical discussion can give us the maturity to see an idea from more and more sides and to make a correct judgement of it.

In this book harsh words are spoken about some of the greatest among the intellectual leaders of mankind, my motive is not, I hope, the wish to belittle them. It springs rather from my conviction that, if our civilization is to survive, we must break with the habit of deference to great men.

The so-called paradox of freedom is the argument that freedom in the sense of absence of any constraining control must lead to very great restraint, since it makes the bully free to enslave the meek.

...the attempt to make heaven on earth invariably produces hell.

The more we learn about the world, and the deeper our learning, the more conscious, specific, and articulate will be our knowledge of what we do not know, our knowledge of our ignorance. For this, indeed, is the main source of our ignorance—the fact that our knowledge can be only finite, while our ignorance must necessarily be infinite.

Popper's tomb.

The Open Society and Its Enemies

Unlimited tolerance must lead to the disappearance of tolerance. If we extend unlimited tolerance even to those who are intolerant, if we are not prepared to defend a tolerant society against the onslaught of the intolerant, then the tolerant will be destroyed, and tolerance with them. In this formulation, I do not imply, for instance, that we should always suppress the utterance of intolerant philosophies; as long as we can counter them by rational argument and keep them in check by public opinion, suppression would certainly be most unwise. But we should claim the right to suppress them if necessary even by force.

Protagoras of Abdera

(Abdera, Macedonia, c.490–early, c.410, BCE)

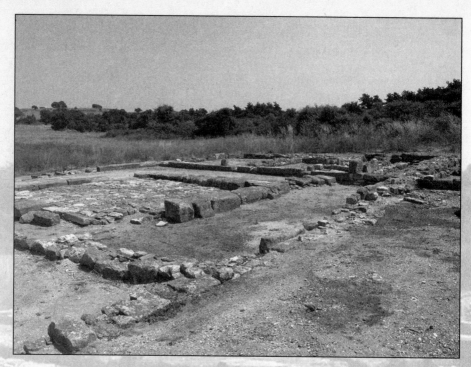

Protagoras is the first sophist on record. He established himself in Athens where it was said he formed friendships with Pericles and Euripides. As with all sophists he was a professional teacher. He was renowned for his eloquence and skill in the art of persuasion.

Three works are attributed to him, although none remain extant: *Concerning the Truth, Antilogiae and Truth,* and *Concerning the Gods.* This last provoked an accusation of impiety causing him to be exiled from Athens. Ironically, the primary sources we have of his thinking come from Plato and Aristotle, his principal opponents.

Recommended reading:

Plato, *Protagoras* (c.390, BCE)

Philostratus, *Lives of the Sophists* (2nd century, CE)

Guthrie, W.K.C., *The Sophists* (1977)

Man is the measure of all things.

There are two sides to every question.

The Athenians are right to accept advice from anyone, since it is
incumbent on everyone to share in that sort of excellence, or else there
can be no city at all.

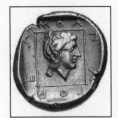

As to gods, I have no way of knowing either that they exist or do not
exist, or what they are like.

...as to the people, they have no understanding, and only repeat what
their rulers are pleased to tell them.

...when [men] meet to deliberate about political virtue, which proceeds
only by way of justice and wisdom, they are patient enough of any man
who speaks of them, as is also natural, because they think that every
man ought to share in this sort of virtue, and that states could not exist
if this were otherwise.

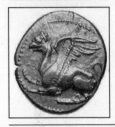

If you will think, Socrates, of the nature of punishment, you will see at
once that in the opinion of mankind virtue may be acquired; no one
punishes the evil-doer under the notion, or for the reason, that he has
done wrong, only the unreasonable fury of a beast acts in that manner.
But he who desires to inflict rational punishment does not retaliate for
a past wrong which cannot be undone; he has regard to the future, and
is desirous that the man who is punished, and he who sees him
punished, may be deterred from doing wrong again.

Coins from Abdera.
Protagoras was an expert in
rhetoric. He was able to
command large sums for his
instruction in grammar and
the use of words. He is
regarded as the inventor of
the professional sophist, or
professor of knowledge.

The previous page shows the
ruins of Abdera, birthplace of
Protagoras and Democritus.

Education and admonition commence in the first years of childhood,
and last to the very end of life. Mother and nurse and father and tutor
are vying with one another about the improvement of the child as soon
as ever he is able to understand what is being said to him: he cannot
say or do anything without their setting forth to him that this is just
and that is unjust; this is honourable, that is dishonourable; this is
holy, that is unholy; do this and abstain from that. And if he obeys, well
and good; if not, he is straightened by threats and blows, like a piece of
bent or warped wood.

Plato, *Protagoras*

After a while the desire of self-preservation gathered men into cities; but when
they were gathered together, having no art of government, they treated one
another badly....Zeus feared that the entire race would be exterminated, and so
he sent Hermes to them, bearing reverence and justice to be the ordering principles of cities and the bonds of friendship and conciliation. Hermes asked Zeus
how he should impart justice and reverence among men: Should he distribute
them as the arts are distributed; that is to say, to a favoured few only. "To all,"
said Zeus; "I should like them all to have a share; for cities cannot exist, if a few
only share in the virtues, as in the arts."

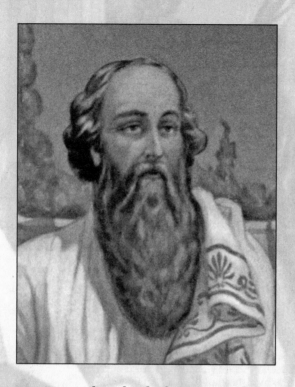

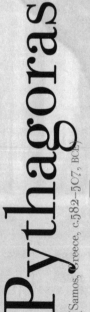

Born on the Island of Samos, Pythagoras traveled to Egypt and Mesopotamia before returning to Greece to found his first school. He was soon forced to flee by the tyrant Polycrates and founded his second school in Magna Graecia (Italy). Men and women of all religions, ethnicity and economic status were welcomed there. The Pythagoreans applied mathematical ideas in their understanding of the cosmos, endowing numbers with a quasi-magical importance.

The famous Pythagorean theorem is still used in geometry and his vision of celestial harmony has inspired thinkers and writers throughout the centuries.

Recommended reading:

📖📖📖 Diogenes Laertius, *Lives of Eminent Philosophers* (1st century BCE)

📖📖 Porphyry, *Life of Pythagoras* (3rd century, BCE)

📖 Iamblichus, *Life of Pythagoras* (3rd century, BCE)

Hermippus also relates another story about Pythagoras. For he says that when he was in Italy, he made a subterraneous apartment... and that Pythagoras came up again after a certain time, lean, and reduced to a skeleton; and that he came into the public assembly, and said that he had arrived from the shades below, and then he recited to them all that had happened during his absence. And they, being charmed by what he told them, wept and lamented, and believed that Pythagoras was a divine being; so that they even entrusted their wives to him, as likely to learn some good from him; and that they too were called Pythagoreans. (Diogenes Laertius)

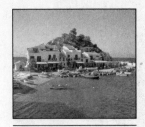

...every man ought so to exercise himself, as to be worthy of belief without an oath. (Diogenes Laertius)

He taught that the soul was immortal and that after death it transmigrated into other animated bodies. After certain specified periods, the same events occur again; that nothing was entirely new; that all animated beings were kin, and should be considered as belonging to one great family. Pythagoras was the first one to introduce these teachings into Greece. (Porphyry)

Pythagoras was born on Samos, an island located in the easternmost part of the Aegean Sea, close to the coast of Asia Minor. According to Greek mythology, Samos was the birthplace of Hera, wife of Zeus.

He soothed the passions of the soul and body by rhythms, songs, and incantations. These he adapted and applied to his friends. He himself could hear the harmony of the Universe, and understood the universal music of the spheres, and of the stars which move in concert with them, and which we cannot hear because of the limitations of our weak nature. (Porphyry)

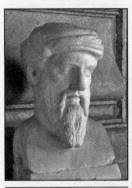

Moreover, he enjoined the following. A cultivated and fruit-bearing plant, harmless to man and beast, should be neither injured nor destroyed. A deposit of money or of teachings should be faithfully preserved by the trustee. There are three kinds of things that deserve to be pursued and acquired; honorable and virtuous things, those that conduce to the use of life, and those that bring pleasures of the blameless, solid and grave kind, of course not the vulgar intoxicating kinds. Of pleasures there were two kinds; one that indulges the bellies and lusts by a profusion of wealth, which he compared to the murderous songs of the Sirens; the other kind consists of things honest, just, and necessary to life, which are just as sweet as the first, without being followed by repentance; and these pleasures he compared to the harmony of the Muses. (Porphyry)

Bust of Pythoagoras. Plato credited Pythagoras with founding a new way of life that distinguished him and his followers from other men.

■ **Diógenes Laertius, *Lives of Eminent Philosophers***

Heraclides Ponticus says, that [Pythagoras] was accustomed to speak of himself in this manner; that he had formerly been Aethalides, and had been accounted the son of Mercury; and that Mercury had desired him to select any gift he pleased except immortality. And that he accordingly had requested that whether living or dead, he might preserve the memory of what had happened to him. While, therefore, he was alive, he recollected everything; and when he was dead, he retained the same memory.

Richard Rorty

(New York, 1931–Palo Alto, California, 2007)

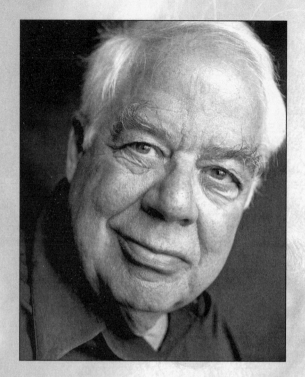

After receiving his doctorate at Yale, Rorty became Professor of Philosophy at Princeton and of the Humanities at the University of Virginia. A successor to the American pragmatism of William James, he is considered to be one of the leading twentieth-century American philosophers.

In agreement with Heidegger and Wittgenstein, Rorty questioned the ability of the philosophic enterprise to attain to an uncontested truth or fundamental absolutes. Instead, he sought a philosophical approach capable of engaging in life, fighting against injustice, and redirecting the American dream toward a more equitable democracy. Though many of his ideas have been called into question, there is no doubt that he revitalized the debate about the public role of philosophy.

Recommended reading:

📖 📖 📖 *Philosophy and the Mirror of Nature* (1979)

📖 📖 *Consequences of Pragmatism* (1982)

📖 *Contingency, Irony, and Solidarity* (1989)

Truth cannot be out there—cannot exist independently of the human mind—because sentences cannot so exist, or be out there. The world is out there, but descriptions of the world are not. Only descriptions of the world can be true or false. The world on its own unaided by the describing activities of humans cannot.

My principal motive is the belief that we can still make admirable sense of our lives even if we cease to have...an ambition of transcendence.

Nowadays, to say that we are clever animals is not to say something philosophical and pessimistic but something political and hopeful— namely, if we can work together, we can make ourselves into whatever we are clever and courageous enough to imagine ourselves becoming. This is to set aside Kant's question "What is man?" and to substitute the question "What sort of world can we prepare for our great grandchildren?"

Philosophers get attention only when they appear to be doing something sinister—corrupting the youth, undermining the foundations of civilization, sneering at all we hold dear. The rest of the time everybody assumes that they are hard at work somewhere down in the sub-basement, keeping those foundations in good repair. Nobody much cares what brand of intellectual duct tape is being used.

What makes us moral beings is that...there are some acts we believe we ought to die rather than commit...But now suppose that one has in fact done one of the things one could not have imagined doing, and finds that one is still alive. At that point, one's choices are suicide, a life of bottomless self-disgust, and an attempt to live so as never to do such a thing again. Dewey recommends the third choice.

Philosophy makes progress not by becoming more rigorous but by becoming more imaginative.

If I had to lay bets, my bet would be that everything is going to go to hell, but, you know, what else have we got except hope?

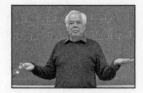

One of Rorty's contributions has been to desacralize the language of philosophy, by considering it to be more inclusive, homologous to literature. Rorty speaks of language games by which he means that philosophy that tends to metaphysics (engaged in the big questions such as what is real or true versus the merely apparent) is doomed to failure wandering down roads that lead nowhere.

As long as we try to project from the relative and conditioned to the absolute and unconditioned, we shall keep the pendulum swinging between dogmatism and skepticism. The only way to stop this increasingly tiresome pendulum swing is to change our conception of what philosophy is good for. But that is not something which will be accomplished by a few neat arguments. It will be accomplished, if it ever is, by a long, slow process of cultural change—that is to say, of change in common sense, changes in the intuitions available for being pumped up by philosophical arguments.

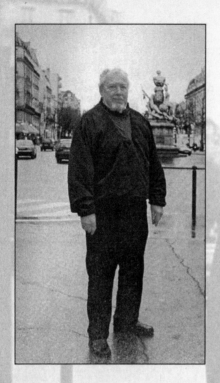

Clément Rosset

(Carteret, France, 1939)

Rosset studied at the prestigious École Normale Supérieure. Afterwards he taught at the University of Montreal and then in Nice. In 1998 he retired from teaching to concentrate on his writings, which are marked by a brilliant and lucid style.

His books are filled with humor and imagination. His early writings celebrate the happiness and joy of existence. Later, Rosset suffered from acute depression, and his thought turned toward a more tragic vision of life. He is the author of an important trilogy, which has become a classic philosophical analysis of the postmodern view of reality.

Recommended reading:

📖 📖 📖 *The Real and Its Double* (1983)

📖 📖 *The Logic of the Worst* (1976)

📖 *The Principle of Cruelty* (1994)

Nothing is more fragile than the human faculty to accept reality, to submit to the imperious prerogative of the real.

...one mysterious point not fully understood about human nature: its intolerance of certainty, an intolerance that leads many people to suffer terrible things in exchange for hope, no matter how vague...

Shadow, reflection, echo, these are the necessary attributes of all real things, whatever their nature...their absence announces the relinquishment of reality.

It would not be so bad to die, if we could assure ourselves that we have lived.

False security is more than the ally of illusion; it is illusion itself.

Simple existence is in itself a cause for rejoicing.

Perfect joy consists in the joy of living, and nothing else.

The vision of the invisible, or rather the suggestion of such vision, does not constitute the material of illusion, but rather material of the creation of poetry.

Here is the true place of anguish: not the impossibility of satisfaction, but the absurdity of wanting it.

Why is there being and not nothing? Why does being have these characteristics? Absurd questions, and even more unwarranted in a world in which causality is a mirage: the world is mute.

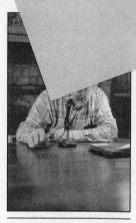

In recent years Rosset has written about the social and literary attitudes toward depression, which he terms "an infirmity of the soul," in contrast to his earlier writings about the joy of existence.

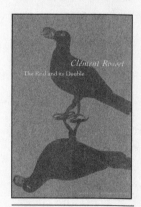

Cover from the English edition of *The Real and Its Double.*

The Principle of Cruelty

Love is without a doubt the most gratifying experience that there is, but it is not, despite a tenacious prejudice to that effect, a true discovery. What I mean to say, is that one experiences something that is already possessed, which explains the paradoxical fact that those thinkers who have spoken most profoundly about love (Schopenhauer, Kierkegaard, or Nietzsche) never experienced it in reality...It is reminiscent of Freud's observation that the love the adult experiences is actually the infant's love of the mother: it is a rediscovery.

153

Jean Jacques Rousseau

(Geneva, Switzerland, 1712–Ermenonville, France, 1778)

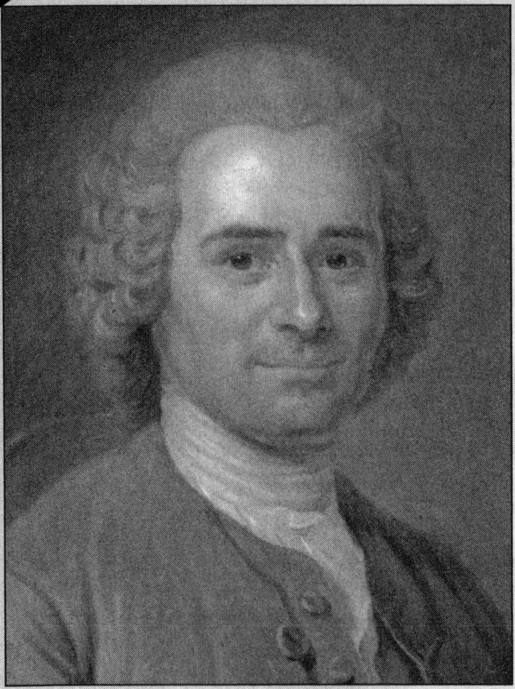

Rousseau's mother died soon after his birth, and he was raised by his father, a watchmaker. At the age of 16 he ran away from Geneva and was taken under the wing of the Baroness Warens in neighboring Savoy. There he began an intense course of study. In 1742 he left for Paris where he became friends with the leading intellectuals of his day and contributed to Diderot's *Encyclopedia*.

Rousseau criticized the doctrine of the progress of civilization. He considered civilization to be the cause of inequality. His conception of the social contract, his defense of the will of the people against the theory of divinely ordained authority, and his arguments in favor of civil liberties caused him to be hailed as the primary theorist of the French Revolution.

Recommended reading:

📖 📖 📖 *The Social Contract* (1762)
Discourse on the Origin and Basis of Inequality among Men (1754)

📖 📖 *Émile* (1762)

📖 *Confessions* (1770)

Women are not made for running; when they flee it is with the intention of being caught.

To understand men, you have to see them in action.

Laws are always useful to those who have and harmful to those who have not.

Youth is the time to study wisdom, age the time to put it into practice.

Man is born free, and yet he is everywhere in chains.

I have learned from my own experience that the source of true happiness lies within us.

No man has any natural authority over his fellow men.

I have resolved on an enterprise that has no precedent and will have no imitator. I want to set before my fellow human beings a man in every way true to nature; and that man will be myself.

Our will is always for our own good, but we do not always see what that is.

If man differs from animals it is because animals are from birth what they will be their entire lives, whereas man through his perfectibility is a dynamic being who is capable of surpassing himself and becoming other than what nature has made him.

Adversity is no doubt a fine teacher, but its lessons are expensive, and often the profit one gains is not worth the cost.

The world of reality has its limits; the world of imagination is boundless.

Civilization is a hopeless race to discover remedies for the evils it produces.

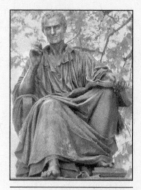

Statue of Rousseau. His ideas were truly revolutionary for his time. The publication of *The Social Contract* caused his expulsion from France.

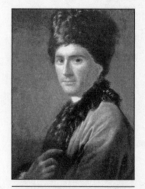

Deprived of his mother in infancy and raised in a poor family, Rousseau dedicated himself to study and was taken under the protection of the Baroness Warens.

Discourse on the Origin and Basis of Inequality among Men

The first man to fence in a bit of land proclaiming: "This is mine," and found others foolish enough to believe him, was the true founder of civil society. What crimes, wars, murders, miseries, and horrors humanity could have been spared if someone had ripped out the fence posts or filled in the ditch and cried out: Watch out for this impostor; you are lost if you forget that the earth and its fruits belong to everyone.

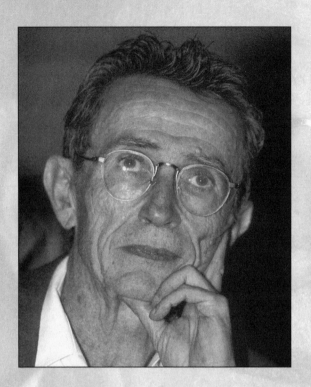

Xavier Rubert de Ventós

(Barcelona, Spain, 1939)

Xavier Rubert de Ventós is Professor of Aesthetics in the School of Architecture at the University of Barcelona and was a founding member of the Barcelona College of Philosophy in 1976. He was elected as a member of parliament for the Socialist Party of Catalonia and then as a representative to the European Parliament.

His writings in Spanish and Catalan have garnered international recognition and won numerous awards, among them the City of Barcelona Prize and the Lletra d'Or Prize for Catalan literature. His provocative and supple texts eschew academicism and philosophical orthodoxies, choosing instead to rely on vivid personal examples.

Recommended reading:

📖 📖 📖 *Self Defeated Man* (1975)

📖 📖 *Heresies of Modern Art* (1975)
The Hispanic Labyrinth (1991)

📖 *God, and Other Inconveniences* (2001)

Brief quotations

I do not want to spend my old age as a practicing intellectual.

The alternative to a good education is ideological indoctrination, just as the alternative to sports is military marches.

I believe that it is much more important to eliminate an old prejudice than to arrive at a new judgment.

If I don't say what I think what is the point of being mad?

But my first theoretical article dealt with what I have later seen is called "the dissonance principle", which might be summarized thus: If you don't do what you believe in, you'll end up believing in what you do.

For me, the gravest sin of all, now and always, is to postulate that man needs to believe in order to remain consistent. Hence my moral aversion to the application of principles and this formulation of "I never." The morality I stand for doesn't include this "never."

If my philosophy has been of any use to me, it's been to situate my monstrous condition within an order of general discourse.

I'm interested in phenomena that, although they are not boundless or incomprehensible, are beyond me in that they are not amenable to reduction by any analysis I might engage in. In this sense, my belonging to a lineage perplexes me more than the things that come out of me, by which I mean, whatever I might call original to me, my own.

Nature and culture increasingly overlap in psychological time and not just in historical time. The latter is what happened, when what was thought to be natural was revealed as cultural. And then we have the contrary, because much of what we believe to be cultural has ended up showing us its socio–biological roots.

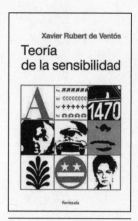

Teoria de la sensibilidad ("Theory of Sensibility") was one of the philosopher's most important early works.

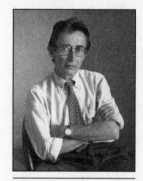

Rubert de Ventós speaks of God, nature, and culture as "resources to fall back on when we try to clarify the enigma of our existence."

Interview

In *Dìos entre otros inconvenientes* ("God and other inconveniences"), I focused on the theme of religion, the "myth", as a crystallization of atavisms that reconstructs—on the symbolic level—instinctive solidarity that has been undermined by the development of "logos." Hence, for example, the thrill associated with physical defenselessness takes on a very different slant when it is linked with religious emotion: atavism is transformed into a sense of the sublime. Nonetheless, given present day circumstances, tragic religions might very well be needed so that we can keep going.

Bertrand Russell

(Trelleck, Wales, 1872–Merionethshire, Wales, 1970)

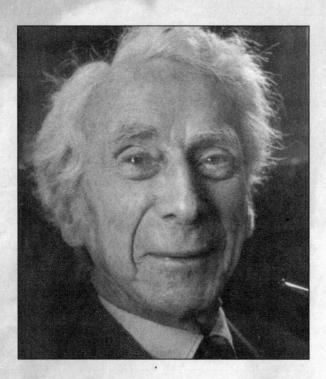

Russell was one of the most relevant and engaged philosophers and mathematicians of the twentieth century. He studied at Cambridge and was on the Board of Governors of Trinity College, Dublin. He opposed the First World War and lost his post at Trinity after being convicted under the Defence of the Realm Act. From 1938 to 1944 he lived in the United States. He was dismissed from his teaching position at the City College of New York after the New York State Supreme Court found him unfit to teach because of his positions on religion and sexual morality. In 1950 he received the Nobel Prize. The committee called him a "champion of humanity and freedom of thought." He was arrested twice at the age of 89 for participation in anti-nuclear demonstrations. At the age of 90 during the Cuban Missile Crisis he wrote letters to both Kennedy and Khrushchev.

Recommended reading:

The Problems of Philosophy (1912)
Principia Mathematica (3 vol.) (1910-1913)

Why I Am Not a Christian and Other Essays (1957)

My Philosophical Development (1959)

YOUR ACTION DESPERATE. THREAT TO HUMAN SURVIVAL. NO CONCEIVABLE JUSTIFICATION. CIVILIZED MAN CONDEMNS IT. WE WILL NOT HAVE MASS MURDER. ULTIMATUM MEANS WAR... END THIS MADNESS. (Telegram to Kennedy during the Cuban Missile Crisis)

We have, in fact, two kinds of morality side by side; one which we preach but do not practice, and another which we practice but seldom preach.

Religion is based, I think, primarily and mainly upon fear. It is partly the terror of the unknown and partly, as I have said, the wish to feel that you have a kind of elder brother who will stand by you in all your troubles and disputes. Fear is the basis of the whole thing—fear of the mysterious, fear of defeat, fear of death. Fear is the parent of cruelty, and therefore it is no wonder if cruelty and religion have gone hand-in-hand. It is because fear is at the basis of those two things.

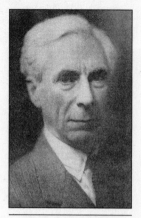

Bertrand Russell began the practice of university sit-ins against war.

Advocates of capitalism are very apt to appeal to the sacred principles of liberty, which are embodied in one maxim: The fortunate must not be restrained in the exercise of tyranny over the unfortunate.

One should respect public opinion insofar as is necessary to avoid starvation and keep out of prison, but anything that goes beyond this is voluntary submission to an unnecessary tyranny.

To modern educated people, it seems obvious that matters of fact are to be ascertained by observation, not by consulting ancient authorities. But this is an entirely modern conception, which hardly existed before the seventeenth century. Aristotle maintained that women have fewer teeth than men; although he was twice married, it never occurred to him to verify this statement by examining his wives' mouths.

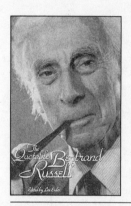

Russell was a proponent of rationalism and social rebellion. His vast work is rich in quotable observations.

Man differs from other animals in one very important respect, and that is that he has some desires which are, so to speak, infinite, which can never be fully gratified, and which would keep him restless even in Paradise. The boa constrictor, when he has had an adequate meal, goes to sleep, and does not wake until he needs another meal. Human beings, for the most part, are not like this.

History of Western Philosophy

Every community is exposed to two opposite dangers: ossification through too much discipline and reverence for tradition...and...dissolution, or subjugation to foreign conquest, through the growth of an individualism and personal independence that makes co-operation impossible. In general, important civilizations start with a rigid and superstitious system, gradually relaxed, and leading, at a certain stage, to a period of brilliant genius, while the good of the old traditional remains and the evil inherent in its dissolution has not yet developed. But as the evil unfolds, it leads to anarchy, thence, inevitably, to a new tyranny, producing a new synthesis secured by a new system of dogma.

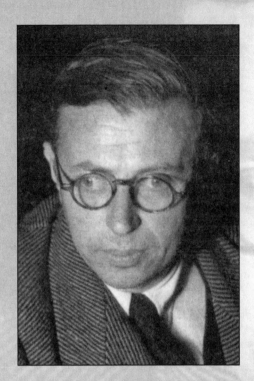

Jean-Paul Sartre

(Paris, France 1905–1980)

Sartre studied philosophy in Paris, in Fribourg, Switzerland, and in Berlin. He became the principal representative of existentialism. At the beginning of the Second World War he was drafted into the army. He was a prisoner of war between 1940 and 1941. Upon his release he returned to teaching and joined the French resistance.

In 1945 he retired from teaching and founded the journal *Les Temps Moderne* with Simone de Beauvoir and other intellectuals. In addition to being a philosopher, Sartre was a novelist and playwright. All of his work displays an unease with political conditions. He was awarded the Nobel Prize for Literature but refused to accept it, saying that it could compromise his integrity as a writer.

Recommended reading:

📖 📖 📖 *Being and Nothingness* (1943)

📖 📖 *Critique of Dialectical Reasoning* (1960)

📖 *No Exit* (1944)

We will freedom for freedom's sake, in and through particular circumstances. And in thus willing freedom, we discover that it depends entirely upon the freedom of others and that the freedom of others depends upon our own.

Nothingness haunts being.

I am condemned to be free.

Life has no meaning a priori...It is up to you to give it a meaning, and value is nothing but the meaning that you choose.

Man cannot will unless he has first understood that he must count on no one but himself; that he is alone, abandoned on earth in the midst of his infinite responsibilities, without help, with no other aim than the one he sets himself, with no other destiny than the one he forges for himself on this earth.

It's quite an undertaking to start loving somebody. You have to have energy, generosity, blindness. There is even a moment right at the start where you have to jump across an abyss: if you think about it you don't do it.

There is no reality except in action.

So that is what hell is. I would never have believed it. You remember: the fire and brimstone, the torture. Ah! the farce. There is no need for torture: Hell is other people.

You and I are real people, operating in a real world. We are not figments of each other's imagination. I am the architect of my own self, my own character, and destiny. It is no use complaining about what I might have been; I am the things I have done and nothing more. We are all free, completely free. We can each do any damn thing we want. Which is more than most of us dare to imagine.

To know what life is worth, you have to risk it once in a while.

The individual's duty is to do what he wants to do, to think whatever he likes, to be accountable to no one but himself, to challenge every idea and every person.

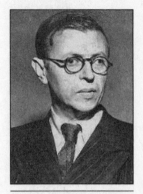

Sartre was in the forefront of intellectuals participating in the protests of 1968. He saw revolution as the only way to regain lost liberty.

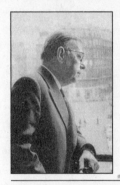

In the course of his political evolution Sartre displayed great sympathies and equally great antipathies. His humanistic socialism caused him to withdraw from the Communist party soon after becoming affiliated with it.

■ *Existentialism Is Humanism*

What do we mean by saying that existence precedes essence? We mean that man first of all exists, encounters himself, surges up in the world—and defines himself afterwards. If man as the existentialist sees him is not definable, it is because to begin with he is nothing. He will not be anything until later, and then he will be what he makes of himself. Thus, there is no human nature, because there is no God to have a conception of it. Man simply is. Not that he is simply what he conceives himself to be, but he is what he wills. Man is nothing else but that which he makes of himself. That is the first principle of existentialism.

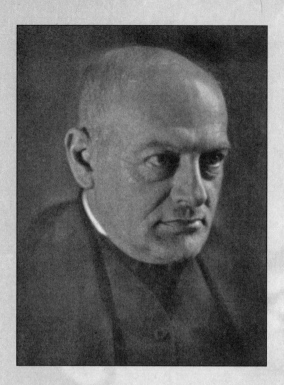

Max Scheler

(Munich, Germany, 1874–Frankfurt, Germany, 1928)

Born to Jewish parents, Scheler converted to Catholicism while in college, calling himself a Nietzschean Catholic. However, he distanced himself from the Church, which, when he fell in love with a student, would not grant him an annulment from his first wife.

In later years he tended toward a more pantheistic worldview. Influenced by Dilthey and Nietzsche he was a disciple of Husserl working with him at the University of Göttingen from 1909–1913. He later he held the Chair in Philosophy at the Universities of Frankfurt and of Cologne. He is considered one of the founders of philosophical anthropology. Pope John Paul II wrote his doctoral dissertation on Scheler's philosophical system.

Recommended reading:

The Human Place in the Cosmos (1928)

The Nature of Sympathy (1913)

Ressentiment (1913-1916)

The highest and ultimate personality values are declared to be independent of contrasts like rich and poor, healthy and sick, etc. The world had become accustomed to considering the social hierarchy, based on status, wealth, vital strength, and power, as an exact image of the ultimate values of morality and personality. The only way to disclose the discovery of a new and higher sphere of being and life, of the "kingdom of God" whose order is independent of that worldly and vital hierarchy, was to stress the vanity of the old values in this higher order.

The precepts "Love your enemies, do good to them which hate you, bless them that curse you"...are born from the Gospel's profound spirit of individualism, which refuses to let one's own actions and conduct depend in any way on somebody else's acts. The Christian refuses to let his acts be mere reactions—such conduct would lower him to the level of his enemy. The act is to grow organically from the person, "as the fruit from the tree.".....What the Gospel demands is not a reaction which is the reverse of the natural reaction, as if it said: "Because he strikes you on the cheek, tend the other"—but a rejection of all reactive activity, of any participation in common and average ways of acting and standards of judgment.

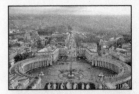

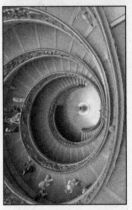

Life is essentially expansion, development, growth in plenitude, and not "self-preservation," as a false doctrine has it. Development, expansion, and growth are not epiphenomena of mere preservative forces and cannot be reduced to the preservation of the "better adapted."

Antiquity believed that the forces of love in the universe were limited. Therefore they were to be used sparingly, and everyone was to be loved only according to his value.

Despite his differences with the Catholic Church teaching, Scheler maintained the primacy of religious and spiritual values over emotional ones.

The medieval peasant prior to the 13th century does not compare himself to the feudal lord, nor does the artisan compare himself to the knight....From the king down to the hangman and the prostitute, everyone is "noble" in the sense that he considers himself as irreplaceable. In the "system of free competition," on the other hand, the notions on life's tasks and their value are not fundamental, they are but secondary derivations of the desire of all to surpass all the others. No "place" is more than a transitory point in this universal chase.

Ressentiment

The process of aging can only be fruitful and satisfactory if the important transitions are accompanied by free resignation, by the renunciation of the values proper to the preceding stage of life. Those spiritual and intellectual values which remain untouched by the process of aging, together with the values of the next stage of life, must compensate for what has been lost. Only if this happens can we cheerfully relive the values of our past in memory, without envy for the young to whom they are still accessible.

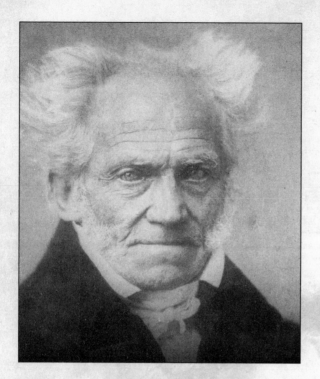

Arthur Schopenhauer

(Danzig, Poland, 1788–Frankfurt am Main, Germany, 1860)

This German philosopher sought to integrate the ideas of Plato and Kant with those of Hinduism and Buddhism in the first attempt to unite Eastern and Western metaphysics.

He studied in Göttingen, Berlin, and Jena and settled in Frankfurt, where he led a solitary life devoted to study. His mother was a writer and that gave him the opportunity to meet important intellectuals of his time, such as Goethe.

He was opposed to the idealistic tendencies of his day, especially those of Hegel. Rather than positing the spiritual nature of all phenomena, he postulated that the will was the ultimate reality.

Recommended reading:

📖 📖 📖 *The World as Will and Representation* (1819)

📖 📖 *Parega and Paralipomena* (1851)

📖 *Letters* (1806-1819)

Man is the only animal to marvel at his own existence.

To question is essentially to suffer, and since to live is to question, life is essentially suffering. The more elevated one's being, the greater the suffering.

At heart man is a terrible and cruel animal. We think of ourselves as domesticated and educated which we conceive of as civilization.

The social instinct is not based upon love of society, but rather on fear of society.

To read good things, one must not read bad things, because life is short and our strength is limited.

Every parting gives a foretaste of death, every reunion a hint of the resurrection.

A man can be himself only so long as he is alone; and if he does not love solitude, he will not love freedom; for it is only when he is alone that he is really free.

The assumption that animals are without rights and the illusion that our treatment of them has no moral significance is a positively outrageous example of Western crudity and barbarity. Universal compassion is the only guarantee of morality.

They tell us that Suicide is the greatest piece of Cowardice...that Suicide is wrong; when it is quite obvious that there is nothing in this world to which every man has a more unassailable title than to his own life and person.

Great men are like eagles: they build their nest on some lofty solitude.

The shortness of life, so often lamented, may be the best thing about it.

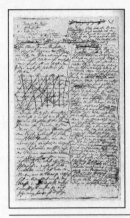

Page from a Schopenhauer manuscript. Famed for his inclination toward a solitary life, his influence extended to Nietzsche, Wagner, and Freud, among others.

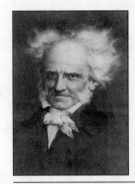

Schopenhauer was a vegetarian and a staunch defender of animal rights.

The World as Will and Representation

There is only one inborn erroneous notion...that we exist in order to be happy....So long as we persist in this inborn error...the world seems to us full of contradictions. For at every step, in great things and small, we are bound to experience that the world and life are certainly not arranged for the purpose of maintaining a happy existence...hence the countenances of almost all elderly persons wear the expression of...disappointment.

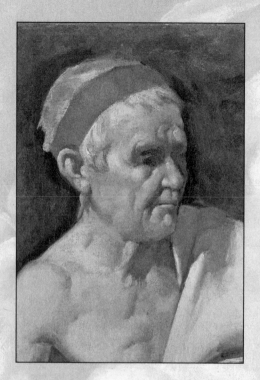

Seneca
(Cordoba, Spain, 4, BCE–Rome, 65, CE)

Seneca was a Roman philosopher born in Cordoba, whose work was marked by a strong emphasis on morals. He studied rhetoric and philosophy in Rome. His total oeuvre comprises moral dialogues, letters, tragedies, and epigrams. His fame as a writer and orator was in ascendance when Gaius Caesar (Caligula) assumed imperial power in 39 CE. He soon fell afoul of the young emperor and was exiled to Corsica.

He returned to Rome in 49, at the request of Agrippina, wife of the Emperor Claudius, and became tutor to her son, Nero. When Nero ascended the throne, Seneca became his close advisor and minister. He retired from public life in 62, and accused by the emperor in 65 of conspiring against him, he committed suicide.

Recommended reading:

📖 📖 📖 *On Providence* (63 CE)

📖 📖 *To Helvia, On Consolation* (42 CE)
On the Constancy of the Wise (55 CE)

📖 *On the Shortness of Life* (55 CE)

The first art of power is to learn to endure hatred.

Fear of war is worse than war itself.

Virtue languishes without an adversary.

What fools these mortals be.

For love of busyness is not industry—it is only the restlessness of a hunted mind.

No man can have a peaceful life who thinks too much about lengthening it.

Nothing is so bitter that a calm mind cannot find comfort in it. Small tablets, because of the writer's skill, have often served for many purposes, and a clever arrangement has often made a very narrow piece of land habitable. Apply reason to difficulties; harsh circumstances can be softened, narrow limits can be widened, and burdensome things can be made to press less severely on those who bear them cleverly.

Withdraw into yourself, as far as you can. Associate with those who will make a better man of you. Welcome those whom you yourself can improve. The process is mutual; for men learn while they teach.

God is near you, with you, and in you. Thus I say, Lucilius: there sits a sacred spirit within us, a watcher of our right and wrong doing, and a guardian...

Man is the rational animal.

All art is but imitation of nature.

Fire tries gold, misfortune tries brave men.

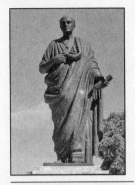

Statue of Seneca in Cordoba located in the eastern section of the city walls.

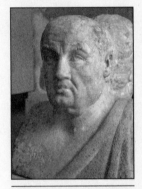

Bust of Lucius Annaeus Seneca. His work devoted to questions of morality exercised a great influence on early Christianity and the medieval Church.

On Providence

We are all chained to fortune: one's chain is gold and wide, another's short and rusty. But what difference does it make? The same prison surrounds all of us, and even those who have bound others are bound themselves; unless perchance you think that a chain on the left side is lighter. Honors bind one man, wealth another; nobility oppresses some, humility others; some are held in subjection by an external power, while others obey the tyrant within; banishments keep some in one place, the priesthood others. All life is slavery. Therefore each one must accustom himself to his own condition and complain about it as little as possible, and lay hold of whatever good is to be found near him.

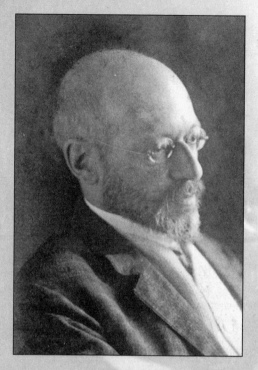

Georg Simmel

(Berlin, Germany, 1858–Strassbourg, Germany, 1918)

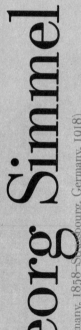

Simmel studied philosophy and law in Berlin and taught at Universities in Berlin and Strassbourg. His work as a historian of philosophy, sociology and culture was enormously influential.

Although he occupied a somewhat marginal position in the academic world, the prestige he enjoyed with his students and other philosophers ranged far beyond the walls of the university. Among those in his debt were Heidegger, Jaspers, Adorno, Benjamin, and Horkheimer. He is considered to be one of the fathers modern sociology along with Max Weber, with whom he founded the German Society for Sociology.

Recommended reading:

On Social Differentiation (1890)
The Philosophy of Money (1900)

Fundamental Questions of Sociology (1917)

The Problems of the Philosophy of History (1905)

Objectivity may also be defined as freedom: the objective individual is bound by no commitments which could prejudice his perception, understanding, and evaluation of the given. The freedom, however, which allows the stranger to experience and treat even his close relationships as though from a bird's-eye view, contains many dangerous possibilities.

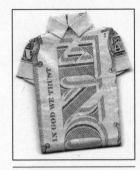

Objectivity does not simply involve passivity and detachment; it is a particular structure composed of distance and nearness, indifference and involvement.

In the stage of first passion, erotic relations strongly reject any thought of generalization: the lovers think that there has never been a love like theirs; that nothing can be compared either to the person loved or to the feelings for that person. An estrangement—whether as cause or as consequence it is difficult to decide—usually comes at the moment when this feeling of uniqueness vanishes from the relationship.

Simmel argued that capitalism becomes a trap when money no longer serves as a means but becomes an end in itself.

The deepest problems of modern life derive from the claim of the individual to preserve the autonomy and individuality of his existence in the face of overwhelming social forces, of historical heritage, of external culture, and of the demands of life.

Punctuality, calculability, exactness are forced upon life by the complexity and extension of metropolitan existence and are not only most intimately connected with its money economy and intellectualist character. These traits must also color the contents of life and favor the exclusion of those irrational, instinctive, sovereign traits and impulses which aim at determining the mode of life from within, instead of receiving the general and precisely schematized form of life from without.

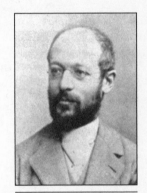

Every relationship between two individuals or two groups will be characterized by the ratio of secrecy that is involved in it.

I understand the task of sociology to be description and determination of the historical-psychological origin of those forms in which interactions take place between human beings. The totality of these interactions, springing from the most diverse impulses, directed toward the most diverse objects, and aiming at the most diverse ends, constitutes "society."

"Useable knowledge" is one of Simmel's basic principals. We acquire knowledge in order to use it.

■ *The Metropolis and Modern Life*

The individual has become a mere cog in an enormous organization of things and powers which tear from his hands all progress, spirituality, and value in order to transform them from their subjective form into the form of a purely objective life....Here in buildings and educational institutions, in the wonders and comforts of space-conquering technology, in the formations of community life, and in the visible institutions of the state, is offered such an overwhelming fullness of crystallized and impersonalized spirit that the personality, so to speak, cannot maintain itself under its impact.

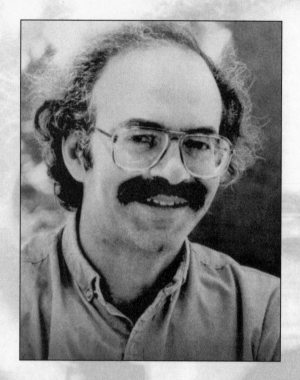

Peter Singer

(Melbourne, Australia, 1946)

Singer studied at the University of Monash in Australia before attending Oxford where he studied the utilitarian philosophers Bentham and Mill. In his landmark publication, *Animal Liberation*, he presented the theory of animal rights and denounced speciesism, the discrimination against other species that he compared to racism.

Singer advocates a philosophy that does not limit itself to theory, an applied or practical philosophy that involves itself in the active struggle against the mistreatment of animals, be it for scientific research or the production of food, fur, or other animal products.

Recommended reading:

Animal Liberation (1975)

The Great Ape Project: Equality beyond Humanity (1993)
Practical Ethics (1979)

Rethinking Life and Death (1994)

All the arguments to prove man's superiority cannot shatter this hard fact: in suffering the animals are our equals.

When we buy new clothes not to keep ourselves warm but to look "well-dressed" we are not providing for any important need. We would not be sacrificing anything significant if we were to continue to wear our old clothes and give the money to famine relief. By doing so, we would be preventing another person from starving. It follows from what I have said earlier that we ought to give money away, rather than spend it on clothes which we do not need to keep us warm. To do so is not charitable, or generous. Nor is it the kind of act which philosophers and theologians have called "supererogatory"—an act which it would be good to do, but not wrong not to do. On the contrary, we ought to give the money away, and it is wrong not to do so.

Science does not stand still, and neither does philosophy, although the latter has a tendency to walk in circles.

We are responsible not only for what we do but also for what we could have prevented.

Hebrew word for "charity" tzedakah, simply means "justice" and as this suggests, for Jews, giving to the poor is no optional extra but an essential part of living a just life.

...chimpanzees, bonobos, gorillas, and orangutans are thinking, self-aware beings, capable of planning ahead, who form lasting social bonds with others and have a rich social and emotional life. The great apes are therefore an ideal case for showing the arbitrariness of the species boundary. If we think that all human beings, irrespective of age or mental capacity, have some basic rights, how can we deny that the great apes, who surpass some humans in their capacities, also have these rights?

If a being suffers there can be no moral justification for refusing to take that suffering into consideration. No matter what the nature of the being, the principle of equality requires that its suffering be counted equally with the like suffering—insofar as rough comparisons can be made—of any other being. So the limit of sentience is the only defensible boundary of concern for the interests of others.

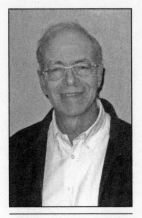

Recent photograph of the philosopher Peter Singer. The philosopher suggests that the Left ought to reread Darwin to recover the apercu in *Origin of Species* that there is an inherent trait in humans that seeks to promote its own interests through cooperation with others.

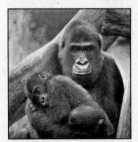

Singer is one of the most prominent activists in the defense of animals.

Animal Liberation

How far down the evolutionary scale shall we go? Shall we eat fish? What about shrimps? Oysters? To answer these questions we must bear in mind the central principle on which our concern for other beings is based...the only legitimate boundary to our concern for the interests of other beings is the point at which it is no longer accurate to say that the other being has interests. To have interests, in a strict, non-metaphorical sense, a being must be capable of suffering or experiencing pleasure. If a being suffers, there can be no moral justification for disregarding that suffering, or for refusing to count it equally with the like suffering of any other being.

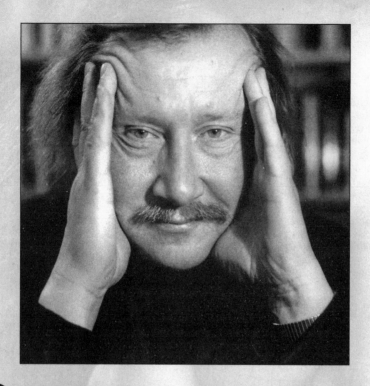

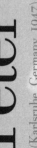

Peter Sloterdijk

(Karlsruhe, Germany, 1947)

Sloterdijk studied philosophy, history, and German literature at the Universities of Hamburg and Munich. He is currently Professor of Philosophy and Aesthetics at the University of Art and Design Karlsruhe. The work for which he is best known, *Critique of Cynical Reason,* has become widely read and argued over in Germany.

He engaged in a celebrated debate with Jürgen Habermas in which the older philosopher leveled the accusation that Sloterdijk employed a fascistic rhetoric in proposing a new genetic selectivity in his book, *Rules for the Human Zoo.* In an open letter, Sloterdijk responded that Habermas had rounded up third parties to attack his position and resorted to an error-ridden text of his remarks.

Recommended reading:

Critique of Cynical Reason (1983)

Spheres (Trilogía, 2003-2006)

Rules for the Human Zoo (1999)

The taming of man has failed. Civilization's potential for barbarism is growing; the everyday bestialization of man is on the increase.

Our lethargic modernity certainly knows how to "think historically," but it has long doubted that it lives in a meaningful history.

Psychologically, present-day cynics can be understood as borderline melancholics, who can keep their symptoms of depression under control and can remain more or less able to work....Their psychic apparatus has become elastic enough to incorporate as a survival factor a permanent doubt about their own activities. They know what they are doing, but they do it because, in the short run, the force of circumstances and the instinct for self-preservation are speaking the same language, and they are telling them that it has to be so.

Because there are no truths that can be taken possession of without a struggle, and because all knowledge must choose a place in the configuration of hegemonic and oppositional forces, the means of establishing knowledge seem to be almost more important than the knowledge itself.

How much truth is contained in something can be best determined by making it thoroughly laughable and then watching to see how much joking around it can take. For truth is a matter that can withstand mockery, that is freshened by any ironic gesture directed at it. Whatever cannot withstand satire is false.

The stakes in this game are not low. Our enterprise is no less than the introduction of an alternative language, and with the language an altered perspective, for a group of phenomena that tradition tended to refer to with such words as 'spirituality', 'piety', 'morality', 'ethics' and 'asceticism'. If the maneuver succeeds, the conventional concept of religion, that ill-fated bugbear from the prop studios of modern Europe, will emerge from these investigations as the great loser. Certainly intellectual history has always resembled a refuge for malformed concepts, and after the following journey through the various stations, one will see through the concept of 'religion' in its failed design, a concept whose crookedness is second only to the hyper-bugbear that is 'culture'.

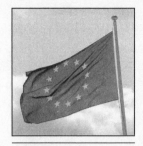

For Sloterdijk the European project is one of the most crucial themes of today's world. The development of the European Union illustrates the history of the tension between the small and great powers.

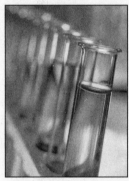

Sloterdijk defends a new vision of a technical-genetic humanity, affirming that "the fantasies of biopolitical selection have the potential for utopias of justice."

Critique of Cynical Reason

In our thinking there is no longer any spark of the uplifting flight of concepts or of the ecstasies of understanding. We are enlightened, we are apathetic. No one talks anymore of a love of wisdom. There is no longer any knowledge whose friend (philos) one could be. It does not occur to us to love the kind of knowledge we have; rather we ask ourselves how we might contrive to live with it without becoming ossified.

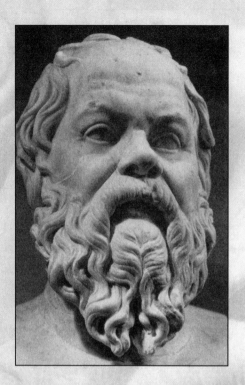

Socrates

(Athens, Greece, 470–399, BCE)

Socrates lived in Athens at its apogee. He was distinguished by his oratorical skill, the force of his arguments, and his celebrated discussions with the sophists. He was the inventor of maieutics, an inductive method of obtaining knowledge that consists in questioning his interlocutors and through the use of logic guiding them to the truth. His disciple Plato elaborated a theory of knowledge upon this foundation.

Socrates did not commit his teachings to writing. Most of what we know of him comes from the works of Plato. Accused of corrupting the youth of Athens, he was condemned to death and committed suicide by imbibing hemlock. He faced his death with admirable composure.

Recommended reading:

📖 📖 📖 Plato, *Apology, Criton, Ion, Protagoras, Symposium, Euthyphro, Phaedo, Republic*

📖 📖 Xenophanes, *Symposium, Apology* (394-387 BCE)

📖 Guthrie, W.K.C., *Socrates* (1972)

We do not know—neither the sophists, nor the orators, nor the artists, nor I—what the True, the Good, and the Beautiful are. But there is this difference between us: although these people know nothing, they all believe they know something; whereas, I, if I know nothing, at least have no doubts about it. As a result, all this superiority in wisdom which the oracle has attributed to me reduces itself to the single point that I am strongly convinced that I am ignorant of what I do not know.

―――――

True knowledge lies in recognizing one's own innocence.

―――――

The unexamined life is not worth living.

―――――

Be kind, for everyone you meet is fighting a hard battle.

―――――

If you don't get what you want, you suffer; if you get what you don't want, you suffer; even when you get exactly what you want, you still suffer because you can't hold on to it forever. Your mind is your predicament. It wants to be free of change. Free of pain, free of the obligations of life and death. But change is law, and no amount of pretending will alter that reality.

―――――

Know thyself.

―――――

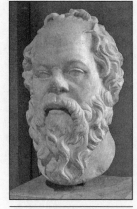

Socrates was the precursor of Plato and Aristotle. Together they produced the essential philosophic legacy of Greece. This bust of Socrates is from the Louvre in Paris.

For this fear of death is indeed the pretense of wisdom, and not real wisdom, being the appearance of knowing the unknown; since no one knows whether death, which they in their fear apprehend to be the greatest evil, may not be the greatest good....this is the point in which, as I think, I am superior to men in general, and in which I might perhaps fancy myself wiser than other men—that whereas I know but little of the world below, I do not suppose that I know...and I will never fear or avoid a possible good rather than a certain evil.

―――――

By all means, marry. If you get a good wife, you'll become happy; if you get a bad one, you'll become a philosopher.

―――――

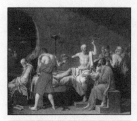

Jacques-Louis David, *The Death of Socrates* (Metropolitan Museum of Art, New York).

If all misfortunes were laid in one common heap whence everyone must take an equal portion, most people would be contented to take their own and depart.

―――――

I was really too honest a man to be a politician and live.

Plato, *The Apology*

Someone will say: And are you not ashamed, Socrates, of a course of life which is likely to bring you to an untimely end? To him I may fairly answer: There you are mistaken: a man who is good for anything ought not to calculate the chance of living or dying; he ought only to consider whether in doing anything he is doing right or wrong—acting the part of a good man or a bad....For wherever a man's place is, whether the place he has chosen or that where he has been placed by a commander. there he ought to remain in the hour of danger; he should not think of death or of anything, but of disgrace.

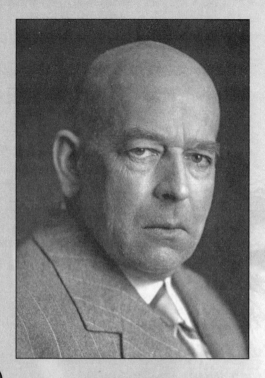

Oswald Spengler

(Bad Blankenburg, Germany, 1880–Munich, Germany, 1936)

Spengler was drawn to the philosophy of Heraclitus. He lectured on Nietzsche and Dilthey and at the end of World War I published *The Decline of the West*, an extremely pessimistic work that argued that civilizations are like organisms that flourish and reach a highpoint and then inevitably come to an end.

He argued that just as the Egyptian and Babylonian Empires perished, so the West was now reaching the downward turn of the cycle. The book gained an avid audience in the United States and Germany, some using it to justify Hitler's National Socialism.

Recommended reading:

📖 📖 📖 *The Decline of the West* (1918)

📖 📖 *Man and Technics* (1932)

📖 *Prussianism and Socialism* (1920)

Today we live so cowed under the bombardment of this intellectual artillery that hardly anyone can attain to the inward detachment that is required for a clear view of the monstrous drama. The will-to-power operating under a pure democratic disguise has finished off its masterpiece so well that the object's sense of freedom is actually flattered by the most thorough-going enslavement that has ever existed.

Today a democrat of the old school would demand, not freedom for the press, but freedom from the press.

Socialism is nothing but the capitalism of the lower classes.

This is our purpose: to make as meaningful as possible this life that has been bestowed upon us...to live in such a way that we may be proud of ourselves, to act in such a way that some part of us lives on.

The question of whether world peace will ever be possible can only be answered by someone familiar with world history. To be familiar with world history means, however, is to know human beings as they have been and always will be. There is a vast difference, which most people will never comprehend, between viewing future history as it will be and viewing it as one might like it to be. Peace is a desire, war is a fact; and history has never paid heed to human desires and ideals.

Every ideology shatters itself on the reality of history.

Philosophy, the love of Wisdom, is at the very bottom defense against the incomprehensible.

One day the last portrait of Rembrandt and the last bar of Mozart will have ceased to be—though possibly a colored canvas and a sheet of notes will remain—because the last eye and the last ear accessible to their message will have gone.

Formerly no one was allowed to think freely; now it is permitted, but no one is capable of it any more. Now people want to think only what they are supposed to want to think, and this they consider freedom.

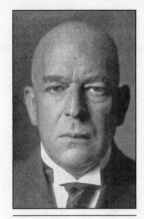

Oswald Spengler. Germany's defeat and its humiliation at the end of the First World War were decisive influences on Spengler's philosophy of history.

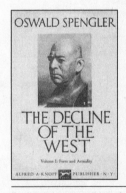

English language edition of one of the fundamental texts of twentieth-century German thought.

Man and Technics

We are born into this time and must bravely follow the path to the destined end. There is no other way. Our duty is to hold on to the lost position, without hope, without rescue, like that Roman soldier whose bones were found in front of a door in Pompeii, who, during the eruption of Vesuvius, died at his post because they forgot to relieve him. That is greatness. That is what it means to be a thoroughbred. The honorable end is the one thing that cannot be taken from a man.

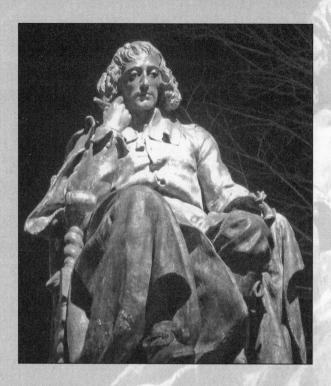

Baruch de Spinoza

(Amsterdam, Holland, 1632–The Hague, Holland, 1677)

Spinoza was born to a Portuguese Jewish family that was forced to convert to Christianity and then emigrate to Holland to escape the Inquisition. The young Spinoza was destined for the rabbinate until his readings in Hobbes and Descartes led him to question his faith. In 1656 he was expelled from the synagogue for his heterodox opinions.

Spinoza earned his living grinding optical lenses while pursuing philosophical investigations in his leisure time. He kept up correspondence with important intellectual figures of his day, provoking intense controversy with the *Tractatus Theologico-Politicus* published anonymously in 1670. Spinoza died of tuberculosis at the age of 44.

Recommended reading:

📖 📖 📖 *The Ethics* (1674)

📖 📖 *Tractatus Theologico-Politicus* (1670)

📖 *Principles of Cartesian Philosophy* (1663)

If men's minds were as easily controlled as their tongues, every king would sit safely on his throne, and government by compulsion would cease; for every subject would shape his life according to the intentions of his rulers, and would esteem a thing true or false, good or evil, just or unjust, in obedience to their dictates.

We feel and know that we are eternal.

As men's habits of mind differ, so that some more readily embrace one form of faith, some another, for what moves one to pray may move another to scoff, I conclude...that everyone should be free to choose for himself the foundations of his creed, and that faith should be judged only by its fruits; each would then obey God freely with his whole heart, while nothing would be publicly honored save justice and charity.

Nature is satisfied with little; and if she is, I am also.

The things which...are esteemed as the greatest good of all...can be reduced to these three headings, to wit : Riches, Fame, and Pleasure. With these three the mind is so engrossed that it cannot scarcely think of any other good.

The ultimate aim of government is not to rule, or restrain, by fear, nor to exact obedience, but, contrariwise, to free every man from fear, that he may live in all possible security ; in other words, to strengthen his natural right to exist and work without injury to himself or others.

If you do not wish to repeat the past, study it.

I have made a ceaseless effort not to ridicule, not to bewail, not to scorn human actions, but to understand them.

Of all the things that are beyond my power, I value nothing more highly than to be allowed the honor of entering into bonds of friendship with people who sincerely love truth. For, of things beyond our power, I believe there is nothing in the world which we can love with tranquility except such men.

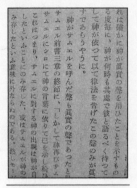

Japanese edition of *Tractatus Theologico-Politicus,* one of Spinoza's essential works.

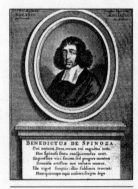

For Spinoza the universe is identical to God. His vision of an impersonal God garnered him the hostility of many of his contemporaries.

The safest way for a state is to lay down the rule that religion is comprised solely in the exercise of charity and justice, and that the rights of rulers in sacred, no less than in secular matters, should merely have to do with actions, but that every man should think what he likes and say what he thinks.

Thales of Miletus

(Miletus, Asia Minor, c.624–546 BCE)

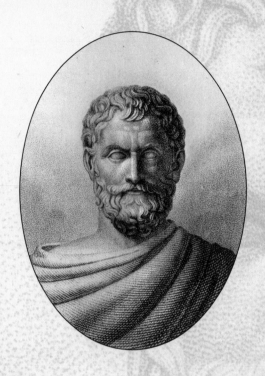

Thales, one of the Seven Sages of Greece, is considered to be the first philosopher in the Western philosophical tradition. He was the first to attempt to find a rational explanation for the universe, its causes, and origins.

The existing references to his life are confused and contradictory; for example, some affirm that he was married and had a son, others that he was a bachelor. Similarly there are many discrepancies about his works: some say he did not write anything at all, others that he was the author of, among other things, a work on nautical astronomy. According to Thales, water is the primal element out of which everything is generated.

Recommended reading:

Diogenes Laertius, *Lives of Eminent Philosophers* (1st century CE)

Kirk, G.S. and J.E. Raven, *The Presocratic Philosophers* (1987)

Barnes, Jonathan, *The Presocratic Philosophers* (1992)

Brief quotations

Avoid doing what you would blame others for doing.

That from which is everything that exists and from which it first becomes and into which it is rendered at last, its substance remaining under it, but transforming in qualities, that they say is the element and principle of things that are....For it is necessary that there be some nature, either one or more than one, from which become the other things of the object being saved...Thales, the founder of this type of philosophy, says that it is water. (Aristotle)

Thales assures us that water is the principle of all things; and that God is that Mind which shaped and created all things from water. (Cicero)

And, he, tis said, did first compute the stars
Which beam in Charles's wain, and guide the bark
Of the Phoenician sailor o'er the sea. (Callimachus)

They say, too, when his mother exhorted him to marry, he said, "No by Jove, it is not yet time." And afterwards, when he was past his youth, and she was again pressing him earnestly, he said, "It is no longer time." (Diogenes Laertius)

It is said that once he was led out of his house by an old woman for the purpose of observing the stars, and he fell into a ditch, on which the old woman said to him "Do you, O Thales, who cannot see what is under your feet, think that you shall understand what is in heaven." (Diogenes Laertius)

And the following is quoted as a saying of his: "God is the most ancient of all things, for he had no birth; the world is the most beautiful thing, for it is the work of God: place is the greatest of all things, for it contains all things: intellect is the swiftest of things, for it runs through everything: necessity is the strongest of things, for it rules everything; time is the wisest of things, for it finds out everything." (Diogenes Laertius)

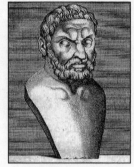

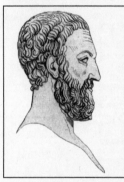

Thales of Miletus cultivated other interests aside from philosophy. As a young man he traveled to Egypt where he studied astronomy and geometry. In later life he took part in building a canal to divert the waters of the Halys River.

Diogenes de Laertius, *Lives of Eminent Philosophers*

He asserted that water was the principle of all things, and that the world had life and was full of daemons. They say, too, that he was the original definer of the seasons of the year, and that it was he who divided the year into three hundred and sixty-five days. And he never had a teacher except during the time he went to Egypt and associated with the priests. Hieronymous also says that he measured the Pyramids: watching their shadow, and calculating when they were of the same size as that was. He lived with Thraybulus the tyrant of Miletus, as we are informed by Minyas.

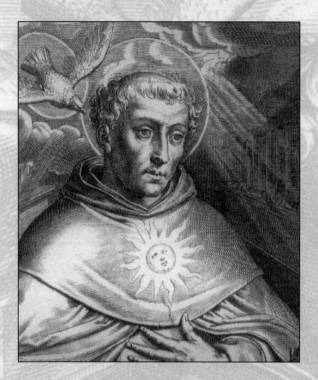

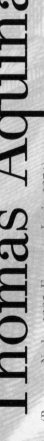

Thomas Aquinas

(Rocaseca, Naples, 1225–Fossanova, Lazio, 1274)

Aquinas was canonized in 1323 and declared Doctor of the Church in 1567. He is without a doubt the most important of all ecclesiastical philosophers. His approach gave birth to the Thomist school of philosophy, which seeks to reconcile faith and reason, reinterpreting Aristotelianism in the service of the Church and incorporating the work of Augustine, Averroes, and Avicenna.

His crowning achievement, *Summa Theologica*, provides five rational proofs of the existence of God. He maintained that the truths of faith are compatible with sensory experience as presented by Aristotle.

Recommended reading:

📖 📖 📖 *Summa Theologica* (1265-1273)

📖 📖 *Summa contra Gentiles* (1261-1264)

📖 Davies, Brian, *The Thought of Thomas Aquinas* (1993)

Because of the diverse conditions of humans, it happens that some acts are virtuous to some people, as appropriate and suitable to them, while the same acts are immoral for others, as inappropriate to them.

By nature all men are equal in liberty, but not in other endowments.

Faith has to do with things that are not seen and hope with things that are not at hand.

The knowledge of God is the cause of things. For the knowledge of God is to all creatures what the knowledge of the artificer is to things made by his art.

Three things are necessary for the salvation of man: to know what he ought to believe; to know what he ought to desire; and to know what he ought to do.

Now the object of the will, i.e., of man's appetite, is the universal good...Hence it is evident that nothing can lull the human will but the universal good. This is to be found, not in any creature, but in God alone; because every creature has goodness by participation. Thus God alone can satisfy the will of a human being.

It is on account neither of God's weakness nor ignorance that evil comes into the world, but rather it is due to the order of his wisdom and the greatness of his goodness that diverse grades of goodness occur in things, many of which would be lacking if no evil were permitted. Indeed, the good of patience would not exist without the evil of persecution; nor the good of preservation of life in a lion if not for the evil of the destruction of the animals on which it lives.

We ought to cherish the body. Our body's substance is not from an evil principle, as the Manicheans imagine, but from God. And therefore, we ought to cherish the body by the friendship of love, by which we love God.

To love is to will the good of the other.

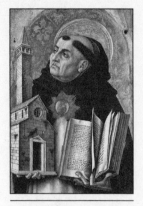

Even though he is now considered a foundational thinker for the Church, he espoused ideas that were revolutionary in his day, such as that knowledge obtained by faith and that obtained by perception are complimentary.

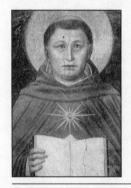

Despite his defense of rationality, Aquinas acknowledged the primacy of faith and the infallibility of the Church.

Summa Theologica

It was necessary for our salvation that there be a knowledge revealed by God, besides philosophical science built up by human reason. Firstly, indeed, because the human being is directed to God, as to an end that surpasses the grasp of his reason....But the end must first be known by men who are to direct their thoughts and actions to the end. Hence it was necessary for the salvation of man that certain truths which exceed human reason should be made known to him by divine revelation.

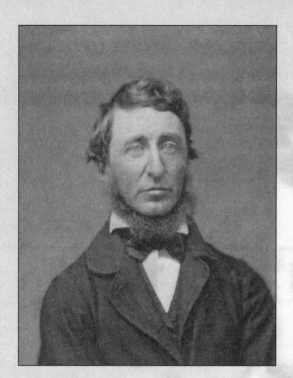

Henry David Thoreau

(Concord, Massachusetts, 1817–1862)

Philosopher, naturalist, political activist, Henry David Thoreau was one of the key figures of nineteenth-century American thought. He is best known for his book *Walden*, the record of a two-year experiment in simple living in a cottage he built himself on Walden Pond.

Thoreau was an ardent opponent of slavery, defending John Brown and supporting the abolitionist writer Wendell Phillips. His work *Civil Disobedience* argued that the citizen had the obligation to resist unjust laws. Thoreau's passionate defense of conscience influenced Gandhi and Martin Luther King in their non-violent struggles for justice.

Recommended reading:

📖 📖 📖 *Walden* (1854)

📖 📖 *Civil Disobedience* (1849)

📖 *The Maine Woods* (1864)

Most of the luxuries and many of the so-called comforts of life are not only not indispensable, but positive hindrances to the elevation of mankind.

———

I heartily accept the motto, "That government is best which governs least"; and I should like to see it acted up to more rapidly and systematically. Carried out, it finally amounts to this, which also I believe—"That government is best which governs not at all"; and when men are prepared for it, that will be the kind of government which they will have.

———

To speak practically and as a citizen, unlike those who call themselves no-government men, I ask for, not at once no government, but at once a better government. Let every man make known what kind of government would command his respect, and that will be one step toward obtaining it.

———

Under a government which imprisons any unjustly, the true place for a just man is also a prison...the only house in a slave State in which a free man can abide with honor.

———

To some extent, mythology is only the most ancient history and biography. So far from being false or fabulous in the common sense, it contains only enduring and essential truth, the I and you, the here and there, the now and then, being omitted.

———

I trust that some may be as near and dear to Buddha, or Christ, or Swedenborg, who are without the pale of their churches. It is necessary not to be Christian to appreciate the beauty and significance of the life of Christ. I know that some will have hard thoughts of me, when they hear their Christ named beside my Buddha, yet I am sure that I am willing they should love their Christ more than my Buddha, for the love is the main thing, and I like him too.

———

The mass of men lead lives of quiet desperation.

———

I went to the woods because I wished to live deliberately, to front only the essential facts of life, and see if I could not learn what it had to teach, and not, when I came to die, discover that I had not lived. I did not wish to live what was not life, living is so dear; nor did I wish to practise resignation, unless it was quite necessary.

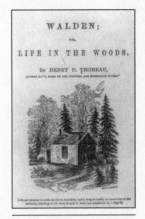

Title page from the first edition of Thoreau's *Walden*.

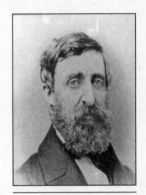

Thoreau was dedicated to the abolitionist cause.

Civil Disobedience

Must the citizen ever for a moment, or in the least degree, resign his conscience to the legislator? Why has every man a conscience, then? I think that we should be men first, and subjects afterward. It is not desirable to cultivate a respect for the law, so much as for the right. The only obligation which I have a right to assume is to do at any time what I think right. It is truly enough said that a corporation has no conscience; but a corporation of conscientious men is a corporation with a conscience. Law never made men a whit more just; and, by means of their respect for it, even the well-disposed are daily made the agents of injustice.

Miguel de Unamuno

(Bilbao, Spain, 1864–Salamanca, Spain, 1936)

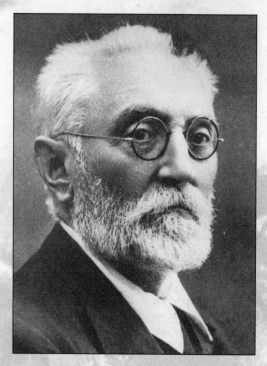

Poet, essayist, and philosopher, Miguel de Unamuno studied philosophy in Madrid and somewhat later became a professor of Greek at the University of Salamanca, in which city he spent the greater part of his life, except for those periods in which he was forced into exile because of his political opinions. Unamuno was a man of intense temperament, polemical, and, at times, contradictory. On the one hand, in 1894 he affiliated himself with the Socialist Party and in 1924 was deported for writing an article critical of King Alphonso XIII. On the other had, the Republican government ended his career as Rector of the University of Salamanca for supporting Franco's rise to power. But he then engaged in a famous debate with one of Franco's generals, Millán Astray, in which he excoriated the nationalist ideology.

Recommended reading:

📖 📖 📖 *The Tragic Sense of Life* (1913)

📖 📖 *Our Lord Don Quixote* (1905)

📖 *The Agony of Christianity* (1926–1931)

It is said that man is a rational animal. I don't know why it is not said that he is an emotional and sentimental animal.

———

No individual, no people, which in a certain sense is an individual as well, can follow a path that ruptures the unity and continuity of his self.

———

Man is an end, not a means.

———

If a philosopher is not a man, he is even less a philosopher; he is a pedant, a shadow of a man.

———

It is not enough to cure the disease, one must know how to cry. Knowing how to cry is perhaps the highest wisdom.

———

To know for the sake of knowing! Truth for truth's sake! This is inhuman.

———

Neither reason nor emotion alone leads to true counsel.

———

Faith in immortality is irrational. And yet, faith, life, and reason are mutually necessary.

———

Reason and faith are enemies, but one cannot have one without the other.

———

Only he who attempts the absurd is capable of achieving the impossible.

———

Faith which does not doubt is dead faith.

———

Some people will believe anything if you whisper it to them.

———

A lot of good arguments are spoiled by some fool who knows what he is talking about.

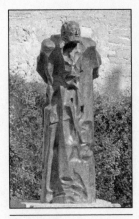

Statue of Unamuno in Salamanca

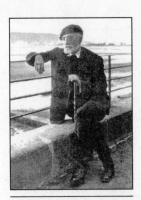

A well-known photograph of the philosopher, essayist, and poet, who was a native of Bilbao.

The Tragic Sense of Life

Homo sum; nihil humani a me alienum puto, said the Latin playwright. And I would rather say, *Nullum hominem a me alienum puto*: I am a man; no other man do I deem a stranger. For to me the adjective *humanus* is no less suspect than its abstract substantive *humanitas*, humanity. Neither "the human" nor "humanity," neither the simple adjective nor the substantivized adjective, but the concrete substantive—man. The man of flesh and bone; the man who is born, suffers, and dies—above all, who dies; the man who eats and drinks and plays and sleeps and thinks and wills; the man who is seen and heard; the brother, the real brother.

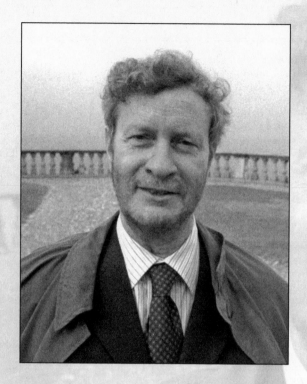

Gianni Vattimo

(Turín, Italy 1936)

Vattimo was a student of Gadamer at the University of Heidelberg. He is currently Professor of Philosophy at the University of Turin. He was influenced by modern German philosophical thinking, above all by Nietzsche and Heidegger. He is considered the leading Italian postmodernist theorist. He coined the term "weak thought" as a corrective to the metaphysical aspirations of traditional philosophy.

Vattimo argues that the modern project of the emancipation of the individual has been undermined by the impact of the complexity of new technology and the pervasive influence of mass media. He has collaborated in diverse Italian journals and is an important figure on the Italian Left.

Recommended reading:

The End of Modernity (1985)

Nihilism and Emancipation (2003)

The Transparent Society (1989)

It is only thanks to God that I am an atheist.

I believe that I believe.

Since Copernicus man has been rolling from the center towards X...the situation in which the human subject explicitly recognizes that the lack of foundation is a constitutive part of its condition (what Nietzsche elsewhere calls 'the death of God').

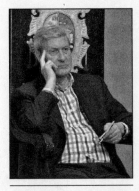

The essence of nihilism is the history in which there is nothing to Being itself.

No, facts are precisely what there is not, only interpretations.

Soviet Communism and Western Capitalism share the same crazy ideology: forced industrialization of society.

Committed to the Italian Left, defender of LGBT rights and in favor of non-dogmatic religion, Gianni Vattimo is one of today's most important philosophers.

I propose hermeneutic communism: non-dogmatic communism, weak communism. Only this can save us.

Ours is an epoch in which the human being has become a determined value.

The death of God—the culminating moment of metaphysics—has become the crisis of humanism.

Postmodernism is characterized not only by something new in respect to modernism, but to a large extent as the dissolution of the category of newness as in the "end of history."

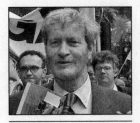

There is no unified history, rather images of proposed pasts and diverse points of view.

Vattimo has asserted that the internet can serve as a non-violent subversion of capitalism.

The Transparent Society

In regards to the idea of the defining rationality of history, minorities—be they ethnic, sexual, religious, cultural or aesthetic—take this to mean, that there is only one repressive and silencing truth that acts to realize humanity. If I am to have a dialogue in a world of dialogues, I have to accept that mine is not the only voice, but dialogue entails a conversation with others. If I profess my system of values—religious, ethnic, political, ethical—in this world of cultural plurality, I need to maintain an acute awareness of historicity, contingency, and the limitation of all systems, starting with my own.

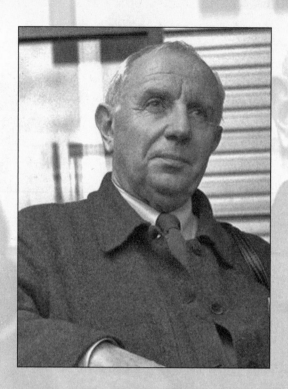

Paul Virilio
(Paris, France, 1932)

Virilio is a philosopher and architect. His father was an Italian communist, his mother was originally from Brittany. Having lived through World War II at a young age, he refers to himself as a "child of war." At the age of eleven, he witnessed the bombing of Nantes, where he and his family had taken refuge, and he says it made of him a relativist. War revealed to him the fragility of apparent reality, leaving in ruins what he conceived of as indestructible.

Virilio is one of the most important essayists on communication, mass media, the audiovisual world, and cybernetics. He is a dissident voice in our "hyperinformation" society.

Recommended reading:

The Aesthetics of Disappearance (1980)

The Information Bomb (1998)

The Administration of Fear (2012)

War was my university. Everything has proceeded from there.

The speed of light does not merely transform the world. It becomes the world. Globalization is the speed of light.

Each time a wall is reached, there is a retreat. And history has just struck the wall of worldwide time. With live transmission, local time no longer creates history. Worldwide time does. In other words, real time conquers real space, space-time. We must reflect on this paradoxical situation which places us in a kind of outside-time. Faced as we are with this time accident, an accident with no equal.

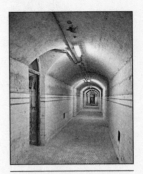

Two attitudes are possible with respect to these new technologies: one declares them a miracle; the other—mine—recognizes that they are interesting while maintaining a critical attitude

In early childhood Virilio was fascinated with the bunker: "little temple without a cult," as he later called it.

A concrete factual reality: meet someone, love that person, make love to that person. Or, the game reality: use the technologies of cybersex to meet that person from a distance, without touching or risk of contamination, contact without contact.

I am an art critic of technologies, a fan worried about the propagandistic and sudden nature of the new technologies. When machines begin to be idolized, social catastrophe is never far behind.

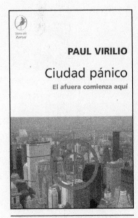

PAUL VIRILIO

Ciudad pánico

El afuera comienza aquí

Resistance is always possible! But we must engage in resistance first of all by developing the idea of a technological culture. However, at the present time, this idea is grossly underdeveloped. For example, we have developed an artistic and a literary culture. Nevertheless, the ideals of technological culture remain underdeveloped and therefore outside of popular culture and the practical ideals of democracy. This is also why society as a whole has no control over technological developments. And this is one of the gravest threats to democracy in the near future.

There are eyes everywhere. No blind spot left. What shall we dream of when everything becomes visible? We'll dream of being blind.

For Virilio the traditional form of war has been replaced by the concentration of media in cities, breeding a new scenario of conflict.

Atomic bomb yesterday, information bomb today, and tomorrow, genetic bomb?

Interview

The first deterrence, nuclear deterrence, is presently being superseded by the second deterrence: a type of deterrence based on what I call 'the information bomb' associated with the new weaponry of information and communications technologies. Thus, in the very near future, and I stress this important point, it will no longer be war that is the continuation of politics by other means, it will be what I have dubbed 'the integral accident' that is the continuation of politics by other means.

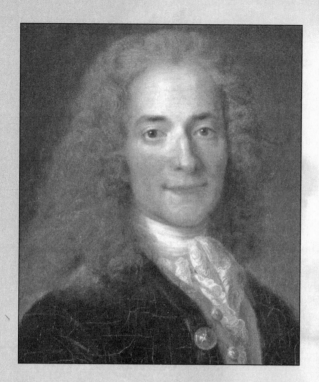

Voltaire

(Paris, France, 1694–1778)

Voltaire was one of the principal representatives of the Enlightenment and a master of polemics. Imprisoned in the Bastille in 1726, he submitted to voluntary exile in Great Britain. There he wrote *Letters Concerning the English Nation*, a fierce critique of the British government, occasioning an order for his arrest. Forced to flee once again he found refuge on the estate of Marquise du Châtelet on the border of Champagne and Lorraine.

In 1749, he traveled to Berlin at the invitation of the Fredrick II, the King of Prussia. A violent rupture with the king led him to return to France. He settled in Geneva, at the chateau of Ferney. There his writings, as acerbic as always, quickly brought him into conflict with the Calvinist inclinations of the Swiss. Shortly before his death in 1778, Voltaire made a triumphant return to Paris.

Recommended reading:

📖 📖 📖 *Treatise on Tolerance* (1767)

📖 📖 *Candide* (1759)

📖 *Philosophical Dictionary* (1764)

I do not agree with what you have to say, but I'll defend to the death your right to say it.

It is better to risk saving a guilty man than to condemn an innocent one.

The best government is a benevolent tyranny tempered by an occasional assassination.

If God did not exist it would be necessary to invent him.

What a pitiful, what a sorry thing to have said that animals are machines bereft of understanding and feeling, which perform their operations always in the same way, which learn nothing, perfect nothing, etc.

Those who can make you believe absurdities, can make you commit atrocities.

The comfort of the rich depends upon an abundant supply of the poor.

Superstition is to religion what astrology is to astronomy: the foolish daughter of a very wise mother. These two daughters, superstition and astrology, have subjugated the world for a long time.

It is forbidden to kill; therefore all murderers are punished unless they kill in large numbers and to the sound of trumpets.

God is a comedian playing to an audience that is too afraid to laugh.

It is dangerous to be right in matters on which the established authorities are wrong.

The human brain is a complex organ with the wonderful power of enabling man to find reasons for continuing to believe whatever it is that he wants to believe.

What is history? The lie that everyone agrees on.

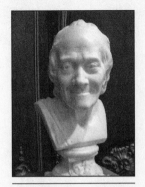

Voltaire advocated secular thinking and anticlericalism, two pillars of the French Revolution.

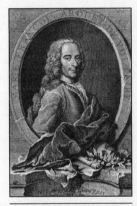

A lucid and critical rationalist, Voltaire was a firm defender of his ideas, attacking absolutism and superstition.

Treatise on Tolerance

This little globe, which is but a point, travels in space like many other globes; we are lost in the immensity. Man, about five feet high, is certainly a small thing in the universe. One of these imperceptible beings says to some of his neighbors, in Arabia or South Africa: "Listen to me, for the God of all these worlds has enlightened me. There are nine hundred million little ants like us on the earth, but my ant-hole alone is dear to God. All the others are eternally reprobated by him. Mine alone will be happy." They would then interrupt me, and ask who was the fool that talked all this nonsense. I should be obliged to tell them that it was themselves. I would then try to appease them, which would be difficult.

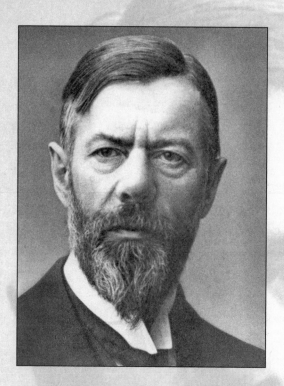

Max Weber

(Erfurt, Germany, 1864–Munich, Germany, 1920)

Weber taught at many universities, spending much of his academic career in Heidelberg. He suffered a severe depression that caused him to suspend teaching from 1898 until 1906. It was during that time that he published his master work, *The Protestant Ethic and the Spirit of Capitalism*, in which he defined modernity as a state of secularization marked by the disenchantment of the world.

Weber argued that sociological phenomena does not depend solely on economic factors (as Marx would have it), but on ideology as well. Accordingly the development of industrial capitalism was a consequent of the Protestant ethic that had dominated most western countries since the rise of Calvinism in the sixteenth and seventeenth centuries.

Recommended reading:

📖 📖 📖 *The Protestant Ethic and the Spirit of Capitalism* (1905)

📖 📖 *Sociology of Religion* (1904-1918)

📖 *Science and Politics* (1919)

194

[Sociology is] the science whose object is to interpret the meaning of social action and thereby give a causal explanation of the way in which the action proceeds and the effects which it produces.

The origin of a rational and inner-worldly ethic is associated in the Occident with the appearance of thinkers and prophets...who developed in a social context which was alien to the Asiatic cultures. This context consisted of the political problems engendered by the bourgeois status-group of the city, without which neither Judaism, nor Christianity, nor the development of Hellenistic thinking are conceivable.

The decisive reason for the advance of the bureaucratic organization has always been its purely technical superiority over any other form of organization.

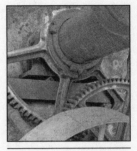

Weber thought that capitalism had broken away from its Protestant roots in favor of a system of mechanical production.

The development of the concept of the calling quickly gave to the modern entrepreneur a fabulously clear conscience—and also industrious workers; he gave to his employees as the wages of their ascetic devotion to the calling and of co-operation in his ruthless exploitation of them through capitalism the prospect of eternal salvation.

We know of no scientifically ascertainable ideals. To be sure, that makes our efforts more arduous than in the past, since we are expected to create our ideals from within our breast in the very age of subjectivist culture

---

The state is that association that claims for itself the monopoly on the use of legitimate violence.

Power is the chance to impose your will within a social context, even when opposed and regardless of the integrity of that chance.

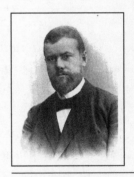

The fate of an epoch that has eaten of the tree of knowledge is that it must...recognize that general views of life and the universe can never be the products of increasing empirical knowledge, and that the highest ideals, which move us most forcefully, are always formed only in the struggle with other ideals which are just as sacred to others as ours are to us.

Collotype of Weber from 1894.

"Objectivity" in Social Science

There is no absolutely "objective" scientific analysis of culture....All knowledge of cultural reality... is always knowledge from particular points of view. ... an "objective" analysis of cultural events, which proceeds according to the thesis that the ideal of science is the reduction of empirical reality to "laws," is meaningless... [because]... the knowledge of social laws is not knowledge of social reality but is rather one of the various aids used by our minds for attaining this end.

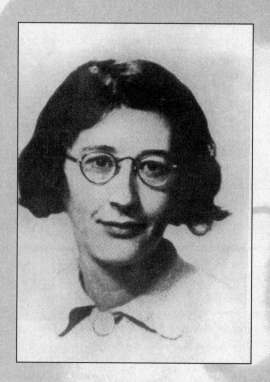

Simone Weil

(Paris, France, 1909–Ashford, England, 1943)

Born to a Jewish family, Simone Weil evinced a passionate interest in philosophy at a young age. She completed her studies at the École Normale Supérieure at the age of 22 and began her teaching career. When she was 25 she asked for leave and spent over a year working in a factory.

She took part in the Spanish Civil War, joining with anarchist groups. In 1940 she fled Paris for Marseilles to escape from the Nazis. Then in 1942 she emigrated to England and in the last stage of her life she converted to Christianity. She died of tuberculosis at the age of 34. Her works, published posthumously, have attracted the attention of philosophers, writers, theologians, and sociologists.

Recommended reading:

Gravity and Grace (1941-42)

Awaiting God (1941-42)

Oppression and Liberty (1934)

At the bottom of the heart of every human being, from earliest infancy until the tomb, there is something that goes on indomitably expecting, in the teeth of all experience of crimes committed, suffered, and witnessed, that good and not evil will be done to him. It is this above all that is sacred in every human being.

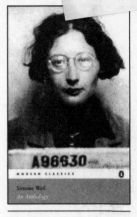

Capitalism has brought about the emancipation of collective humanity with respect to nature. But this collective humanity has itself taken on with respect to the individual the oppressive function formerly exercised by nature.

Imaginary evil is romantic and varied; real evil is gloomy, monotonous, barren, boring. Imaginary good is boring; real good is always new, marvelous, intoxicating.

The thought of Simone Weil turned toward mysticism. She was not baptized because she did not feel herself to be worthy of such an honor.

Just as a vagrant accused of stealing a carrot from a field stands before a comfortably seated judge who keeps up an elegant flow of queries, comments, and witticisms while the accused is unable to stammer a word, so truth stands before an intelligence which is concerned with the elegant manipulation of opinions.

Human history is simply the history of the servitude which makes men—oppressed and oppressors alike—the plaything of the instruments of domination they themselves have manufactured, and thus reduces living humanity to being the chattel of inanimate chattels.

We can know only one thing about God—that he is what we are not. Our wretchedness alone is an image of this. The more we contemplate it, the more we contemplate him.

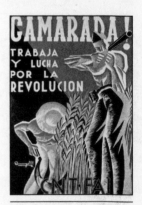

A hurtful act is the transference to others of the degradation which we bear in ourselves.

In struggling against anguish one never produces serenity; the struggle against anguish only produces new forms of anguish.

The only way into truth is through one's own annihilation; through dwelling a long time in a state of extreme and total humiliation.

Weil was one of the first intellectuals to participate in the Spanish Civil War.

Evil, when we are in its power, is not felt as evil, but as a necessity, even a duty.

The Power of Words

What a country calls its vital economic interests are not the things which enable its citizens to live, but the things which enable it to make war; petrol is much more likely than wheat to be a cause of international conflict. International politics are wholly involved in this vicious cycle...What is called national security is an imaginary state of affairs in which one would retain the capacity to make war while depriving all other countries of it. It amounts to this, that a self-respecting nation is ready for anything, including war, except for a renunciation of its option to make war.

Ludwig Wittgenstein

(Vienna, Austria, 1889–Cambridge, England, 1951)

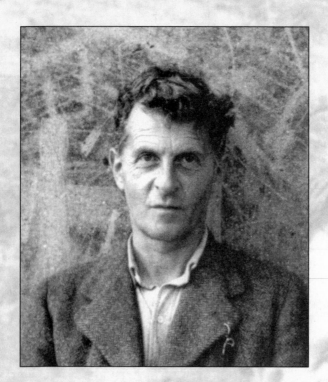

Wittgenstein was one of the most influential thinkers of the twentieth century. He is recognized for his important contributions to analytic philosophy. He was a student of Bertram Russell at Trinity College. With his famous work, *Tractatus logico-philosophicus* he sought a definitive solution to all philosophical problems.

However, later on in his *Philosophical Investigations*, he retracted many of his previous conclusions. He declined to receive treatment for cancer and according to his student Elisabeth Anscombe, his last words were "I have had a marvelous life."

Recommended reading:

📖 📖 📖 *Tractatus logico-philosophicus* (1921)

📖 📖 *Philosophical Investigations* (1953)

📖 *The Blue and Brown Books* (1958)

Philosophy is a battle against the bewitchment of our intelligence by means of language.

If anyone is unwilling to descend into himself, because this is too painful, he will remain superficial in his writing....If I perform to myself, then it's this that the style expresses. And then the style cannot be my own. If you are unwilling to know what you are, your writing is a form of deceit.

The problems are solved, not by giving new information, but by arranging what we have known since long.

The limits of my language are the limits of my mind. All I know is what I have words for.

We feel that even if all possible scientific questions be answered, the problems of life have still not been touched at all.

An honest religious thinker is like a tightrope walker. He almost looks as though he were walking on nothing but air. His support is the slenderest imaginable. And yet it really is possible to walk on it.

The world is everything that is the case.

What do I know about God and the purpose of life? I know that this world exists. That I am placed in it like my eye in its visual field. That something about it is problematic, which we call its meaning. This meaning does not lie in it but outside of it. That life is the world. That my will penetrates the world. That my will is good or evil. Therefore that good and evil are somehow connected with the meaning of the world. The meaning of life, i.e. the meaning of the world, we can call God. And connect with this the comparison of God to a father.

What we cannot speak about we must pass over in silence.

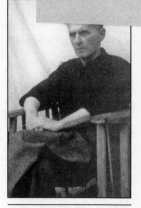

Wittgenstein was a mathematician as well as a philosopher.

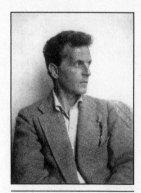

During a heated discussion with Karl Popper in Cambridge Wittgenstein challenged him to formulate just one moral proposition.

Tractatus logico-philosophicus

Death is not an event in life: we do not live to experience death. If we take eternity to mean not infinite temporal duration but timelessness, then eternal life belongs to those who live in the present. Our life has no end in just the way in which our visual field has no limits.

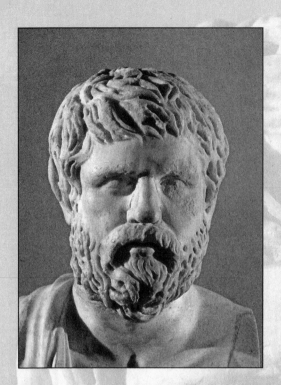

Xenophanes

(Colophon, Asia Minor, c. 570–c. 475 BCE)

Xenophanes was an ancient Greek philosopher, poet and theologian and author of the first work on epistemology. Many consider him to be the creator of the earliest theory of human consciousness.

He was the first philosopher to consider the limits of philosophy itself. He denied that consciousness was the product of direct experience. He mocked at the Greek tendency to anthropomorphize its gods and considered myths of their wanton behavior to be immoral. Rather he espoused the idea of one God who could in no way be compared to human beings. His work comes down to us only through fragments preserved in the works of other Greek philosophers.

Recommended reading:

Diogenes Laertius, *Lives of Eminent Philosophers* (1st century CE)

Kirk, G.S., Raven, J.E., *The Presocratic Philosophers* (1987)

Jonathan Barnes, *The Presocratic Philosophers* (1992)

One god, greatest among gods and humans, like mortals neither in form nor in thought.

Homer and Hesiod have attributed to the gods everything that is blameworthy and disgraceful among humans: theft and adultery and mutual trickery...but humans suppose that gods have been born and wear clothes like theirs and have voice and body.

And so no man has seen anything clearly nor will anyone know about the gods and what I say about everything, for if one should by chance speak about what has come to pass even as it is, still he himself does not know, but opinion is stretched over all.

But if cattle and horses and lions had hands or could paint with their hands and create works such as men do, horses like horses and cattle like cattle also would depict the gods' shapes and make their bodies of such a sort as the form they themselves have.

Indeed not from the beginning did gods intimate all things to mortals, but as they search in time they discover better.

The upper limit of the earth is seen here at our feet, pushing up against the air, but that below goes on without limit.

All things which come into being and grow are earth and water.

The sea is the source of water and the source of wind; for neither would blasts of wind arise in the clouds and blow out from within them, except for the great sea, nor would the streams of rivers nor the rain-water in the sky exist but for the sea ; but the great sea is the begetter

Xenophon said that the sun is formed of constantly burning clouds. (Aecius)

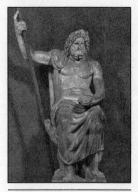

Xenophanes engaged in an important polemic against the anthropomorphic representation of god as depicted in Greek mythology. He argued that Hesiod and Homer had endowed the gods with the worst qualities of men, and proposed instead the existence of a single, undivided God whose nature was radically different from that of men.

Xenophanes conceived of God as all-seeing, all-hearing, all-knowing, uncreated and immortal. However, he considered phenomena to be strictly material originating from a combination of water and earth, wet and dry, and he thought that it was everywhere the same, homogeneous and unvarying.

Hippolytus, *Refutation of All Heresies*

And Xenophanes is of opinion that there had been a mixture of the earth with the sea, and that in process of time it was disengaged from the moisture...that in the midst of earth, and in mountains, shells are discovered; and also in Syracuse he affirms was found in the quarries the print of a fish and of seals...and in Melita parts of all sorts of marine animals. And he says that these were generated when all things originally were embedded in mud, and that an impression of them was dried in the mud, but that all men had perished when the earth, being precipitated into the sea, was converted into mud; then, again, that it originated generation, and that this overthrow occurred to all worlds.

María Zambrano

(Vélez Málaga, Spain, 1904–Madrid, 1991)

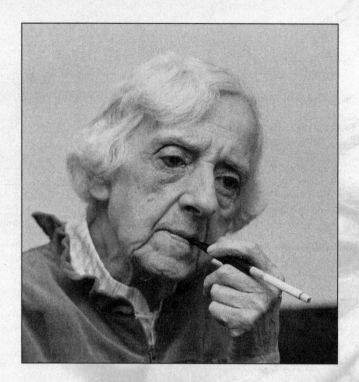

Zambrano studied philosophy in Madrid where she attended classes given by Ortega y Gasset and participated in many of the important political events of the day. She was friends with leading Spanish poets Cernuda, Jorge Guillén and Miguel Hernánadez, and later on with Octavio Paz, Albert Camus, and René Char.

A supporter of the Republic, she was exiled to Paris and then moved to Mexico, Havana, and finally Puerto Rico, where she taught at the university.

In 1981 she received the Prince of Asturias Prize and returned to Madrid in 1984, after 45 years in exile. In 1988 she was awarded the Cervantes Prize for Literature.

Recommended reading:

Man and the Divine (1955)
Philosophy and Poetry (1939)

Toward a Knowledge of the Soul (1950)

The Individual and Democracy (1957)

By Utopia I understand irreducible beauty, and even the sword of destiny of an angel who leads us toward that which we know is impossible.

————

Despite the fact that for some fortunate mortals, poetry and thought may have been given at the same time and in parallel, despite that for others yet more fortunate, poetry and thought may have been able to be merged in a single expressive form, the truth is that thought and poetry have been in serious confrontation throughout the length of our culture. Each of them wants for itself eternally the soul where it nests. And that double pull may be the cause of certain misallocated vocations and endless anxiety drowning in sterility.

————

"In the beginning was the word," the logos, the creative and ordering word, which puts into motion and legislates. With these words, Christian reason comes to grapple with Greek philosophic reason.

————

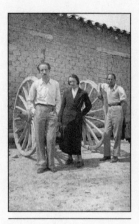

During the years of Spain's Second Republic Zambrano met the poet Luis Cernuda, who also was forced into exile.

All words require an alienation from the reality to which they refer; every word is also a liberation for whomever speaks it. Whoever speaks, even if it is only of appearances, is not completely a slave; whoever speaks, even if it be of the most varied multiplicity, has already attained a certain fortune in unity, whether it be imbibed as pure astonishment, caught in what changes and flows, it states no certainties, but its statement shall be a song.

————

"All men have a natural desire to know," says Aristotle at the beginning of his *Metaphysics*...Also, assuming that in effect all people need this wisdom, the question we apply to philosophy immediately presents itself. That if everyone needs you, why do so few attain you?

————

Existence, marvelous life which cannot be saved, travels towards the dead and when old age arrives—"white hair crowns my head"—desire has not disappeared, nor anything that has matured in my soul. No other life appears behind the burning fire of desire. Only mortality and intoxication.

————

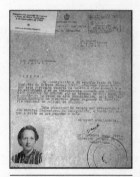

Entry card for Zambrano into Cuba on a Spanish tourist visa.

The poet extracts the humiliation of not being what groans in him, takes nothing from nothingness itself and gives it name and face. The poet does not wish of things which are, that some exist and others do not obtain this privilege, yet instead works so that everything that there is and is not, shall attain being. The poet does not fear nothingness.

Philosophy and Poetry

And it is painful to say that Plato did not know how to extend justice to the poet. The poet does not know what he says and, nevertheless, has a conscience, a sort of conscience. A special, private lucidity of the poet without which how many pages Plato might not have written. And if the poet has gained anything throughout the ages it is this lucidity, this awakened consciousness, constantly more awake and lucid as the modern poets testify, as is testified by the father of them all, Baudelaire.

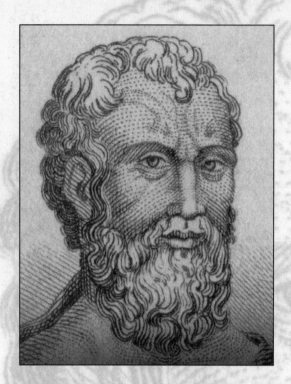

Zeno of Elea

(Elea, Campania, Italy, c. 490–c.430)

He is remembered for his paradoxes and aporias (irresolvable philosophical or logical propositions). Beyond this Zeno maintained the positions of his teacher Parmenides, denying the reality of motion and the plurality of beings.

According to Diogenes Laertius, Heraclides recounted that Zeno was imprisoned for trying to overthrow the tyrant Nearches. When Nearches interrogated him, he drew near him and bit him and would not let go until he was stabbed. Finally Zeno bit off his own tongue and spat it in the tyrant's face. This emboldened his fellow citizens who rose up and stoned the tyrant. Laertius also quotes Hermippus who stated that Zeno was put into a mortar and stoned to death.

Recommended reading:

Diogenes Laertius, *Lives of Eminent Philosophers* (1st century BCE)

Kirk, G.S. and J.E. Raven, *The Presocratic Philosophers* (1987)

Plato, *Parmenides* (4th century, BCE)

His chief doctrines were, that there were several worlds, and that there was no vacuum; that the nature of all things consisted of hot and cold, and dry and moist, these elements interchanging their substances with one another; that man was made out of earth, and that his soul was a mixture of the before-named elements in such a way that no one of them predominated. (Diogenes Laertius)

If I accede to Parmenides there is nothing left but the One; if I accede to Zeno, not even the One is left. (Seneca the Younger)

[The Achilles paradox] is that the slowest runner never will be overtaken by the fastest; for it is necessary for the one chasing to come first to where the one fleeing started from, so that it is necessary for the slower runner always to be ahead some.

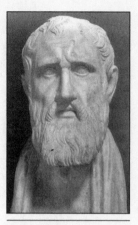

Zeno questioned the apparent plurality of reality, considering the universe as a unique unity.

If there are many things, it is necessary that they be just so many as they are and neither greater than themselves nor fewer. But if they are just as many as they are, they will be limited. If there are many things, the things that are are unlimited; for there are always others between these entities, and again others between those. And thus the things that are unlimited. (Simplicius)

Zeno's reasoning, however, is fallacious, when he says that if everything when it occupies an equal space is at rest, and if that which is in locomotion is always in a now, the flying arrow is therefore motionless. This is false; for time is not composed of indivisible nows any more than any other magnitude is composed of indivisibles. (Aristotle)

The truth is, that these writings of mine were meant to protect the arguments of Parmenides against those who make fun of him and seek to show the many ridiculous and contradictory results which they suppose to follow from the affirmation of the one. My answer is addressed to the partisans of the many, whose attack I return with interest by retorting upon them that their hypothesis of the being of many, if carried out, appears to be still more ridiculous than the hypothesis of the being of one.

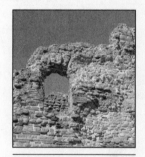

The ruins of Elea are situated in Campania on the coast of Italy. The Greek settlement was founded there in 540 BCE.

Plato, *Parmenides*

Socrates: You (Parmenides) say in your poem that the all is one, and you give splendid and excellent proofs for that; Zeno says that it is not many and gives a vast array of very grand proofs of his own. So, with one of you saying "one," and the other saying "not many," and with each of you speaking in a way that suggests you've said nothing the same—although you mean practically the same thing—what you've said you appear to have said over the heads of the rest of us.

205

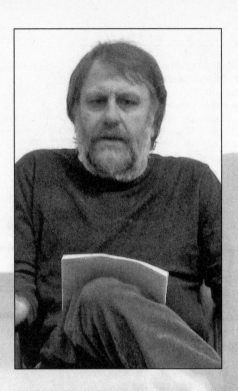

Slavoj Zizek

(Lublijana, Slovenia, 1949)

Slovaj Zizek enjoys great prestige in the academic world and is one of the most interesting personalities in contemporary culture. He studied philosophy and psychoanalysis at the University of Paris. He is a researcher at the Institute of Sociology at the University of Lublijana and has been invited to teach at many universities and institutions.

The footprints of Marx, Hegel, and Lacan can be easily discerned in his work. The last of these inspired him to undertake a singular account of our modern world in psychoanalytic terms. He touches upon subjects such as fundamentalism versus tolerance and current political conflicts as well as mass media and Hollywood.

Recommended reading:

📖 📖 📖 *The Sublime Object of Ideology* (1989)

📖 📖 *Everything You Always Wanted to Know about Lacan...But Were Afraid to Ask Hitchcock* (1993)

📖 *The Metastases of Enjoyment* (1994)

There is no such thing as the Communist big Other, there's no historical necessity or teleology directing and guiding our actions.

———

Cinema is the ultimate pervert art. It doesn't give you what you desire—it tells you how to desire.

———

We feel free because we lack the very language to articulate our unfreedom.

———

The problem for us is not whether our desires are satisfied or not. The problem is how do we know what we desire.

———

A German officer visited Picasso in his Paris studio during the Second World War. There he saw Guernica and, shocked at the modernist "chaos" of the painting, asked Picasso: "Did you do this?" Picasso calmly replied: "No, you did this!"

———

Liberals always say about totalitarians that they like humanity, as such, but they have no empathy for concrete people, no? OK, that fits me perfectly. Humanity? Yes, it's OK—some great talks, some great arts. Concrete people? No, 99% are boring idiots.

———

The same philanthropists who give millions for AIDS or education in tolerance have ruined the lives of thousands through financial speculation and thus created the conditions for the rise of the very intolerance that is being fought. In the 1960s and '70s it was possible to buy soft-porn postcards of a girl clad in a bikini or wearing an evening gown; however, when one moved the postcard a little bit or looked at it from a slightly different perspective, her clothes magically disappeared to reveal the girl's naked body. When we are bombarded by the heartwarming news of a debt cancellation or a big humanitarian campaign to eradicate a dangerous epidemic, just move the postcard a little to catch a glimpse of the obscene figure of the liberal communist at work beneath.

———

"Hello, glad to be here, but just don't expect to get from me what you will never get from me. You will not get from me big, glad news...no, things are going pretty bad, I think."—@ Creative Time Summit 4: Confronting Inequity.

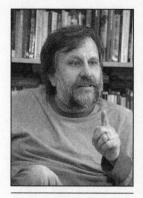

A prestigious philosopher, Zizek revitalized psychoanalysis. He is fully committed to his political ideas. He ran for president in Slovenia in 1990.

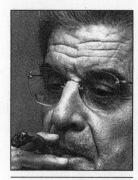

Zizek dismisses the intellectual elitism characteristic of many contemporary philosophers. He prefers to speak in a "popular" idiom. For example, he discusses the difficult writings of Lacan (above) with reference to the works of Hitchcock and Stephen King.

Against Human Rights

Liberal attitudes towards the other are characterized both by respect for other- ness, openness to it, and an obsessive fear of harassment. In short, the other is welcomed insofar as its presence is not intrusive, insofar as it is not really the other. Tolerance thus coincides with its opposite. My duty to be tolerant towards the other effectively means that I should not get too close to him or her, not intrude into his space....This is increasingly emerging as the central human right of advanced capitalist society: the right...to be kept at a safe distance from others.